Study Guide for

STRUCTURE & FUNCTION OF THE BODY

Fourteenth Edition

Prepared by
Linda Swisher, RN, EdD

ELSEVIER
MOSBY

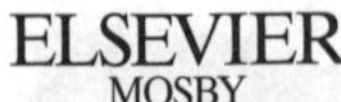

MOSBY

3251 Riverport Lane
St. Louis, Missouri 63043

Study Guide for Structure & Function of the Body ISBN: 978-0-323-07723-1

ISBN: 978-0-323-07723-1

Executive Editor: Kellie White
Managing Editor: Rebecca Swisher
Publishing Services Manager: Deborah Vogel
Project Manager: Brandilyn Tidwell
Design Direction: Margaret Reid

Printed in the United States of America

Last digit is the print number: 9 8 7 6 5 4 3 2 1

Preface

TO THE INSTRUCTOR

This study guide is designed to help your students master basic anatomy and physiology. It works in two ways.

First, the section of the preface titled "To the Student" contains detailed information about the following topics:

- How to achieve good grades in anatomy and physiology
- How to read the textbook
- How to use the exercises in this study guide
- How to use visual memory as a learning tool
- How to use mnemonic devices as learning aids
- How to prepare for an examination
- How to take an examination
- How to find out why questions were missed on an examination

Second, the study guide itself contains features that facilitate learning. These features include the following:

1. LEARNING OBJECTIVES, designed to break down the information to be mastered into smaller, more manageable units. The questions in this study guide have been developed to help the student master the learning objectives that are identified at the beginning of each chapter in the text. The guide is also sequenced to correspond to key areas of each chapter. A variety of questions has been prepared to cover the material effectively and to expose the student to several different approaches to learning.
2. CROSSWORD PUZZLES, WORD FINDS, and UNSCRAMBLE THE WORDS to encourage the use of new vocabulary words and emphasize the proper spelling of these terms in an entertaining manner.
3. OPTIONAL APPLICATION QUESTIONS, particularly targeted for the health occupations student but appropriate for any student of anatomy and physiology because they are based entirely on information contained within the chapter.
4. DIAGRAMS, with key features marked by numbers for identification. Students can easily check their work by comparing the diagram in the workbook with the equivalent figure in the text.
5. PAGE NUMBER REFERENCES, found in the "Answers to Chapter Exercises" section. Each answer is cross-referenced with the page in the text where the information supporting that answer is found. Additionally, questions are grouped by specific topics that correspond to sections of the text. Following each major section of the study guide are references to specific areas of the text that will help students who are having difficulty with a particular grouping of questions. These references will point the students to the part of the text on which they should focus their study. These references are of great assistance to both instructor and student because remedial work is made easier and more effective when the area of weakness is identified accurately.
6. ONE LAST QUICK CHECK, found at the end of each chapter. Students can determine how successfully they have retained the information from each section test in the chapter by taking this sample test of questions reviewing all areas of the text.

These features should make mastery of the material contained in this text and study guide a rewarding experience for both instructor and student.

TO THE STUDENT

How to Achieve Good Grades in Anatomy and Physiology

This study guide is designed to help you succeed in learning anatomy and physiology. Before you begin using the study guide, read the following suggestions. Understanding effective study techniques and having good study habits will help you become a more successful student.

How to Read the Textbook

Keep up with the reading assignments. Read the textbook assignment before the instructor covers the material in a lecture. If you have failed to read the assignment beforehand, you will not grasp what the instructor is talking about in lecture. When you read, do the following:

1. As you finish reading a sentence, ask yourself if you understand it. If you do not, put a question mark in the margin by that sentence. If the instructor does not clear up the problem in a lecture, ask him or her to explain it to you.
2. Make sure you can perform all of the learning objectives in the text. A learning objective is a specific task that you are expected to be able to do after you have read a chapter. The objectives set specific goals and break down learning into small steps. They emphasize the key points that the author is making in the chapter.
3. Underline the text and make notes in the margin to highlight key ideas, to mark something you need to reinforce at a later time, or to indicate things that you do not understand.
4. If you come to a word you do not understand, look it up. Write the word on one side of an index card, and write its definition on the other. Carry these cards with you, and when you have a spare minute, use them like flash cards (like you may have done when you were learning your multiplication tables). Learn how to properly pronounce and spell the word. If you do not know how to spell or pronounce a word, you will have a hard time remembering it.
5. Carefully study each diagram and illustration as you progress through the text. Many students ignore these aids, but the author included them to help you understand the material.
6. Summarize what you read. After you finish a paragraph, try to restate the main ideas. Do this again when you finish the chapter. In your mind, identify and review the main concepts of the chapter, then check to see if you are correct. In short, be an active reader. Do not just stare at a page or read it superficially.

Finally, approach each unit of learning with a positive mental attitude. Motivation and perseverance are prime factors in your effort to achieve successful grades. The combination of your instructor, the text, the study guide, and your dedicated work will lead to your success in anatomy and physiology.

How to Use the Exercises in This Study Guide

After you have read a chapter and learned all the new vocabulary it contains, begin working with the study guide. Read the overview of the chapter, which summarizes the main points.

Familiarize yourself with the "Topics for Review" section of the overview, which emphasizes key objectives that were outlined in the text. Complete the questions and diagrams in the study guide. The questions have been sequenced to follow the chapter outline and headings, and they are divided into small sections to facilitate learning. A variety of questions is offered throughout the study guide to help you cover the material effectively. The following examples are among the exercises that have been included to assist you.

Multiple Choice Questions

Multiple choice questions will offer you many options to select from, but only one answer will be correct. There are two types of multiple choice questions that you may not be familiar with that have been included in this study guide:

How to Prepare for an Examination

Prepare for an examination far in advance. Actually, your preparation for an examination should begin on the first day of class. Keeping up with your daily assignments makes the final preparation for an examination much easier. You should begin your final preparation at least three nights before a test. Last-minute studying usually means poor results and limited retention of the material. The following suggestions may help you improve your test results:

1. Make sure that you understand and can perform all of the learning objectives for the chapter on which you are being tested.
2. Review the appropriate questions in this study guide. Reviewing is something that you should do after every class and at the end of every study session. It is important to keep going over the material until you have a thorough understanding of the chapter and a rapid recall of its contents. If review becomes a daily habit, studying for the actual examination will not be difficult. Go through each question in the study guide and write down an answer. Do the same for the exercises in which you label each structure on a diagram. If you have already done this as part of your daily review, cover the answers with a piece of paper and quiz yourself again.
3. Check the answers that you have written down against the correct answers in the back of the study guide. Go back and study the areas in the text that refer to questions that you answered incorrectly and then try to answer those questions again. If you still cannot answer a question or label a structure correctly, ask your instructor for additional help.
4. As you read a chapter, ask yourself what questions you would ask if you were writing an evaluation for that unit. You will most likely ask yourself many of the questions that will show up on your examination.
5. Get a good night's sleep before the test. Staying up late and upsetting your biorhythms will only make you less efficient during the test.

How to Take an Examination

The Day of the Test

1. Get up early enough to avoid rushing. Eat appropriately. Your body needs fuel, but a heavy meal just before a test is not a good idea.
2. Keep calm. Briefly look over your notes. If you have properly prepared for the test, there will be no need for last-minute cramming.
3. Make sure that you have everything you need to take the test such as pens, pencils, test sheets, and so forth.
4. Allow enough time to get to the examination site. Missing your bus, getting stuck in traffic, or being unable to find a parking space will not put you in a good frame of mind to do well on the examination.

During the Examination

1. Pay careful attention to the instructions for the test.
2. Note any corrections.
3. Budget your time so that you will be able to finish the test.
4. Ask the instructor for clarification if you do not understand a question or an instruction.
5. Concentrate on your own test and do not allow yourself to be distracted by others in the room.

Hints for Taking a Multiple Choice Test

1. Read each question carefully. Pay attention to each word.
2. Eliminate obviously wrong answers and then carefully consider those that remain.
3. Go through the test once and quickly answer the questions you are sure about; then go back over the test and answer the rest of the questions.
4. Fill in the answer spaces completely. Delete any evidence of a prior answer if you make a mistake an providing a new answer.

5. If you must guess, stick with your first hunch. Most often students will change right answers to wrong ones.
6. If you will not be penalized for guessing, do not leave any blanks.

Hints for Taking an Essay Test

1. Budget time for each question.
2. Write legibly, if the test is handwritten, and try to spell words correctly.
3. Be concise, complete, and specific. Do not be repetitious or long-winded.
4. Organize your answer in an outline. This will help you to keep your thoughts organized, and it will also help the person who is grading the test.
5. Answer each question as thoroughly as you can, but leave some room for possible additions.

Hints for Taking a Laboratory Practical Examination

Students often have a hard time with this kind of test. Visual memory is very important in this situation. To put it simply, you must be able to identify every structure you have studied. If you are unable to identify a structure, then you will be unable to answer any questions about that structure.

Examples that may appear on this sort of examination include the following:

1. Identification of a structure, organ, or feature.
2. Description of the function of a structure, organ, or feature.
3. Description of the sequence in which air flow, passage of food, elimination of urine, etc., occurs.
4. Disease questions such as: "If a thyroid fails, what condition might result?" or "What disease might occur if the pancreas is not functioning properly?"

How to Find Out Why Questions Were Missed on an Examination

After the Examination

Go over your test after it has been scored to see what you missed and why you missed it. You can pick up important clues that will help you on future evaluations. Ask yourself these questions:

1. Did I miss questions because I did not read them carefully?
2. Did I miss questions because I had gaps in my knowledge?
3. Did I miss questions because I did not understand certain scientific words?
4. Did I miss questions because I did not have a good visual memory of things?

Be sure to go back and review the things you did not know. Chances are good that these topics will come up again on another examination in the future. You should have an understanding of these topics before progressing further in the course.

Your grades in other classes will also improve when you apply these study methods to other courses. Learning should be fun. With these helpful hints and this study guide, you should be able to achieve the grades you desire in anatomy and physiology class. Good luck!

Acknowledgments

I wish to express my appreciation to the staff of Elsevier, Inc., and especially to Tom Wilhelm, Jeff Downing, and Rebecca Swisher. My continued admiration and thanks to Gary Thibodeau and Kevin Patton. Your dedication to science education has given countless students an appreciation for the wonderment of the human body, inspired our future scientists, and contributed to the improvement of health care providers. Finally, this book is dedicated in memory of my beloved husband Bill—my beautiful connection to the past, and to my grandchildren Billy, Maddie, and Heather—the sunshine of my life and my link to the future.

Linda Swisher, RN, EdD

Contents

CHAPTER 1

An Introduction to Structure and Function of the Body

Command of terminology is necessary for a student to be successful in any area of science. This chapter defines the terms and concepts basic to the field of anatomy and physiology. A firm foundation in these language skills will assist you with all future chapters.

The study of anatomy and physiology involves the structure and function of an organism and the relationship of its parts. It begins with a basic organization of the body into different structural levels. Beginning with the smallest level (the cell) and progressing to the largest, most complex level (the system), this chapter familiarizes you with the terminology and the levels of organization necessary to facilitate the study of the body as parts or as a whole.

It is also important to be able to identify and describe specific body areas or regions as you progress in this field. The anatomical position is used as a reference position when the body is dissected into planes, regions, or cavities. The terms defined in this chapter allow you to describe the areas efficiently and accurately.

Finally, the process of homeostasis is reviewed. This state of relative constancy in the chemical composition of body fluids is necessary for good health. In fact, the very survival of the body depends on the successful maintenance of homeostasis.

TOPICS FOR REVIEW

Before progressing to Chapter 2, you should have an understanding of the structural levels of organization; the planes, regions, and cavities of the body; the terms used to describe these areas; and the concept of homeostasis as it relates to the survival of the species.

THE SCIENTIFIC METHOD

Complete these statements regarding research.

1. A systematic approach to discovery is known as the scientific theory.
2. A tentative explanation in research is known as the hypothosis.
3. The testing of a hypothesis is experiment.
4. A group getting a drug is the independent variable.
5. A group getting a substitute is the dependent variable.

METRIC SYSTEM

Write T for true and F for false.

_____ 6. There is a subtle shift toward the conversion of English measurements to the metric system.

__F__ 7. A centimeter is 39.37 inches.

__T__ 8. A pound is equivalent to 454 grams.

__T__ 9. An inch equals approximately 2.5 cm.

_____ 10. A centron is another name for a micrometer.

STRUCTURAL LEVELS OF ORGANIZATION

Match the term on the left with the proper selection on the right.

__D__	11. Organism	A.	Many cells that act together to perform a common function
__E__	12. Cells	B.	The most complex units that make up the body
__A__	13. Tissue	C.	A group of several different kinds of tissues arranged to perform a special function
__B__	14. Organ	D.	Denotes a living thing
__B__	15. Systems	E.	The smallest "living" units of structure and function in the body

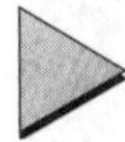

If you have had difficulty with this section, review pages 1-5.

ANATOMICAL POSITION

Match the term on the left with the proper selection on the right.

__C__	16. Body	A.	At the sides
__A__	17. Arms	B.	Face upward
__E__	18. Feet	C.	Erect
__D__	19. Prone	D.	Face downward
__B__	20. Supine	E.	Forward

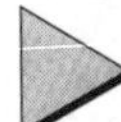

If you have had difficulty with this section, review page 5.

ANATOMICAL DIRECTIONS

Planes or Body Sections

Fill in the crossword puzzle.

Across
21. Lower or below
22. Horizontal plane
23. Toward the midline of the body

Down
24. Upper or above
25. Front (abdominal side)
26. Toward the side of the body
27. Farthest from the point of origin of a body point

Circle the correct answer.

28. The stomach is (superior or inferior) to the diaphragm.
29. The nose is located on the (anterior or posterior) surface of the body.
30. The lungs lie (medial or lateral) to the heart.
31. The elbow lies (proximal or distal) to the forearm.
32. The skin is (superficial or deep) to the muscles below it.
33. A midsagittal plane divides the body into (equal or unequal) parts.
34. A frontal plane divides the body into (anterior and posterior or superior and inferior) sections.
35. A transverse plane divides the body into (right and left or upper and lower) sections.
36. A coronal plane may also be referred to as a (sagittal or frontal) plane.

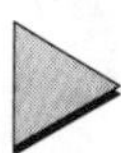 *If you have had difficulty with this section, review pages 5-7.*

BODY CAVITIES

Select the correct term from the choices given and insert the letter in the answer blank.

(A) Ventral cavity (B) Dorsal cavity

A 37. Thoracic
B 38. Cranial
A 39. Abdominal
A 40. Pelvic
A 41. Mediastinum
B 42. Spinal
A 43. Pleural

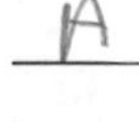
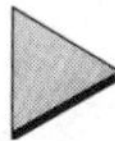 *If you have had difficulty with this section, review pages 7-11.*

BODY REGIONS

Circle the one that does not belong.

44. Axial Head Trunk Extremities
45. Axillary Cephalic Brachial Antecubital
46. Frontal Orbital Plantar Nasal
47. Carpal Crural Plantar Pedal
48. Cranial Occipital Tarsal Temporal

If you have had difficulty with this section, review pages 11-12.

THE BALANCE OF BODY FUNCTIONS

Fill in the blanks.

49. ____________ depends on the body's ability to maintain or restore homeostasis.
50. *Homeostasis* is the term used to describe the relative constancy of the body's ____________.
51. The basic type of homeostatic control system in the body is called a ____________ ____________.
52. Homeostatic control mechanisms are categorized as either ____________ or ____________ feedback loops.
53. Negative feedback loops tend to ____________ conditions.
54. Positive feedback control loops are ____________.
55. Changes and functions that occur during the early years are called ____________ ____________.
56. Changes and functions that occur after young adulthood are called ____________ ____________.

If you have had difficulty with this section, review pages 12-15.

UNSCRAMBLE THE WORDS

Unscramble the circled letters and fill in the statement.

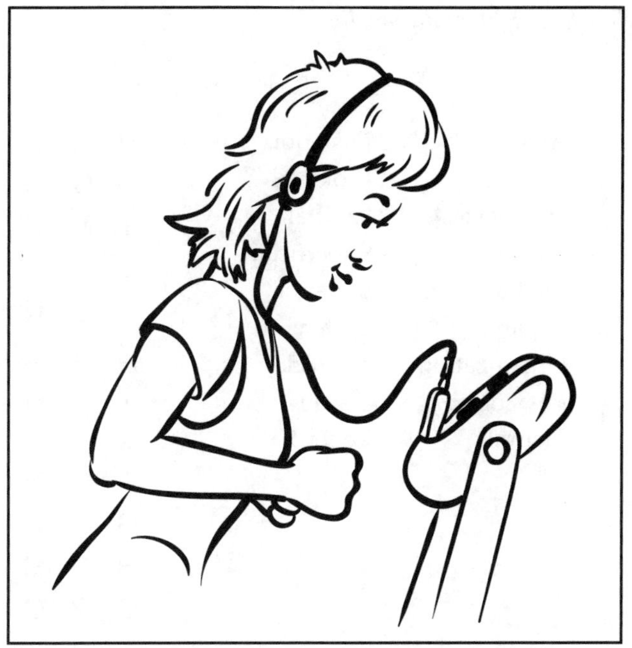

57. **LXAAI**

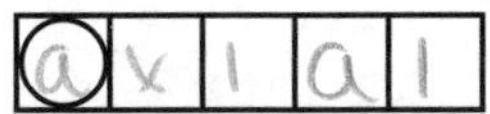

58. **YYGPHIOOSL**

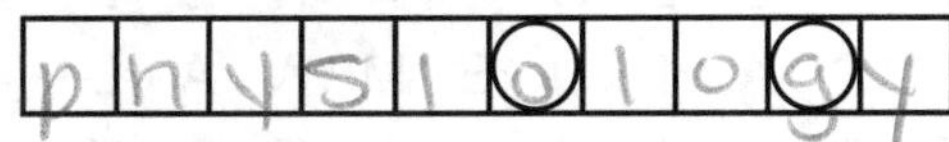

59. **NORLATF**

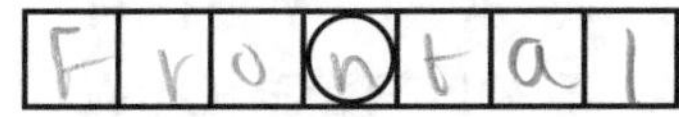

60. **ASRODL**

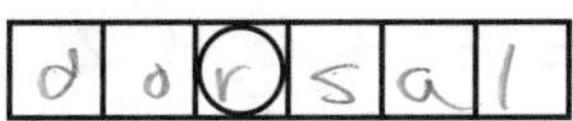

What was Becky's favorite music?

61.

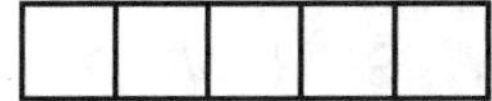

APPLYING WHAT YOU KNOW

62. Wanda has had an appendectomy. The nurse is preparing to change the dressing. She knows that the appendix is located in the right iliac inguinal region and that the distal portion extends at an angle into the hypogastric region. Place an X on the diagram where the nurse will place the dressing.
63. Mrs. Wiedeke noticed a lump in her breast. Dr. Reeder noted on her chart that a small mass was located in the left breast medial to the nipple. Place an X where Mrs. Wiedeke's lump is located.
64. Heather was injured in a bicycle accident. X-ray films revealed that she had a fracture of the right patella. A cast was applied from the distal femoral region and to the pedal region. Place an X where Heather's cast begins and another where it ends.

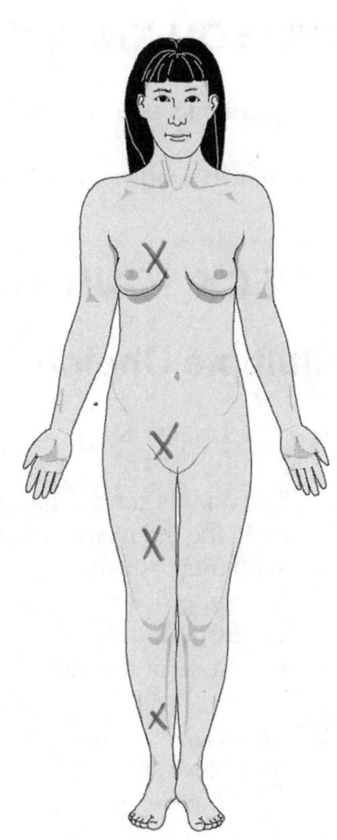

65. WORD FIND

Can you find 18 terms from this chapter in the box of letters? Words may be spelled top to bottom, bottom to top, right to left, left to right, or diagonally.

Anatomy	Posterior
Atrophy	Proximal
Homeostasis	Sagittal
Medial	Superficial
Mediastinum	Superior
Organ	System
Organization	Thoracic
Physiology	Tissue
Pleural	Ventral

N H L T E B W N G N M M Y X A
O O H A V U U C L W E P N G L
I M U N I T S A I D E M W A L
T E R T V C T S I C J S R T K
A O N O P T I A I W A T Y R H
Z S Q S I R L F A T N R G O W
I T W G P R O I R E T S O P F
N A A Z J E E X V E E H L H Z
A S N L M C T P I C P D O Y T
G I C A Y U O X U M N U I V P
R S M R T N U K B S A Y S V M
O R C U R O I R B S Q L Y U G
L H X E M P M E T S Y S H V S
U W L L Q D U Y Y N E E P J B
Q N Z P K D B O D C G I N J A

DID YOU KNOW?

Many animals produce tears but only humans weep as a result of emotional stress.

Men notice subtle signs of sadness in a face only 40% of the time; women pick up on them 90% of the time.

CHECK YOUR KNOWLEDGE

Multiple Choice

Select the best answer.

1. The body's continuous ability to respond to changes in the environment and to maintain relative constancy in the internal environment is called:
   A. Homeostasis
   B. Superficial
   C. Structural levels
   D. None of the above

2. The regions frequently used by health professionals to locate pain or tumors divide the abdomen into four basic areas called:
   A. Planes
   B. Cavities
   C. Pleural
   D. Quadrants

3. Which of the following organs or structures does *not* lie within the mediastinum?
   A. Aorta
   B. Liver
   C. Esophagus
   D. Trachea

4. A lengthwise plane running from front to back that divides the body into right and left sides is called:
   A. Transverse
   B. Coronal
   C. Frontal
   D. Sagittal

5. A study of the functions of living organisms and their parts is called:
   A. Physiology
   B. Chemistry
   C. Biology
   D. None of the above

6. The thoracic portion of the ventral body cavity is separated from the abdominopelvic portion by a muscle called the:
   A. Latissimus dorsi
   B. Rectus femoris
   C. Diaphragm
   D. Pectoralis

7. An organization of varying numbers and kinds of organs arranged together to perform a complex function is called a:
   A. Cell
   B. Tissue
   C. System
   D. Region

8. The plane that divides superior from inferior is known as the _____________ plane.
   A. Transverse
   B. Sagittal
   C. Frontal
   D. None of the above

9. Which one of the following structures does *not* lie within the abdominal cavity?
   A. Spleen
   B. Most of the small intestine
   C. Urinary bladder
   D. Stomach

10. Which of the following is an example of an upper abdominal region?
   A. Right iliac region
   B. Left hypochondriac region
   C. Left lumbar region
   D. Hypogastric region

11. The dorsal body cavity contains components of the:
   A. Reproductive system
   B. Digestive system
   C. Respiratory system
   D. Nervous system

12. What organ is *not* found in the pelvic cavity?
    A. Bladder
    B. Stomach
    C. Rectum
    D. Colon

13. Many cells acting together to perform a common function exist at the ______________ level of organization.
    A. Organ
    B. Chemical
    C. Tissue
    D. System

14. A plane that divides the body into __________ and __________ portions is a coronal plane.
    A. Anterior and posterior
    B. Upper and lower
    C. Right and left
    D. Superficial and deep

15. If your reference point is "nearest the trunk of the body" rather than "farthest from the trunk of the body," where does the elbow lie in relation to the wrist?
    A. Anterior
    B. Posterior
    C. Distal
    D. Proximal

16. In the anatomical position:
    A. The dorsal body cavity is anterior to the ventral body cavity
    B. The palms face toward the back of the body
    C. The body is erect
    D. All of the above

17. The buttocks are often used as intramuscular injection sites. This region can be called:
    A. Sacral
    B. Buccal
    C. Cutaneous
    D. Gluteal

18. In the human body, the chest region:
    A. Can be referred to as the *thoracic cavity*
    B. Is a component of the ventral body cavity
    C. Contains the mediastinum
    D. All of the above

19. Which of the following is *not* a component of the axial subdivision of the body?
    A. Upper extremity
    B. Neck
    C. Trunk
    D. Head

20. A synonym for medial is:
    A. Toward the side
    B. In front of
    C. Midline
    D. Anterior

Matching

Select the most appropriate answer in column B for each item in column A. There is only one correct answer for each item.

Column A	Column B
_____ 21. Ventral	A. Equal
_____ 22. Skin	B. Cutaneous
_____ 23. Transverse	C. Lung
_____ 24. Anatomy	D. Extremities
_____ 25. Superficial	E. Respiratory
_____ 26. Pleural	F. Anterior
_____ 27. Appendicular	G. Structure
_____ 28. Posterior	H. Surface
_____ 29. Midsagittal	I. Back
_____ 30. System	J. Horizontal

DORSAL AND VENTRAL BODY CAVITIES

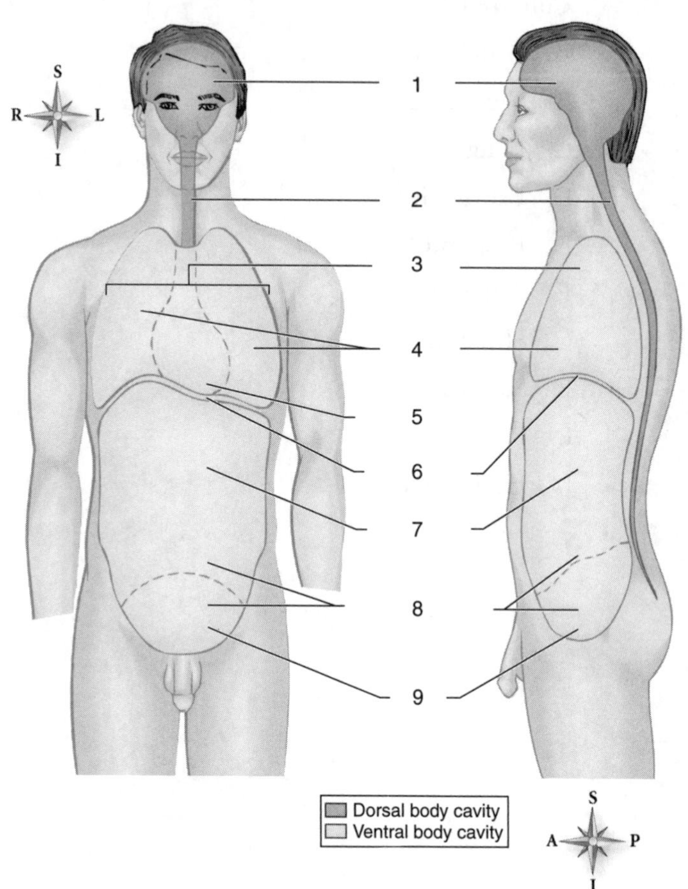

1. cranial cavity
2. spinal cavity
3. thoracic cavity
4. pleural cavities
5. mediastinum
6. diaphragm
7. abdominal cavity
8. abdominopelvic cavity
9. pelvic cavity

DIRECTIONS AND PLANES OF THE BODY

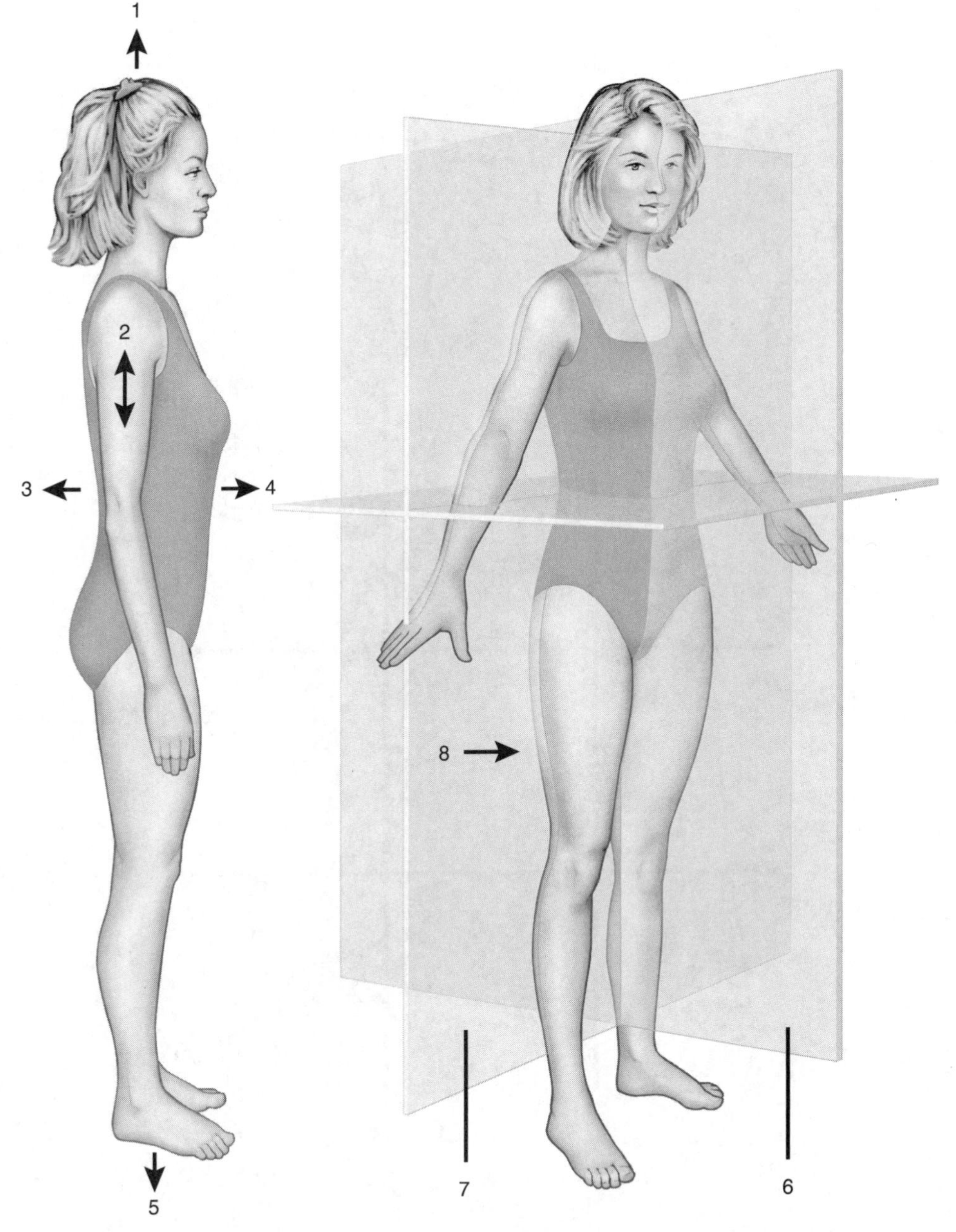

1. superior
2. proximal
3. posterior
4. anterior
5. inferior
6. sagittal plane
7. frontal plane
8. lateral

REGIONS OF THE ABDOMEN

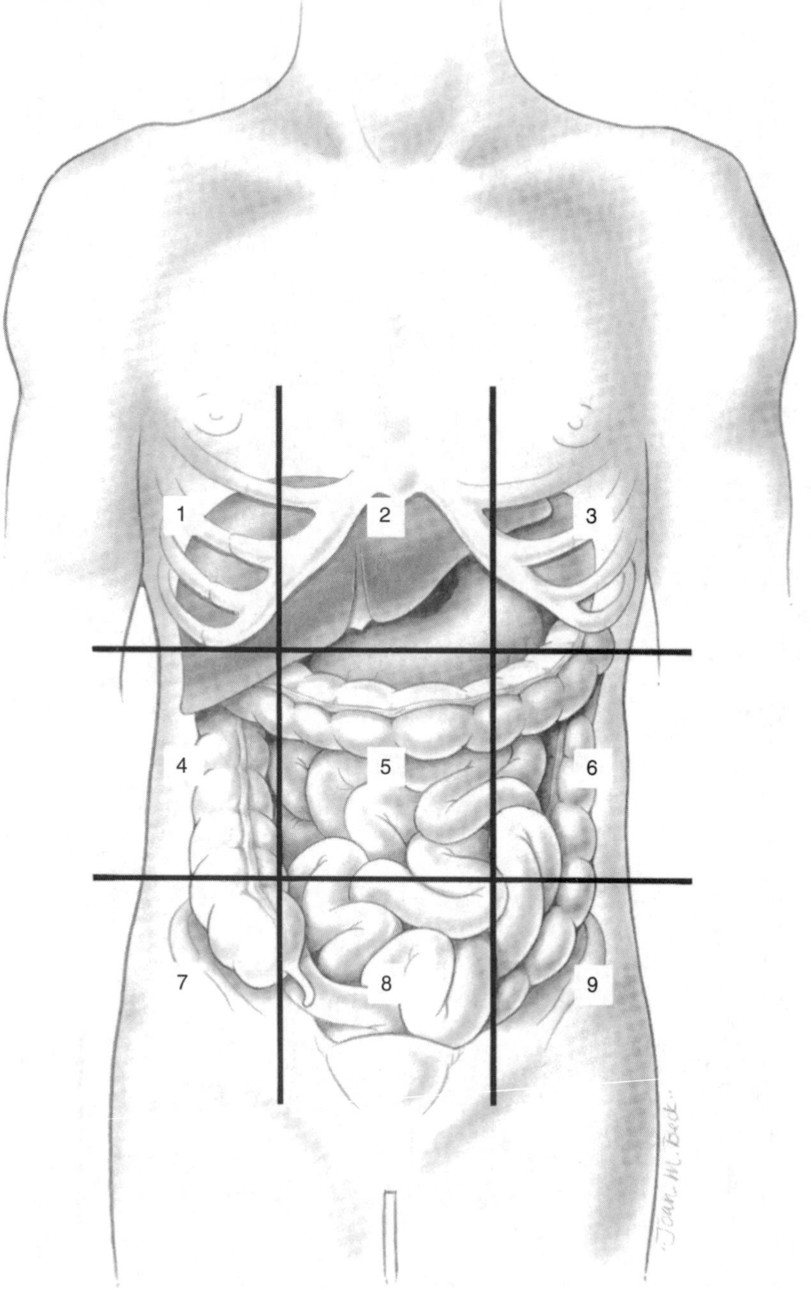

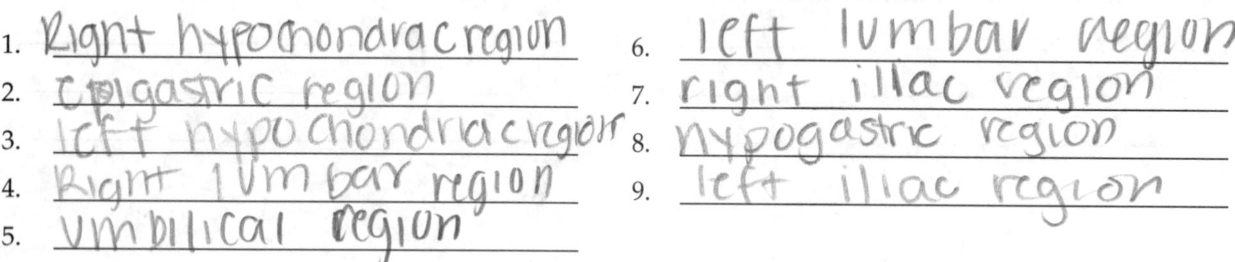

1. Right hypochondrac region
2. epigastric region
3. left hypochondriac region
4. Right lumbar region
5. umbilical region
6. left lumbar region
7. right illac region
8. hypogastric region
9. left iliac region

CHAPTER 2

Chemistry of Life

Although anatomy can be studied without knowledge of chemistry, it is hard to imagine an understanding of physiology without a basic comprehension of chemical reactions in the body. Trillions of cells make up the various levels of organization in the body. Our health and survival depends upon the proper chemical maintenance in the cytoplasm of our cells.

Chemists use the terms *elements* or *compounds* to describe all of the substances (matter) in and around us. Distinguishing these two terms is the fact that an element cannot be broken down. A compound, on the other hand, is made up of two or more elements and has the ability to be broken down into the elements that form it.

Organic and inorganic compounds are equally important to us. Without organic compounds such as carbohydrates, proteins, and fats, and inorganic compounds such as water, we could not sustain life.

Because we cannot see many of the chemical reactions that take place daily in our bodies, it is sometimes difficult to comprehend the principles involved in initiating them. Chemicals are responsible for directing virtually all of our bodily functions. It is, therefore, important to master the fundamental concepts of chemistry.

TOPICS FOR REVIEW

Before progressing to Chapter 3, you should have an understanding of the basic chemical reactions in the body and the fundamental concepts of biochemistry.

LEVELS OF CHEMICAL ORGANIZATION

Multiple Choice

Select the best answer.

1. Which of the following is *not* a subatomic particle?
   A. Proton
   B. Electron
   C. Isotope
   D. Neutron

2. Electrons move about within certain limits called:
   A. Energy levels
   B. Orbitals
   C. Chemical bonding
   D. Shells

3. The number of protons in the nucleus is an atom's:
   A. Atomic mass
   B. Atomic energy level
   C. Atomic number
   D. None of the above

4. The number of protons and neutrons combined is the atom's:
   A. Atomic mass
   B. Atomic energy level
   C. Orbit
   D. Chemical bonding

5. Which of the following is *not* one of the major elements present in the human body?
   A. Oxygen
   B. Carbon
   C. Nitrogen
   D. Iron

6. Atoms usually unite with each other to form larger chemical units called:
   A. Energy levels
   B. Mass
   C. Molecules
   D. Shells

7. Substances whose molecules have more than one element in them are called:
   A. Compounds
   B. Orbitals
   C. Elements
   D. Neutrons

True or False

In the space provided, write T for true and F for false.

_____ 8. Matter is anything that occupies space and has mass.

_____ 9. Most chemicals in the body are in the form of electrons.

_____ 10. At the core of each atom is a nucleus composed of positively charged protons and uncharged neutrons.

_____ 11. Orbitals are arranged into energy levels depending on their distance from the nucleus.

_____ 12. The formula for a compound contains symbols for the elements in each molecule.

If you have had difficulty with this section, review pages 19-21.

CHEMICAL BONDING

Multiple Choice

Select the best answer.

13. Ionic bonds are chemical bonds formed by the:
    A. Sharing of electrons between atoms
    B. Donation of protons from one atom to another
    C. Donation of electrons from one atom to another
    D. Acceptance of protons from one atom to another

14. Molecules that form ions when dissolved in water are called:
    A. Covalent bonds
    B. Electrolytes
    C. Isotopes
    D. Ionic bonds

15. When atoms share electrons, a(n) ____________ forms.
    A. Covalent bond
    B. Electrolyte
    C. Ionic bond
    D. Isotope

16. Covalent bonds:
    A. Break apart easily in water
    B. Are not easily broken
    C. Donate electrons
    D. None of the above

17. Hydrogen bonds:
    A. Do *not* form new molecules
    B. Are strong bonds
    C. Have a negative effect on body water
    D. Separate neighboring molecules, allowing them to act more effectively in other areas of the body

18. If a molecule "dissociates" in water, it:
    A. Has taken on additional ions
    B. Has eliminated ions
    C. Separates to form free ions
    D. Forms a covalent bond

If you have had difficulty with this section, review pages 21-23.

INORGANIC CHEMISTRY

Identify each term with its corresponding description or definition.

A. Aqueous solution
B. Water
C. ATP
D. Base
E. Solvent
F. pH
G. Dehydration synthesis
H. Inorganic
I. Weak acid
J. Hydrolysis
K. Strong acid
L. Reactants

_____ 19. A type of compound

_____ 20. Compound most essential to life

_____ 21. Dissolves solutes

_____ 22. Water plus common salt

_____ 23. Reactants combine only after (H) and (O) atoms removed

_____ 24. Combine to form a larger product

_____ 25. The reverse of dehydration synthesis

_____ 26. Yields energy for muscle contraction

_____ 27. Alkaline compound

_____ 28. A measure of the H^+ concentration

_____ 29. Easily dissociates to form H^+ ions

_____ 30. Dissociates very little

If you have had difficulty with this section, review pages 23-26.

ORGANIC CHEMISTRY

Select the best answer.

(A) Carbohydrate (B) Lipid (C) Proteins (D) Nucleic acid

_____ 31. Monosaccharide

_____ 32. Triglyceride

_____ 33. DNA

_____ 34. Cholesterol

_____ 35. Amino acid

_____ 36. Glycogen

_____ 37. Sucrose

_____ 38. Phospholipid

_____ 39. Contains C, O, H, and N

_____ 40. RNA

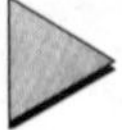

If you have had difficulty with this section, review pages 26-31.

CHEMISTRY OF LIFE

Fill in the crossword puzzle.

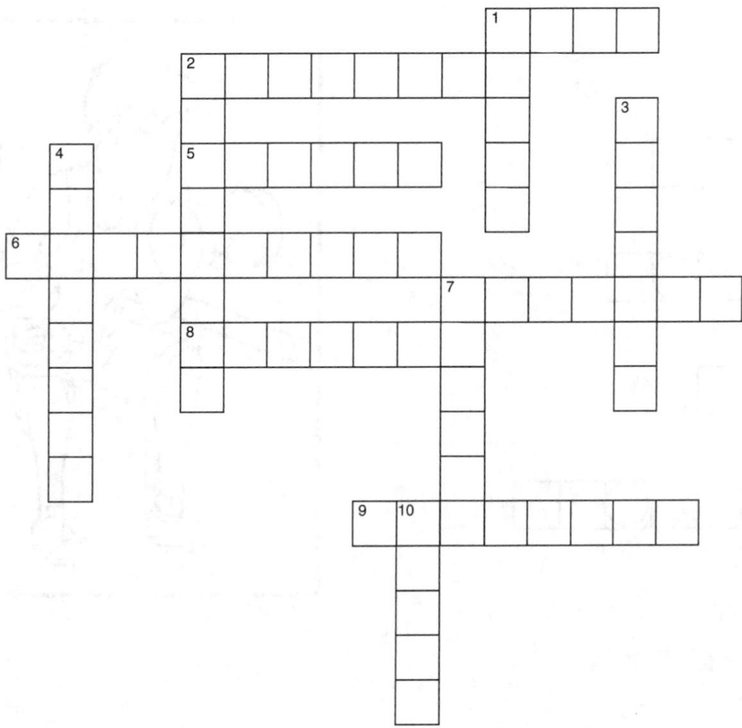

Across
1. Below 7.0 on pH scale
2. Bond formed by sharing electrons
5. Occupies space and has mass
6. Reverse of dehydration synthesis
7. Substances composed of one type of atom
8. Uncharged subatomic particle
9. Subatomic particle

Down
1. Combine to form molecules
2. Substances whose molecules have more than one element
3. Amino acid
4. Polysaccharide
7. Chemical catalyst
10. Fat

UNSCRAMBLE THE WORDS

Take the circled letters, unscramble them, and fill in the statement.

41. **TMATRE**

42. **SETLMENE**

43. **CLSMOEUEL**

44. **NAGRIOC**

45. **RLECETOLYET**

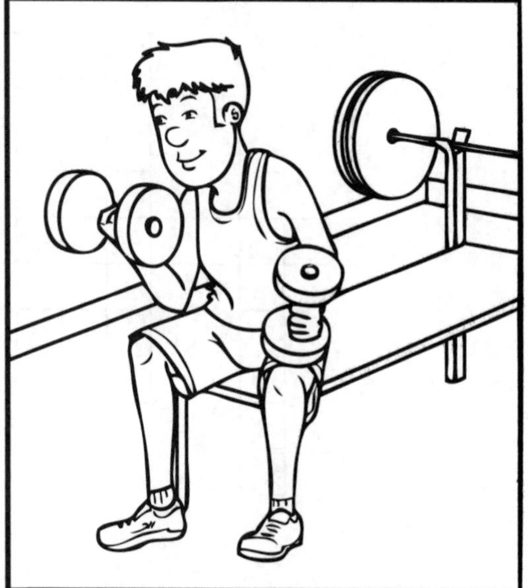

Why Bill worked out each day.

46.

APPLYING WHAT YOU KNOW

47. Sandy just finished preparing a meal of pan-fried hamburgers for her family. While the frying pan was still hot, she poured the liquid grease into a metal container to cool. Later she noticed that the liquid oil had solidified as it cooled. Explain the chemistry of why the now room-temperature fat was solid.

48. Carol was gaining weight, yet she was eating very little. Her physician suspected hypothyroidism and suggested a test that measures radiation emitted by the thyroid when radioactive iodine is introduced into the gland. Describe what the radiologist will do to evaluate Carol's thyroid function.

49. WORD FIND

Can you find 12 terms from this chapter in the box of letters? Words may be spelled top to bottom, bottom to top, right to left, left to right, or diagonally.

Alkaline	Electrolyte
Atomic mass	Molecule
Base	Nucleic acid
Carbohydrate	Proton
Dehydration	Reactant
Dissociation	Solvent

```
E T A R D Y H O B R A C E
T B H S I H L I N A T O D
B N E H S G O U L P O T E
R Z A M S F R K U S M T H
P R O T O N A I E C I X Y
B R N U C L E I C A C I D
C A F T I A E W G G M W R
L E S N A B E C E E A E A
G Q E E T E A R U S S F T
Q R P V I B Y K I L S W I
E T Y L O R T C E L E B O
S B U O N E S P N B R B N
O P J S T D J M O L U H D
```

DID YOU KNOW?

After a vigorous workout, your triglycerides fall 10–20% and your HDL increases by the same percentage for 2–3 hours.

When hydrogen burns in the air, water is formed.

CHECK YOUR KNOWLEDGE

Fill in the Blanks

1. ____________________ is the field of science devoted to studying the chemical aspects of life.
2. Atoms are composed of protons, electrons, and ____________________.
3. The farther an orbital extends from the nucleus, the ____________________ its energy level.
4. Substances can be classified as ____________________ or ____________________.
5. Chemical bonds form to make atoms more ____________________.
6. A(n) ____________________ is an electrically charged atom.
7. Few ____________________ compounds have carbon atoms in them and none have C-C or C-H bonds.
8. ______________ ____________________ is a reaction in which water is lost from the reactants.
9. Chemists often use a(n) ______________ ________________ to represent a chemical reaction.

10. High levels of ____________________ in the blood make the blood more acidic.

11. ____________________ are compounds that produce an excess of H^+ ions.

12. ____________________ maintain pH balance by preventing sudden changes in the H^+ ion concentration.

13. ____________________ literally means "carbon" and "water."

14. ____________________ is a steroid lipid.

15. Collagen and keratin are examples of ____________________ proteins.

Multiple Choice

Select the best answer.

16. Two atoms that have the same atomic number but different atomic masses are ______________ of the same element.
    A. Isotopes
    B. Compounds
    C. Molecules
    D. Hydrogen bonds

17. An example of an ionic bond is:
    A. NaCl
    B. Ca
    C. O
    D. P

18. The "internal sea" of the body is:
    A. Blood
    B. Aqueous solution
    C. Water
    D. Urine

19. An example of a polysaccharide is a(n):
    A. Triglyceride
    B. Enzyme
    C. Steroid
    D. Glycogen

20. ATP serves the body by:
    A. Metabolizing excess proteins in the blood
    B. Filtering harmful bacteria out of the blood
    C. Making energy available to cellular processes
    D. Serving as a catalyst for chemical reactions in the urine filtration process

CHAPTER 3

Cells and Tissues

Cells are the smallest structural units of living things. Therefore, because we are living, we are made up of a mass of cells. Human cells, which vary in shape and size, can only be seen under a microscope. The three main parts of a cell are the cytoplasmic membrane, the cytoplasm, and the nucleus. As you review this chapter, you will be amazed at the resemblance of cells to the body as a whole. You will identify miniature circulatory systems, reproductive systems, digestive systems, power plants (much like muscular systems), and many other structures that will aid in your understanding of these body systems in future chapters.

Cells, just like humans, require water, food, gases, the elimination of wastes, and numerous other substances and processes in order to survive. The movement of these substances into and out of cells is accomplished by two primary methods: passive transport processes and active transport processes. In passive transport processes, no cellular energy is required to effect movement through the cell membrane. However, in active transport processes, cellular energy is required to provide movement through the cell membrane. The cellular energy required for this movement is obtained from adenosine triphosphate (ATP)

The study of cell reproduction completes the chapter's overview of cells. A basic explanation of DNA, "the hereditary molecule," provides a proper respect for the capability of the cell to transmit physical and mental traits from generation to generation. Reproduction of the cell, mitosis, is a complex process requiring several stages. These stages are outlined and diagrammed in the text to facilitate learning.

This chapter concludes with a discussion of tissues and reviews the four main types of tissues: epithelial, connective, muscle, and nervous. Knowledge of the characteristics, location, and function of these tissues is necessary to complete your understanding of the next structural level of organization.

TOPICS FOR REVIEW

Before progressing to Chapter 4, you should have an understanding of the structure and function of the smallest living unit in the body—the cell. Your review should also include the methods by which substances move through the cell membrane and the stages that occur during cell reproduction. As you finish this chapter, you should have an understanding of tonicity and body tissues and the function they perform in the body.

CELLS

Match the term on the left with the proper selection on the right.

Group A

____ 1. Cytoplasm
____ 2. Plasma membrane
____ 3. Cholesterol
____ 4. Nucleus
____ 5. Centrioles

A. Component of plasma membrane
B. Controls reproduction of the cell
C. "Living matter"
D. Function during cell division
E. Surrounds and serves as a boundary for cells

Group B

____ 6. Ribosomes
____ 7. Endoplasmic reticulum
____ 8. Mitochondria
____ 9. Lysosomes
____ 10. Golgi apparatus

A. "Power plants"
B. "Digestive bags"
C. "Chemical processing and packaging center"
D. "Protein factories"
E. "Smooth and rough"

Fill in the blanks.

11. The numerous small structures that function like organs in a cell are called ____________.

12. A procedure performed prior to transplanting an organ from one individual to another is ____________ ____________.

13. Fine, hairlike extensions found on the exposed or free surfaces of some cells are called ____________.

14. The process that uses oxygen to break down glucose and other nutrients to release energy required for cellular work is called ____________ ____________.

15. ____________ are usually attached to rough endoplasmic reticulum and produce enzymes and other protein compounds.

16. The ____________ provide energy-releasing chemical reactions that go on continuously.

17. The organelles that can digest and destroy microbes that invade the cell are called ____________.

18. Mucus is an example of a product manufactured by the ____________ ____________.

19. These rod-shaped structures, ____________, play an important role during cell division.

20. ____________ ____________ in the nucleus are made of proteins around which are wound segments of the long, threadlike molecules called *DNA*.

If you have had difficulty with this section, review pages 36-44.

MOVEMENT OF SUBSTANCES THROUGH CELL MEMBRANES

Select the best answer.

21. The energy required for active transport processes is obtained from:
    A. ATP
    B. DNA
    C. Diffusion
    D. Osmosis

22. An example of a passive transport process is:
    A. Permease system
    B. Phagocytosis
    C. Pinocytosis
    D. Diffusion

23. Movement of substances from a region of high concentration to a region of low concentration is known as:
    A. Active transport
    B. Passive transport
    C. Cellular energy
    D. Concentration gradient

24. Osmosis is the ____________________ of water across a selectively permeable membrane when some of the solutes cannot cross the membrane.
    A. Filtration
    B. Equilibrium
    C. Active transport
    D. Diffusion

25. ________________________ involves the movement of solutes across a selectively permeable membrane by the process of diffusion.
    A. Osmosis
    B. Filtration
    C. Dialysis
    D. Phagocytosis

26. An example of diffusion is:
    A. Osmosis
    B. An ion pump
    C. Filtration
    D. Phagocytosis

27. ________________ always occurs down a hydrostatic pressure gradient.
    A. Osmosis
    B. Filtration
    C. Dialysis
    D. Facilitated diffusion

28. The uphill movement of a substance through a living cell membrane is:
    A. Osmosis
    B. Diffusion
    C. Active transport process
    D. Passive transport process

29. An example of an active transport process is:
    A. Ion pump
    B. Phagocytosis
    C. Pinocytosis
    D. All of the above

30. An example of a cell that uses phagocytosis is the:
    A. White blood cell
    B. Red blood cell
    C. Muscle cell
    D. Bone cell

31. A solution that contains a higher concentration of salt than living red blood cells would be:
    A. Hypotonic
    B. Hypertonic
    C. Isotonic
    D. Homeostatic

32. A red blood cell becomes engorged with water and will eventually lyse, releasing hemoglobin into the solution. This solution is _______________ to the red blood cell.
    A. Hypotonic
    B. Hypertonic
    C. Isotonic
    D. Homeostatic

If you have had difficulty with this section, review pages 44-49.

CELL REPRODUCTION

Circle the one that does not *belong.*

33. DNA	Adenine	Uracil	Thymine
34. Complementary base pairing	Guanine	Telophase	Cytosine
35. Anaphase	Specific sequence	Gene	Base pairs
36. RNA	Ribosome	Thymine	Uracil
37. Translation	Protein synthesis	mRNA	Interphase
38. Cleavage furor	Anaphase	Prophase	2 daughter cells
39. "Resting"	Prophase	Interphase	DNA replication
40. Identical	2 nuclei	Telophase	Metaphase
41. Metaphase	Prophase	Telophase	Gene

If you have had difficulty with this section, review pages 49-54.

TISSUES

42. *Fill in the missing areas of the chart.*

TISSUE	LOCATION	FUNCTION
	Epithelial	
1. Simple squamous	1A. Alveoli of lungs	1A. diffusion of respiratory gases
	1B. Lining of blood and lymphatic vessels	1B. diffusion, filtration, osmosis
2. Stratified squamous	2A. surface of mouth & esophagus lining	2A. Protection
	2B. surface of skin (epidermis)	2B. Protection
3. Simple columnar	3. surface layer of lining of stomach, intestines, respiratory tract	3. Protection, secretion, absorption
4. stratified transitional	4. Urinary bladder	4. Protection
5. Pseudostratified	5. surface lining of trachea	5. Protection
6. Simple cuboidal	6. Glands; kidney tubules	6. secretion / absorption
	Connective	
1. Areolar	1. area between tissues & organs	1. Connection
2. Adipose (fat)	2. Under skin	2. Protection; insulation
3. Dense fibrous	3. Tendons; ligaments; fascia, scar tissue	3. flexible but strong connection
4. Bone	4. skeleton	4. Support, protection
5. Cartilage	5. disks between vertebrea	5. Firm but flexible support
6. Blood	6. Blood vessels	6. transportation
7. hematopoietic	7. Red bone marrow	7. Blood cell formation
	Muscle	
1. Skeletal (striated voluntary)	1. muscles that attach to bone	1. Movement of bones
2. cardiac (striated involuntary)	2. Wall of heart	2. Contraction of heart
3. Smooth (nonstriated involuntary or visceral)	3.	3. Movement of substances along ducts; change in diameter of pupils and shape of lens; "gooseflesh"
	Nervous	
1.	1. brain, spinal cord, nerves	1. Irritability, conduction

If you have had difficulty with this section, review pages 54-64 and Tables 3-6, 3-7, and 3-8.

UNSCRAMBLE THE WORDS

Take the circled letters, unscramble them, and fill in the statement.

43. **L S A N T A R O I T N**

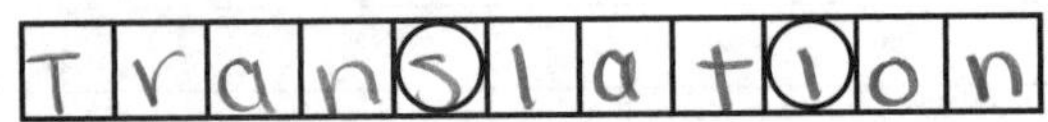

44. **P T R A E S I N H E**

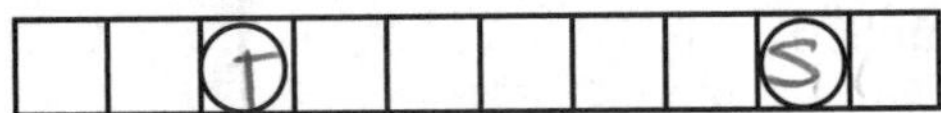

45. **N E E G**

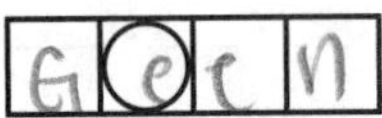

46. **O O S S S M I**

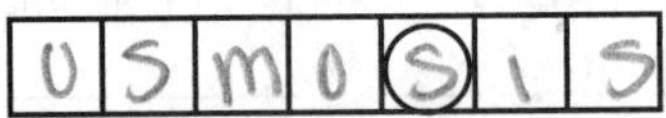

47. **N D F S I F U O I**

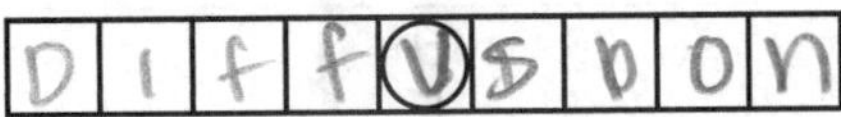

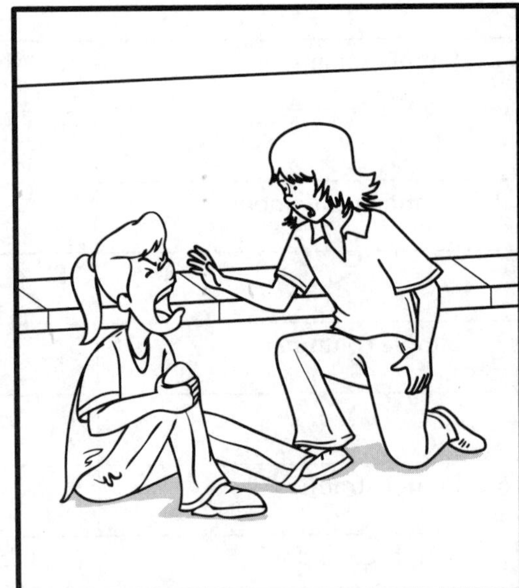

What Madison's friend gave her when she tripped and fell.

48. 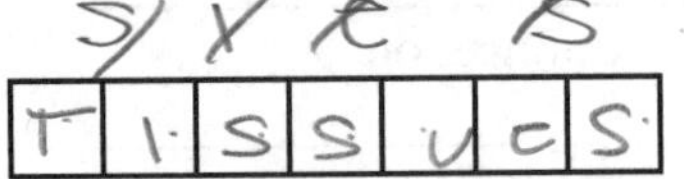

APPLYING WHAT YOU KNOW

49. Mr. Fee's boat had capsized, and he was stranded on a deserted shoreline for 2 days without food or water. When he was found, it was discovered that he had swallowed a great deal of seawater. He was taken to the emergency room in a state of dehydration. In the space below, draw the appearance of Mr. Fee's red blood cells as they would appear to the laboratory technician.

hyper tonic

50. The nurse was instructed to dissolve a pill in a small amount of liquid medication. As she dropped the capsule into the liquid, she was interrupted by the telephone. On her return to the medication cart, she found the medication completely dissolved and apparently was scattered evenly throughout the liquid. This phenomenon did not surprise her since she was aware from her knowledge of cell transport that osmosis had created this distribution.

51. Ms. Bence has emphysema. She has been admitted to the hospital and is receiving oxygen per nasal cannula. Emphysema destroys the tiny air sacs in the lungs. These tiny air sacs, called *alveoli*, provide what function for Ms. Bence?

52. Merrily was 5′4″ and weighed 115 lbs. She appeared very healthy and fit, yet her doctor advised her that she was "overfat." What might be the explanation for this assessment?

no musdc all fat.

53. WORD FIND

Can you find 16 terms from this chapter? Words may be spelled top to bottom, bottom to top, right to left, left to right, or diagonally.

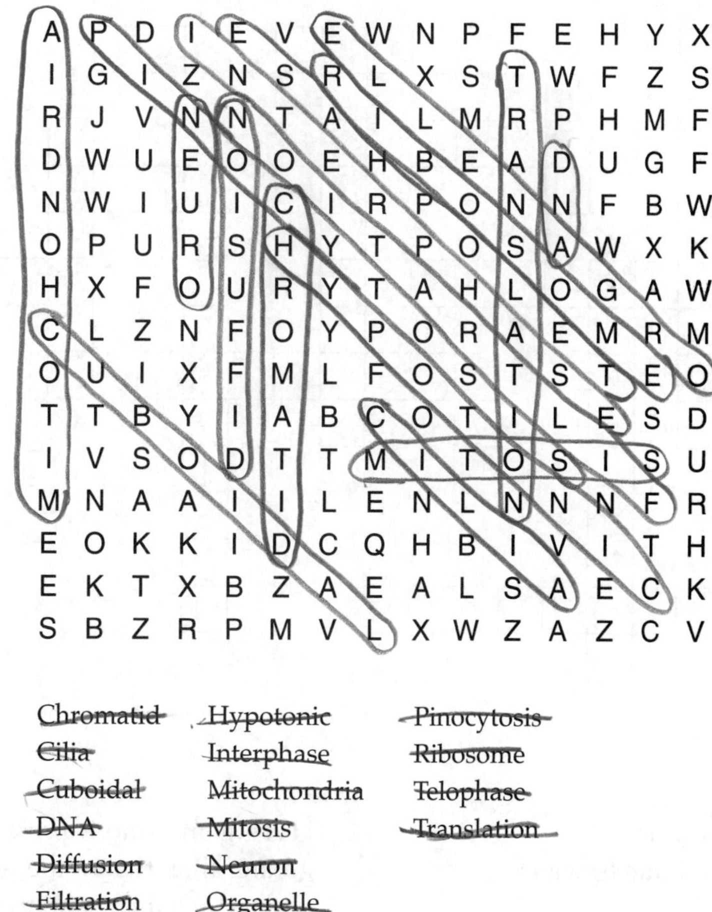

Chromatid	Hypotonic	Pinocytosis
Cilia	Interphase	Ribosome
Cuboidal	Mitochondria	Telophase
DNA	Mitosis	Translation
Diffusion	Neuron	
Filtration	Organelle	

DID YOU KNOW?

The largest single cell in the human body is the female sex cell, the ovum. The smallest single cell in the human body is the male sex cell, the sperm.

Other than your brain cells, 50,000,000 of the cells in your body will have died and been replaced with others in the time it took you to read this sentence.

The longest living cells in the body are brain cells, which can live an entire lifetime.

Only 5% of eligible donors across the nation donate blood, but the number of transfusions nationwide increases by 9% every year.

CELLS AND TISSUES

Fill in the crossword puzzle.

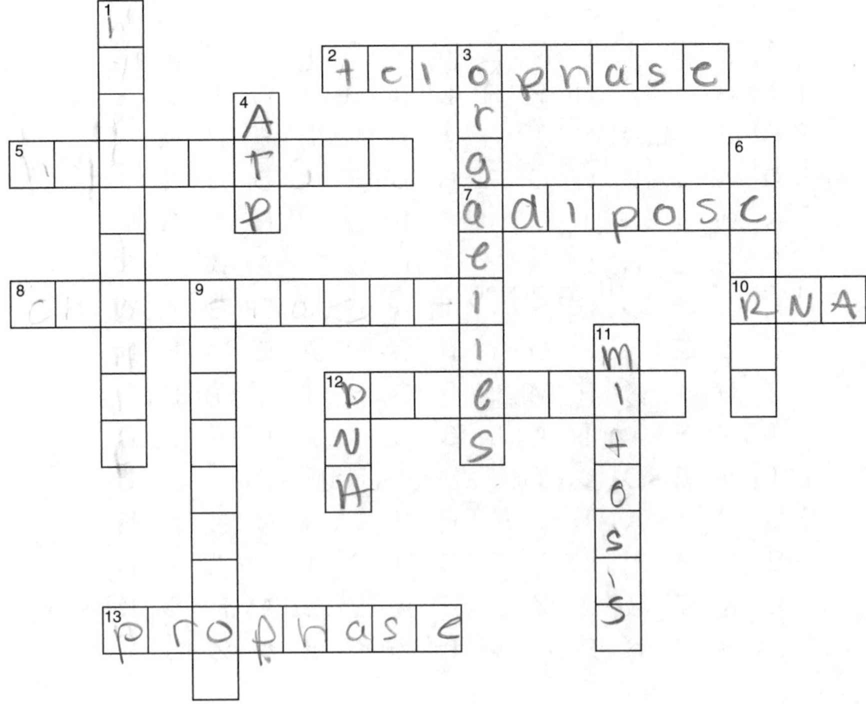

Across

2. Last stage of mitosis
5. Shriveling of cell due to water withdrawal
7. Fat
8. Cartilage cell
10. Ribonucleic acid (abbreviation)
12. Specialized example of diffusion
13. First stage of mitosis

Down

1. Having an osmotic pressure greater than that of the solution with which it is compared
3. Cell organ
4. Energy source for active transport
6. Nerve cell
9. Occurs when substances scatter themselves evenly throughout an available space
11. Reproduction process of most cells
12. Chemical "blueprint" of the body (abbreviation)

CHECK YOUR KNOWLEDGE

Multiple Choice

Select the best answer.

1. The internal living material of cells is/are the:
   A. Cytoplasm
   B. Plasma membrane
   C. Nucleus
   D. Centrioles

2. The "protein factories" of the cell are the:
   A. Mitochondria
   B. Ribosomes
   C. Lysosomes
   D. Golgi apparatus

3. The process of enzymes using oxygen to break down glucose and other nutrients to release energy required for cellular work is:
   A. Chemical processing
   B. Cellular respiration
   C. Apoptosis
   D. Passive transport

4. Two of these rod-shaped structures exist in every cell.
   A. Centrioles
   B. Cilia
   C. Ribosomes
   D. Lysosomes

5. Adenosine triphosphate is the chemical substance that provides the energy required for:
   A. Passive transport
   B. Osmosis
   C. Active transport
   D. Dialysis

6. A solution that contains a lower concentration of salt than living red blood cells would be:
   A. Hypotonic
   B. Hypertonic
   C. Isotonic
   D. Homeostatic

7. It is the sequence of base pairs in each gene of each chromosome that determines:
   A. Anaphase
   B. Thymine
   C. Translation
   D. Heredity

8. The specific and visible stages of cell division are preceded by a period called:
   A. Anaphase
   B. Interphase
   C. Prophase
   D. Metaphase

9. Which of the following is *not* an example of muscle tissue?
   A. Smooth
   B. Skeletal
   C. Hemopoietic
   D. Cardiac

10. Stratified squamous epithelium assists the body by providing:
    A. Anchors for our bones
    B. Support for the body
    C. Contractility
    D. Protection against invasion by microorganisms

Matching

Select the most correct answer from column B for each statement in column A. (Only one answer is correct.)

Column A

F 11. Endoplasmic reticulum
G 12. Flagellum
J 13. Chromosomes
A 14. Passive transport
C 15. Active transport
B 16. Isotonic
I 17. Transcription
H 18. Anaphase
D 19. Telophase
E 20. Connective tissue

Column B

A. Phagocytosis
B. 0.9% NaCl solution
C. Osmosis
D. Cell division complete
E. Blood
F. Rough and smooth
G. Tail of the sperm cell
H. Cleavage furrow
I. Messenger RNA
J. DNA

CELL STRUCTURE

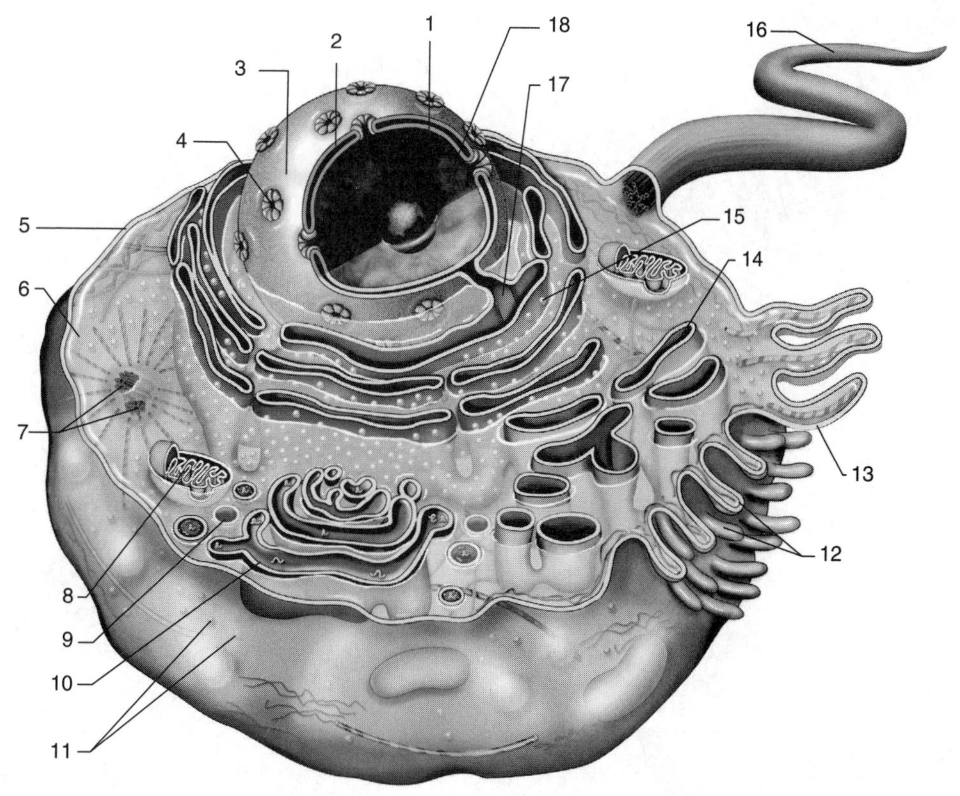

1. nucleolus
2. nuclear envelope
3. nucleus
4. nuclear pores
5. plasma membrane
6. cytoplasm
7. centrioles
8. mitochondria
9. lysosomes
10. golgi apparatus
11. free ribosomes
12. microvilli
13. cilia
14. smooth ER
15. ribosome
16. flagellum
17. rough ER
18. chromatin

MITOSIS

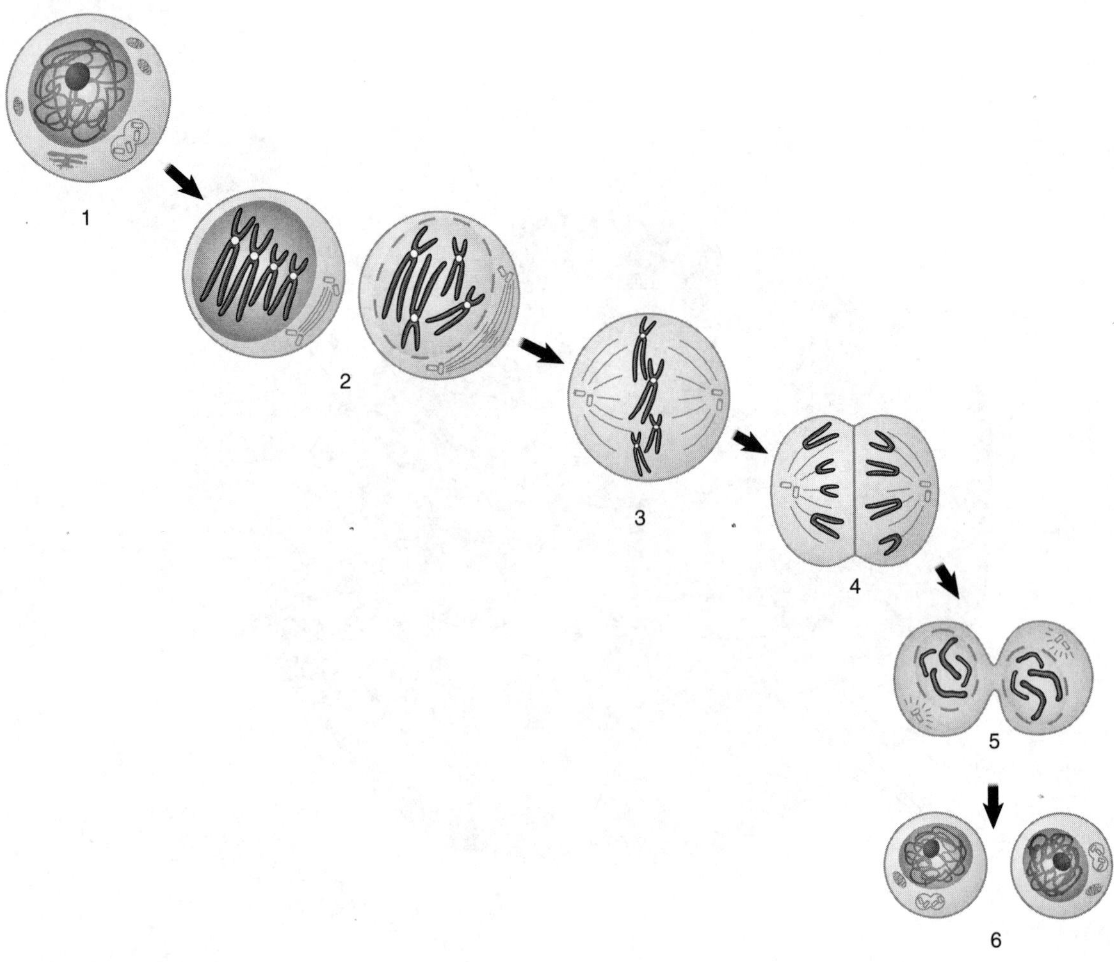
1
2
3
4
5
6

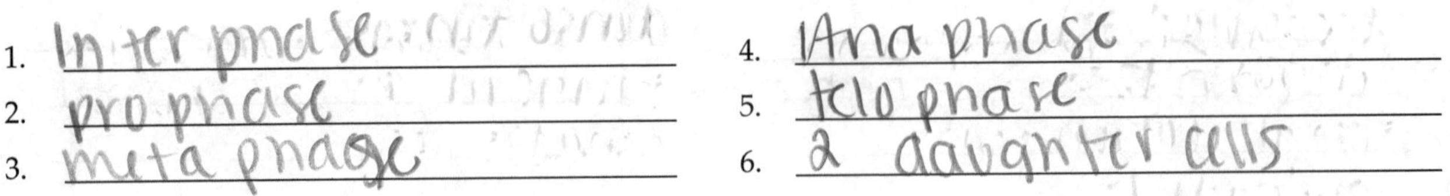
1. In ter phase
2. pro phase
3. meta phage
4. Ana phase
5. telo phase
6. 2 daughter cells

TISSUES

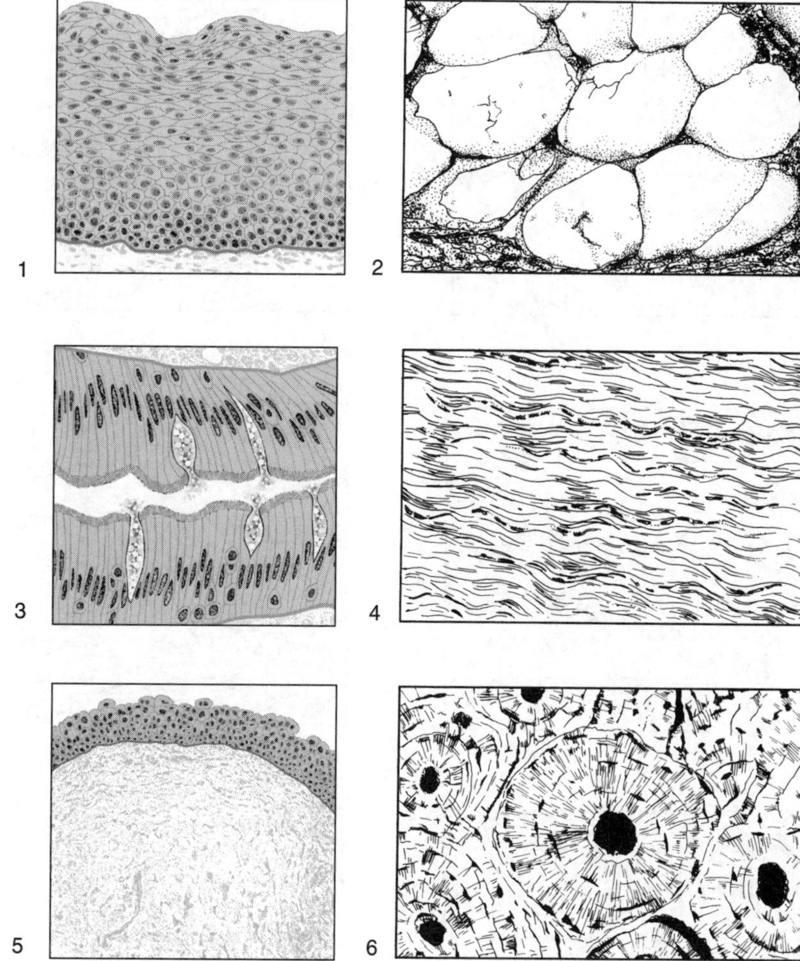

1. stratified squmosepithelium
2. adipose tissue
3. simple columnar epithelium
4. dense fibrous connective tissue
5. stratified transitional epithelium
6. bone tissue

(Continued next page.)

TISSUES *(CONT.)*

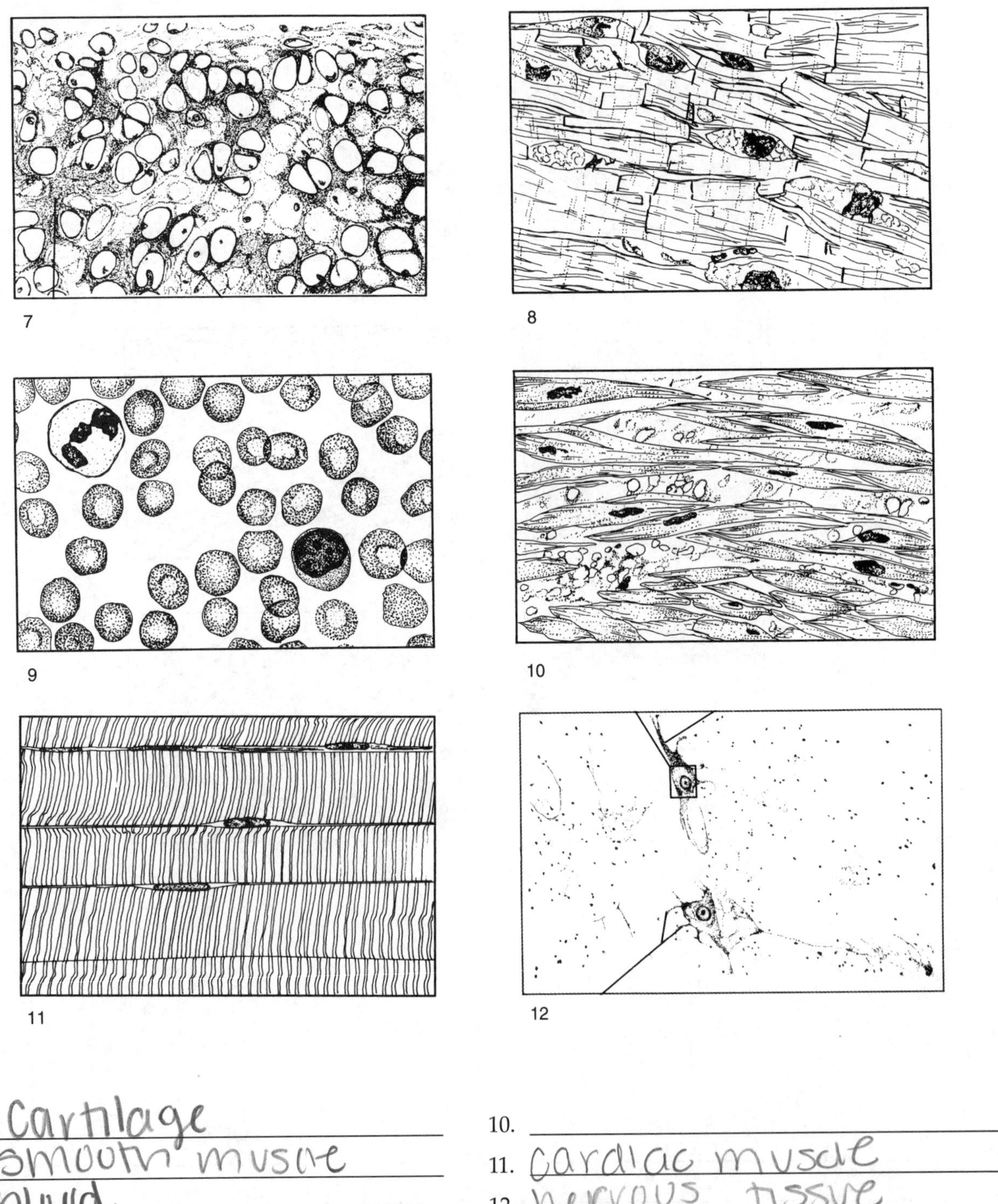

7. cartilage
8. smooth muscle
9. blood.
10.
11. cardiac muscle
12. nervous tissue

CHAPTER 4

Organ Systems of the Body

A smooth-running automobile is the result of many systems harmoniously working together. The engine, the fuel system, the exhaust system, the brake system, and the cooling system are but a few of the many complex structural units that the automobile as a whole relies on to keep it functioning smoothly. So it is with the human body. We, too, depend on the successful performance of many individual systems working together to create and maintain a healthy human being.

When you have completed your review of the 11 major organ systems and the organs that make up these systems, you will find your understanding of the performance of the body as a whole much more meaningful.

TOPICS FOR REVIEW

Before progressing to Chapter 5, you should have an understanding of the 11 major organ systems and be able to identify the organs that are included in each system.

ORGAN SYSTEMS OF THE BODY

Match the term on the left with the proper selection on the right.

Group A

_____	1. Integumentary	A. Hair
_____	2. Skeletal	B. Spinal cord
_____	3. Muscular	C. Hormones
_____	4. Nervous	D. Tendons
_____	5. Endocrine	E. Joints

Group B

_____	6. Circulatory	A. Esophagus
_____	7. Lymphatic	B. Ureters
_____	8. Urinary	C. Larynx
_____	9. Digestive	D. Genitalia
_____	10. Respiratory	E. Spleen
_____	11. Reproductive	F. Capillaries

Circle the one that does not *belong.*

12. Pharynx	Trachea	Mouth	Alveoli
13. Uterus	Rectum	Gonads	Prostate
14. Veins	Arteries	Heart	Pancreas
15. Pineal	Bladder	Ureters	Urethra
16. Cardiac	Smooth	Joints	Voluntary
17. Pituitary	Brain	Spinal cord	Nerves
18. Cartilage	Joints	Ligaments	Tendons
19. Hormones	Pituitary	Pancreas	Appendix
20. Thymus	Nails	Hair	Oil glands
21. Esophagus	Pharynx	Mouth	Trachea
22. Thymus	Spleen	Tonsils	Liver

Fill in the missing areas.

SYSTEM	ORGANS	FUNCTION
23. Integumentary	Skin, nails, hair, sense receptors, sweat glands, oil glands	
24. Skeletal		Support, movement, storage of minerals, blood formation
25. Muscular	Muscles	
26.	Brain, spinal cord, nerves	Communication, integration, control, recognition of sensory stimuli
27. Endocrine		Secretion of hormones; communication, integration, control
28. Circulatory	Heart, blood vessels	
29. Lymphatic		Transportation, immunity
30.	Kidneys, ureters, bladder, urethra	Elimination of wastes, electrolyte balance, acid-base balance, water balance
31. Digestive		Digestion of food, absorption of nutrients
32.	Nose, pharynx, larynx, trachea, bronchi, lungs	Exchange of gases in the lungs, regulation of acid-base balance
33. Reproductive		Survival of species; production of sex cells, fertilization, development, birth; nourishment of offspring; production of hormones

If you have had difficulty with this section, review pages 71-83.

UNSCRAMBLE THE WORDS

Take the circled letters, unscramble them, and fill in the statement.

34. **R T A H E**

☐☐☐◯☐

35. **I E P L N A**

☐☐◯◯☐☐

36. **E E N V R**

☐☐☐◯☐

37. **S U H E S O P G A**

☐◯◯☐☐☐◯☐

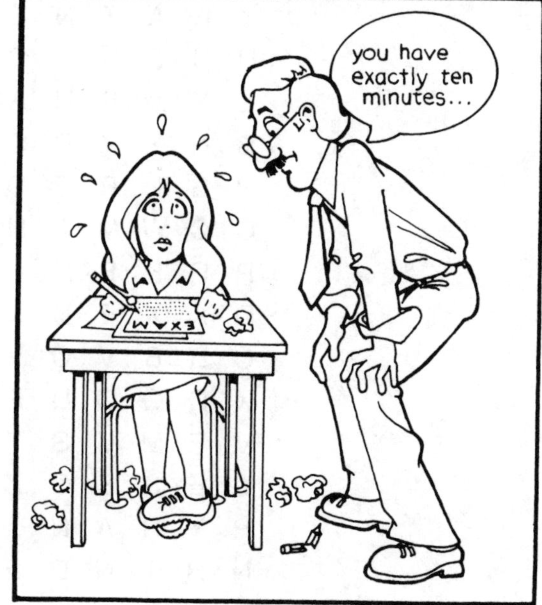

The more thoroughly you review this chapter, the less ________________ you will be during your test.

38.

☐☐☐☐☐☐☐

APPLYING WHAT YOU KNOW

39. Myrna was 15 years old and had not yet started menstruating. Her family physician decided to consult two other physicians, each of whom specialized in a different system. Specialists in the areas of ________________________ and ________________________ were consulted.
40. Brian was admitted to the hospital with second- and third-degree burns that covered 50% of his body. He was placed in isolation, so when Jenny went to visit him, she was required to wear a hospital gown and mask. Why was Brian placed in isolation? Why was Jenny required to wear special attire?

41. WORD FIND

Can you find 11 organ systems? Words may be spelled top to bottom, bottom to top, right to left, left to right, or diagonally.

Y	R	A	T	N	E	M	U	G	E	T	N	I	R	F
H	N	E	R	V	O	U	S	K	I	R	J	M	G	T
L	Y	M	P	H	A	T	I	C	I	S	Y	Y	U	I
B	N	X	Y	R	O	T	A	L	U	C	R	I	C	W
P	E	L	R	E	O	M	J	M	S	O	M	M	P	S
C	C	W	M	A	N	D	L	A	T	E	L	E	K	S
R	R	K	E	M	L	I	U	A	A	V	V	U	K	N
D	K	X	P	D	J	U	R	C	J	I	R	Q	E	M
C	D	B	V	C	V	I	C	C	T	T	K	W	C	X
X	R	Q	Q	D	P	H	C	S	O	I	X	P	A	Z
M	F	M	U	S	Y	D	E	V	U	D	V	Y	K	E
U	E	S	E	C	Z	G	T	Q	D	M	N	E	K	O
P	Y	R	A	N	I	R	U	C	T	C	N	E	W	H
N	H	T	N	D	E	P	S	I	X	A	Q	O	I	E

Circulatory
Digestive
Endocrine
Integumentary
Lymphatic
Muscular
Nervous
Reproductive
Respiratory
Skeletal
Urinary

DID YOU KNOW?

Muscles comprise 40% of your body weight. Your skeleton, however, only accounts for 18% of your body weight.

Every person has a unique tongue print.

MATCHING

Select the most correct answer from column B for each statement in column A. (Only one answer is correct.)

Column A	Column B
_____ 11. Oil glands	A. Endocrine
_____ 12. Blood vessels	B. Urinary
_____ 13. Tonsils	C. Integumentary
_____ 14. Vas deferens	D. Circulatory
_____ 15. Ureters	E. Respiratory
_____ 16. Appendix	F. Digestive
_____ 17. Vulva	G. Male reproductive
_____ 18. Larynx	H. Lymphatic
_____ 19. Brain	I. Female reproductive
_____ 20. Thyroid	J. Nervous

CHAPTER 5

Integumentary System and Body Membranes

More of our time, attention, and money are spent on this system than any other one. Every time we look into a mirror, we become aware of the integumentary system as we observe our skin, hair, nails, and the appendages that give luster and comfort to this system. The discussion of the skin begins with the structure and function of the two primary layers—the epidermis and the dermis. It continues with an examination of the appendages of the skin, which include the hair, receptors, nails, sebaceous glands, and sudoriferous glands. Your study of skin concludes with a review of one of the most serious and frequent threats to the skin—burn injury. An understanding of the integumentary system provides you with an appreciation of the danger that severe burns pose to this system.

Membranes are thin, sheetlike structures that cover, protect, anchor, or lubricate body surfaces, cavities, and organs. The two major categories of membranes are epithelial and connective. Each type is located in specific areas of the body and is vulnerable to specific disease conditions. Knowledge of the location and function of these membranes prepares you for the study of their relationship to other systems and to the body as a whole.

TOPICS FOR REVIEW

Before progressing to Chapter 6, you should have an understanding of the skin and its appendages. Your review should include the classification of burns and the method used to estimate the percentage of body surface area affected by burn injury. Knowledge of the types of body membranes, their location, and their function is also necessary as you complete your study of this chapter.

CLASSIFICATION OF BODY MEMBRANES

Select the best answer.

(A) Cutaneous (B) Serous (C) Mucous (D) Synovial

B 1. Pleura
D 2. Lines joint spaces
___ 3. Respiratory tract
A 4. Skin
B 5. Peritoneum
A 6. Contains no epithelium
___ 7. Urinary tract
C 8. Lines body surfaces that open directly to the exterior

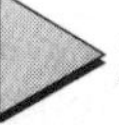

If you have had difficulty with this section, review pages 89-92.

THE SKIN

Match the term on the left with the proper selection on the right.

Group A

Answer	Term	Selection
D	9. Integumentary system	A. Outermost layer of skin
A	10. Epidermis	B. Deeper of the two layers of skin
B	11. Dermis	C. Hypodermis
C	12. Subcutaneous	D. The skin is the primary organ
E	13. Cutaneous membrane	E. Composed of dermis and epidermis

Group B

Answer	Term	Selection
A	14. Keratin	A. Protective protein
D	15. Melanin	B. Blue-gray color of skin resulting from a decrease in oxygen
E	16. Stratum corneum	C. Parallel rows of tiny bumps
C	17. Dermal papillae	D. Brown pigment
B	18. Cyanosis	E. Outer layer of epidermis

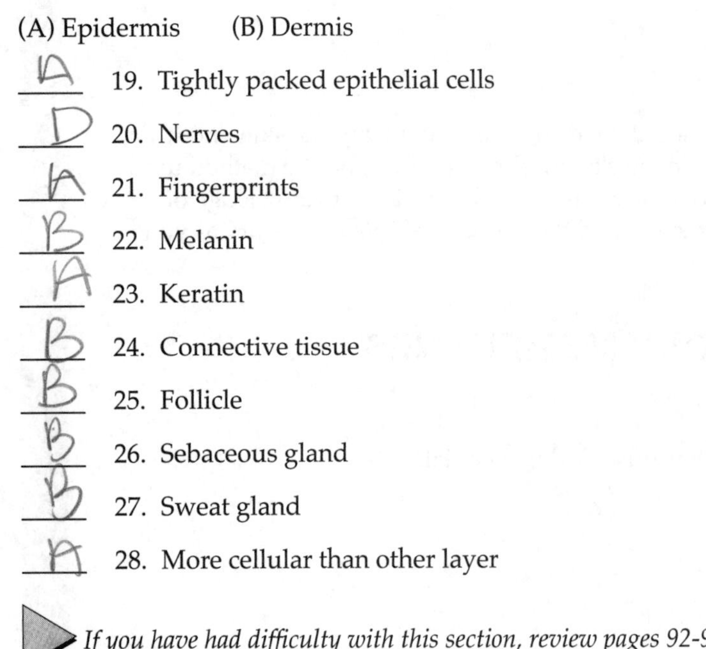

Select the correct term from the choices given and write the letter in the answer blank.

(A) Epidermis (B) Dermis

A 19. Tightly packed epithelial cells

D 20. Nerves

A 21. Fingerprints

B 22. Melanin

A 23. Keratin

B 24. Connective tissue

B 25. Follicle

B 26. Sebaceous gland

B 27. Sweat gland

A 28. More cellular than other layer

If you have had difficulty with this section, review pages 92-95.

Fill in the blanks.

29. The three most important functions of the skin are ____________, ____________ ____________, and ____________ ____________ ____________.

30. ____________ prevents the sun's ultraviolet rays from penetrating the interior of the body.

31. The hair of a newborn infant is called ____________.

32. Hair growth begins from a small cap-shaped cluster of cells called the ____________ ____________.

33. The nail body nearest the root has a crescent-shaped white area known as the ____________ or "little moon."

34. The ____________ ____________ muscles produce "goose pimples."

35. Meissner's corpuscle is generally located rather close to the skin's surface and is capable of detecting sensations of ____________ ____________.

36. The most numerous, important, and widespread sweat glands in the body are the ____________ sweat glands.

37. The ____________ sweat glands are found primarily in the axilla and in the pigmented skin areas around the genitals.

38. ____________ has been described as "nature's skin cream."

Circle the correct answer.

39. A first-degree burn (will or will not) blister.

40. A second-degree burn (will or will not) scar.

41. A third-degree burn (will or will not) have pain immediately.

42. According to the "rule of nines," the body is divided into (9 or 11) areas of 9%.

43. Destruction of the subcutaneous layer occurs in (second or third) -degree burns.

If you have had difficulty with this section, review pages 93-102.

UNSCRAMBLE THE WORDS

Take the circled letters, unscramble them, and fill in the statement.

44. **PIDEEMIRS**

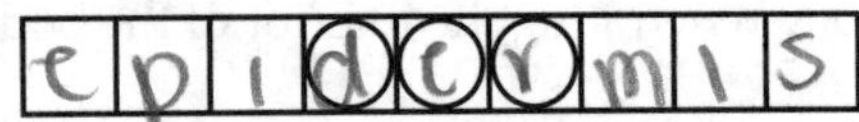

45. **REKTAIN**

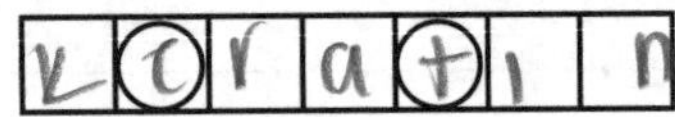

46. **AHIR**

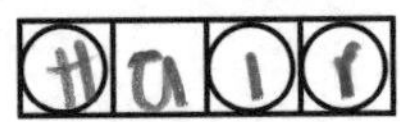

47. **UGONAL**

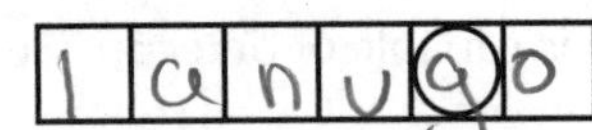

48. **DRTONIDEHYA**

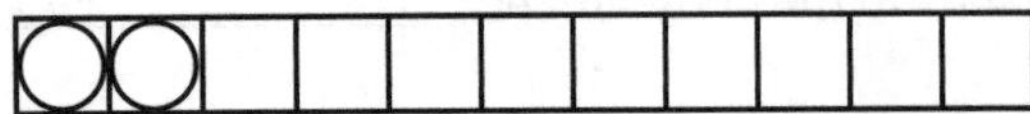

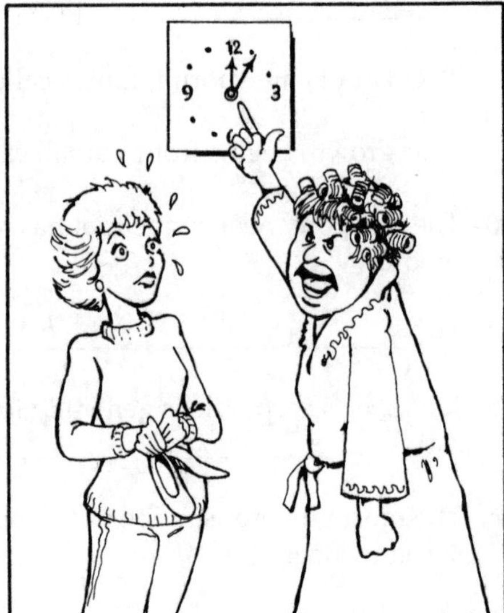

What Amanda's mother gave her after every date.

49.

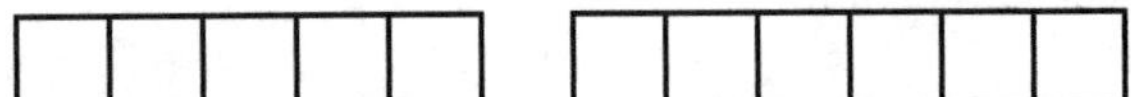

APPLYING WHAT YOU KNOW

50. Mr. Ziven was admitted to the hospital with second- and third-degree burns. Both arms, anterior trunk, right anterior leg, and genital region were affected by the burns. The doctor quickly estimated that ______% of Mr. Ziven's body had been burned.
51. Mrs. Shearer complained to her doctor that she had severe pain in her chest and feared that she was having a heart attack. An electrocardiogram revealed nothing unusual, but Mrs. Shearer insisted that every time she took a breath she experienced pain. What might be the cause of Mrs. Shearer's pain?

Pleurisy

52. After investigating the scene of the crime, Officer Halas announced that he had found dermal papillae that would help solve the case. What did he mean?

53. WORD FIND

Can you find the 15 terms from this chapter in the box of letters? Words may be spelled top to bottom, bottom to top, right to left, left to right, or diagonally.

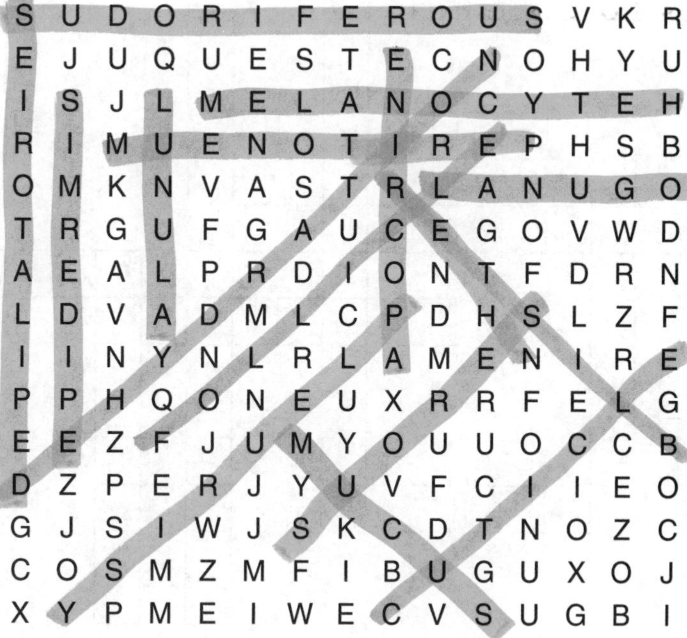

Apocrine
Blister
Cuticle
Dehydration
Depilatories
Epidermis
Follicle
Lanugo
Lunula
Melanocyte
Mucus
Peritoneum
Pleurisy
Serous
Sudoriferous

DID YOU KNOW?

Because the dead cells of the epidermis are constantly being worn and washed away, we get a new outer skin layer every 27 days.

In your lifetime, you will shed 40 pounds of skin.

Blype is the skin that peels off after a bad sunburn.

Your fingernails will grow 84 feet in your lifetime.

SKIN/BODY MEMBRANES

Fill in the crossword puzzle.

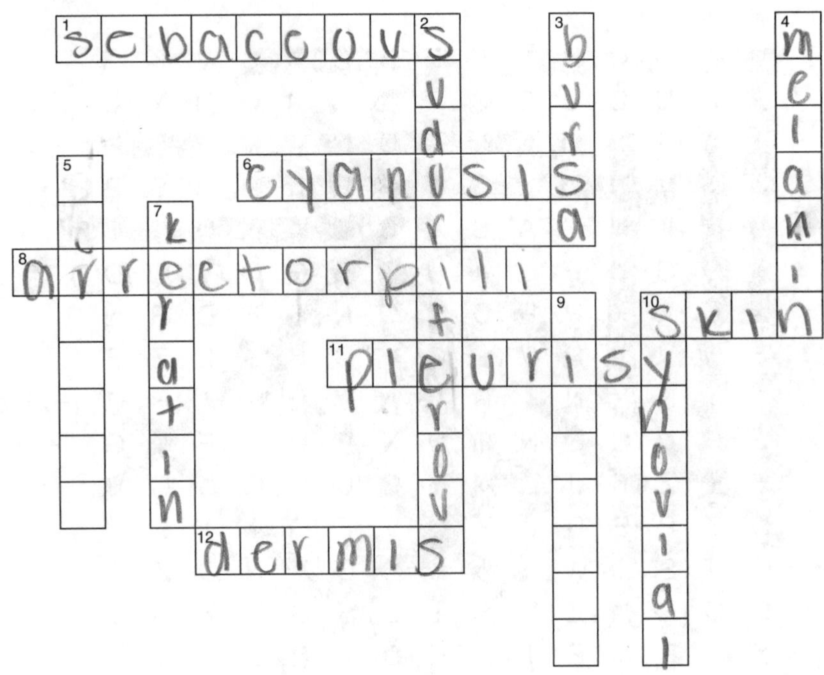

Across

1. Oil gland
6. Bluish gray color of skin due to decreased oxygen
8. "Goose pimples" (two words)
10. Cutaneous
11. Inflammation of the serous membrane that lines the chest and covers the lungs
12. Deeper of the two primary skin layers

Down

2. Sweat gland
3. Cushionlike sac found between moving body parts
4. Brown pigment
5. Forms the lining of serous body cavities
7. Tough waterproof substance that protects body from excess fluid loss
9. Covers the surface of organs found in serous body cavities
10. Membrane that lines joint spaces

LONGITUDINAL SECTION OF THE SKIN

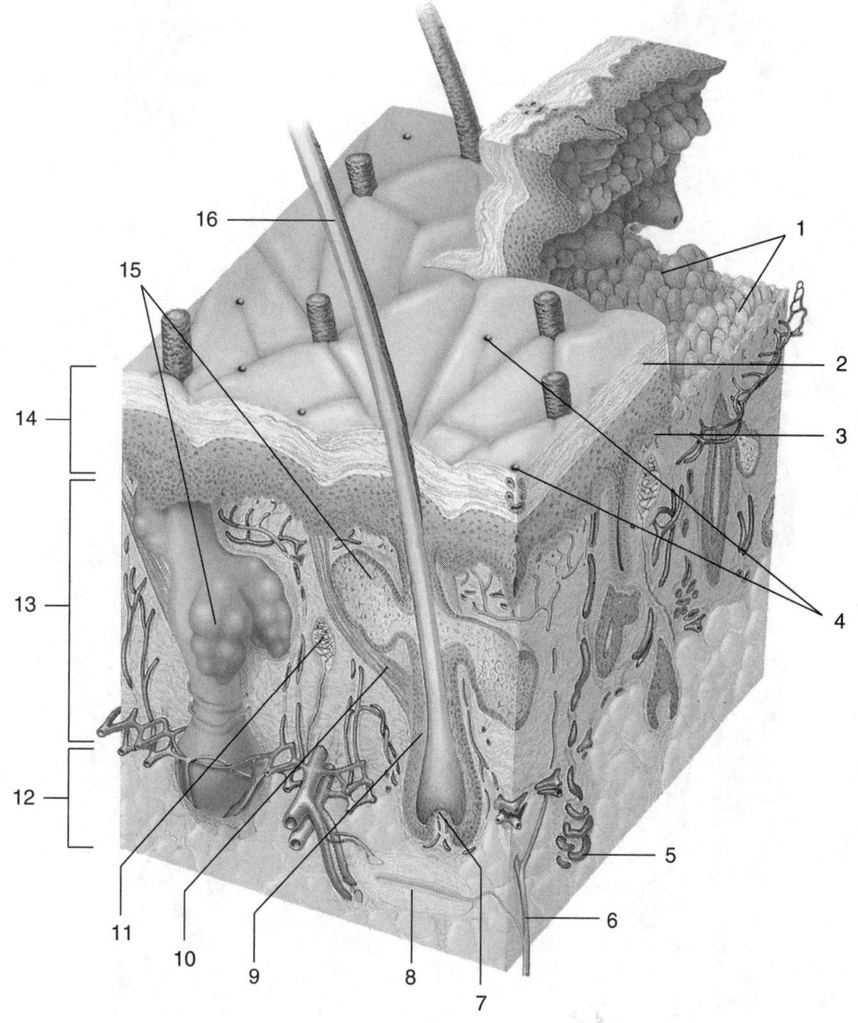

1. dermal papilla
2. stratum corneum
3. stratum germinativum
4. open sweat ducts
5. sweat glands
6. nerves
7. papilla of hair
8. lamellar corpuscle
9. hair follicle
10. arrector pili musle
11. tactile corpuscle
12. subutaneous
13. dermis
14. epidermis
15. sebaceous gland
16. hair shaft

"RULE OF NINES" FOR ESTIMATING SKIN SURFACE BURNED

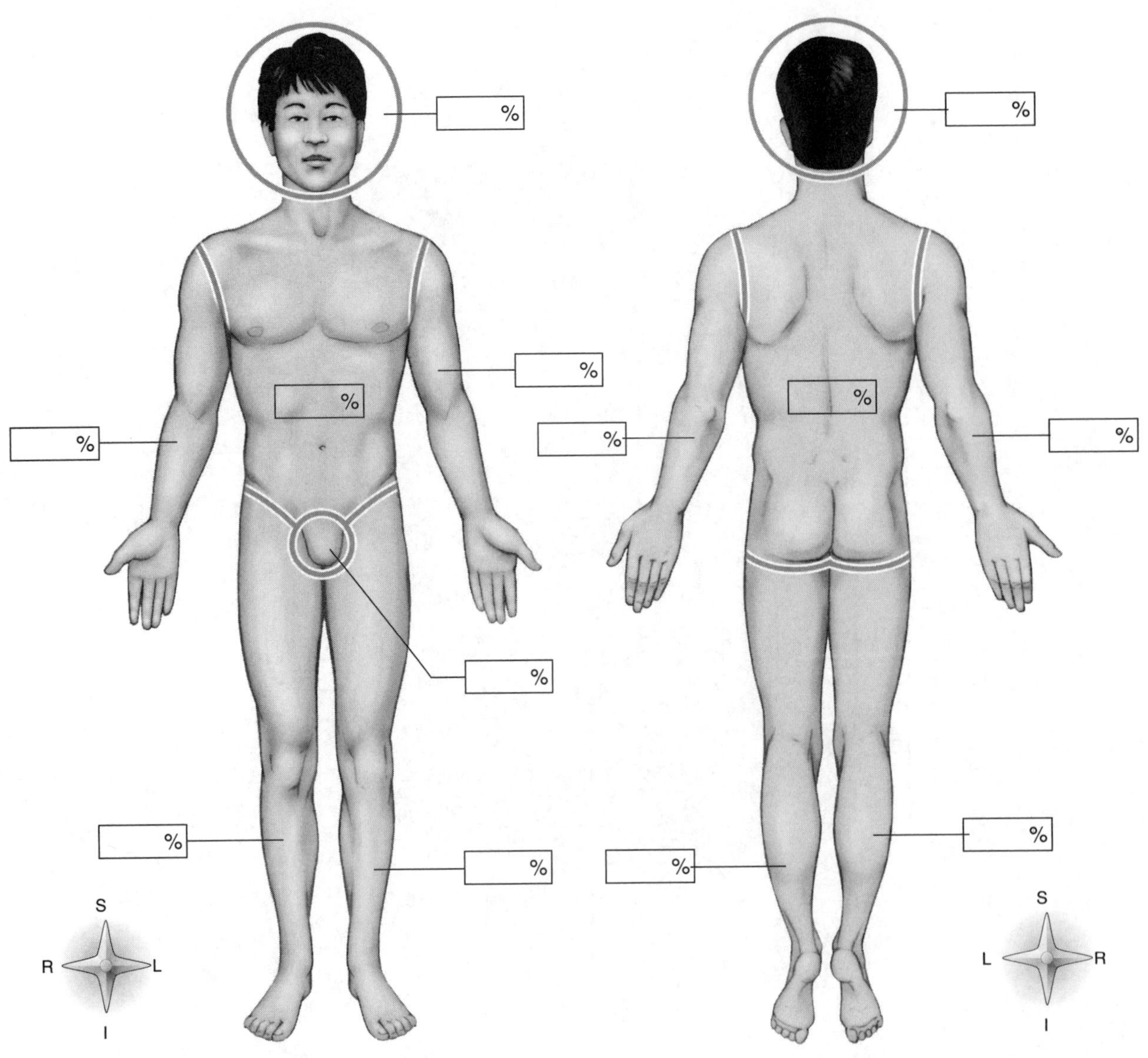

CHAPTER 6

The Skeletal System

How strange we would look without our skeleton! It is the skeleton that provides us with the rigid, supportive framework that gives shape to our bodies. But this is just the beginning, since it also protects the organs beneath it, maintains homeostasis of blood calcium, produces blood cells, and assists the muscular system in providing movement for us.

After reviewing the microscopic structure of bone and cartilage, you will understand how skeletal tissues are formed, their differences, and their importance in the human body. Your microscopic investigation will make the study of this system easier as you logically progress from this view to macroscopic bone formation and growth and visualize the structure of the long bones.

The skeleton is divided into two main divisions: the axial skeleton and the appendicular skeleton. All of the 206 bones of the human body may be classified into one of these two categories. And, although we can divide the bones neatly by this system, we are still aware that subtle differences exist between men's and women's skeletons. These structural differences provide us with insight to the differences in function between men and women.

Finally, three types of joints exist in the body: synarthroses, amphiarthroses, and diarthroses. It is important to have knowledge of these joints and to understand how movement is facilitated by these various articulations.

TOPICS FOR REVIEW

Before progressing to Chapter 7, you should familiarize yourself with the functions of the skeletal system, the structure and function of bone and cartilage, bone formation and growth, and the types of joints found in the body. Additionally, your understanding of the skeletal system should enable you to identify the two major subdivisions of the skeleton, the bones found in each area, and any differences that exist between men's and women's skeletons.

FUNCTIONS OF THE SKELETAL SYSTEM
TYPES OF BONES
STRUCTURE OF LONG BONES

Fill in the blanks.

1. There are ______________________ types of bones.

2. The ______________ ______________ is the hollow area inside the diaphysis of a bone.

3. A thin layer of cartilage covering each epiphysis is the ______________ ______________.

4. The ______________ lines the medullary cavity of long bones.

5. ______________ is used to describe the process of blood cell formation.

6. Blood cell formation is a vital process carried on in ______________ ______________ ______________.

7. The ______________ is a strong fibrous membrane covering a long bone except at joint surfaces.

8. Osteoporosis occurs most frequently in ______________ ______________ ______________.

9. Bones serve as a safety-deposit box for ______________, a vital substance required for normal nerve and muscle function.

10. As muscles contract and shorten, they pull on bones and thereby ______________ them.

If you have had difficulty with this section, review pages 108-111 and page 115.

MICROSCOPIC STRUCTURE OF BONE AND CARTILAGE

Match the term on the left with the proper selection on the right.

Group A

_____ 11. Trabeculae — A. Outer covering of bone

_____ 12. Compact — B. Dense bone tissue

_____ 13. Spongy — C. Fibers embedded in a firm gel

_____ 14. Periosteum — D. Needlelike threads of spongy bone

_____ 15. Cartilage — E. Ends of long bones

Group B

_____ 16. Osteocytes — A. Connect lacunae

_____ 17. Canaliculi — B. Cartilage cells

_____ 18. Lamellae — C. Structural unit of compact bone

_____ 19. Chondrocytes — D. Bone cells

_____ 20. Haversian system — E. Ring of bone

If you have had difficulty with this section, review pages 111-113.

BONE FORMATION AND GROWTH

If the statement is true, write "T" in the answer blank. If the statement is false, correct the statement by circling the incorrect term and inserting the correct term in the answer blank.

______________ 21. When the skeleton forms in a baby before birth, it consists of cartilage and fibrous structures.

_______________ 22. The diaphyses are the ends of the bone.

_______________ 23. Bone-forming cells are known as osteoclasts.

_______________ 24. It is the combined action of osteoblasts and osteoclasts that sculpts bones into their adult shapes.

_______________ 25. The stresses placed on certain bones during exercise decrease the rate of bone deposition.

_______________ 26. The epiphyseal plate can be seen in both external and cutaway views of an adult long bone.

_______________ 27. The shaft of a long bone is known as the articulation.

_______________ 28. Cartilage in the newborn becomes bone when it is replaced with calcified bone matrix deposited by osteoblasts.

_______________ 29. When epiphyseal cartilage becomes bone, growth begins.

_______________ 30. The epiphyseal cartilage is visible, if present, on x-ray films.

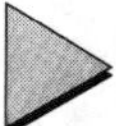

If you have had difficulty with this section, review pages 113-116.

DIVISIONS OF SKELETON

Select the best answer.

31. Which one of the following is *not* a part of the axial skeleton?
    A. Scapula
    B. Cranial bones
    C. Vertebra
    D. Ribs
    E. Sternum

32. Which one of the following is *not* a cranial bone?
    A. Frontal
    B. Parietal
    C. Occipital
    D. Lacrimal
    E. Sphenoid

33. Which of the following statements is *not* true?
    A. A baby is born with a straight spine.
    B. In the adult, the sacral and thoracic curves are convex.
    C. The normal curves of the adult spine provide greater strength than a straight spine.
    D. A curved structure has more strength than a straight one of the same size and materials.

34. True ribs:
    A. Attach to the cartilage of other ribs
    B. Do not attach to the sternum
    C. Attach directly to the sternum without cartilage
    D. Attach directly to the sternum by means of cartilage

35. The bone that runs along the lateral side of your forearm is the:
    A. Humerus
    B. Ulna
    C. Radius
    D. Tibia

36. The shinbone is also known as the:
    A. Fibula
    B. Femur
    C. Tibia
    D. Ulna

37. The bones in the palm of the hand are called:
    A. Metatarsals
    B. Tarsals
    C. Carpals
    D. Metacarpals

38. Which one of the following is *not* a bone of the upper extremity?
    A. Radius
    B. Clavicle
    C. Humerus
    D. Ilium

39. The heel bone is known as the:
    A. Calcaneus
    B. Talus
    C. Metatarsal
    D. Phalanges

40. The mastoid process is part of the ___________ bone.
    A. Parietal
    B. Temporal
    C. Occipital
    D. Frontal

41. When a baby learns to stand, the ______________ area of the spine becomes concave.
    A. Lumbar
    B. Thoracic
    C. Cervical
    D. Coccyx

42. Which bone is the "funny" bone?
    A. Radius
    B. Ulna
    C. Humerus
    D. Carpal

43. There are _______ pairs of true ribs.
    A. 14
    B. 7
    C. 5
    D. 3

44. The 27 bones in the wrist and the hand allow for more:
    A. Strength
    B. Dexterity
    C. Protection
    D. Red blood cell production

45. The longest bone in the body is the:
    A. Tibia
    B. Fibula
    C. Femur
    D. Humerus

46. Distally, the _______________ articulates with the patella.
    A. Femur
    B. Fibula
    C. Tibia
    D. Humerus

47. The __________ bones form the cheekbones.
    A. Mandible
    B. Palatine
    C. Maxillary
    D. Zygomatic

48. In a child, there are five of these bones. In an adult, they are fused into one.
    A. Pelvic
    B. Lumbar vertebrae
    C. Sacrum
    D. Carpals

49. The spinal cord enters the cranium through a large hole (foramen magnum) in the _________ bone.
    A. Temporal
    B. Parietal
    C. Occipital
    D. Sphenoid

Circle the one that does not *belong.*

50. Cervical	Thoracic	Coxal	Coccyx
51. Pelvic girdle	Ankle	Wrist	Axial
52. Frontal	Occipital	Maxilla	Sphenoid
53. Scapula	Pectoral girdle	Ribs	Clavicle
54. Malleus	Vomer	Incus	Stapes
55. Ulna	Ilium	Ischium	Pubis
56. Carpal	Phalanges	Metacarpal	Ethmoid
57. Ethmoid	Parietal	Occipital	Nasal
58. Anvil	Atlas	Axis	Cervical

If you have had difficulty with this section, review pages 116-127.

DIFFERENCES BETWEEN A MAN'S AND A WOMAN'S SKELETON

Choose the correct answer.

(A) Male (B) Female

_____ 59. Funnel-shaped pelvis

_____ 60. Broader-shaped pelvis

_____ 61. Osteoporosis occurs more frequently

_____ 62. Larger overall bone structure

_____ 63. Wider pelvic inlet

If you have had difficulty with this section, review pages 127-128.

BONE MARKINGS

From the choices given, match the bone with the identifying marking. There may be more than one marking for some of the bones.

A. Mastoid
B. Pterygoid process
C. Foramen magnum
D. Sella turcica
E. Mental foramen
F. Conchae
G. Xiphoid process
H. Glenoid cavity
I. Olecranon process
J. Ischium
K. Acetabulum
L. Symphysis pubis
M. Ilium
N. Greater trochanter
O. Medial malleolus
P. Calcaneus
Q. Acromion process
R. Frontal sinuses
S. Condyloid process
T. Tibial tuberosity

_____ 64. Occipital

_____ 65. Sternum

_____ 66. Coxal

_____ 67. Femur

_____ 68. Ulna

_____ 69. Temporal

_____ 70. Tarsals

_____ 71. Sphenoid

_____ 72. Ethmoid

_____ 73. Scapula

_____ 74. Tibia

_____ 75. Frontal

_____ 76. Mandible

If you have had difficulty with this section, review pages 117-127.

JOINTS (ARTICULATIONS)

Circle the correct answer.

77. Freely movable joints are (amphiarthroses or diarthroses).

78. The sutures in the skull are (synarthrotic or amphiarthrotic) joints.

79. All (diarthrotic or amphiarthrotic) joints have a joint capsule, a joint cavity, and a layer of cartilage over the ends of the two joining bones.

80. (Ligaments or tendons) grow out of periosteum and attach two bones together.

81. The (articular cartilage or epiphyseal cartilage) absorbs jolts.

82. Gliding joints are the (least movable or most movable) of the diarthrotic joints.

83. The knee is the (largest or smallest) joint.

84. Hinge joints allow motion in (2 or 4) directions.

85. The saddle joint at the base of each of our thumbs allows for greater (strength or mobility).

86. When you rotate your head, you are using a (gliding or pivot) joint.

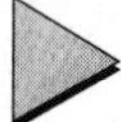
If you have had difficulty with this section, review pages 128-136.

UNSCRAMBLE THE BONES

Take the circled letters, unscramble them, and fill in the statement.

87. **E T V E R R B A E**

88. **B P S U I**

89. **S C A L U P A**

90. **I M D B A L N E**

91. **A P N H G A E L S**

What the fat lady wore to the ball.

92.

APPLYING WHAT YOU KNOW

93. Mrs. Perine had advanced cancer of the bone. As the disease progressed, Mrs. Perine required several blood transfusions throughout her therapy. One day she asked the doctor to explain the reason for the transfusions. What explanation might the doctor give to Mrs. Perine?

94. Dr. Kennedy, an orthopedic surgeon, called the admissions office of the hospital to advise that within the next hour he would be admitting a patient with an epiphyseal fracture. Without any other information, the patient is assigned to the pediatric ward. What prompted this assignment?

95. Mrs. Van Skiver, age 70, noticed when she went in for her physical examination that she was a half-inch shorter than she had been on her last visit. Dr. Veazey suggested she begin a regimen of dietary supplements of calcium and vitamin D, and he also gave Mrs. Van Skiver a prescription for sex hormone therapy. What bone disease did Dr. Veazey suspect?

96. WORD FIND

Can you find 14 terms from this chapter in the box of letters? Words may be spelled top to bottom, bottom to top, right to left, left to right, or diagonally.

A	R	T	I	C	U	L	A	T	I	O	N	N	U	T
M	M	L	T	N	I	N	G	U	I	H	J	N	C	G
P	R	P	E	R	I	O	S	T	E	U	M	A	N	B
H	V	P	G	U	A	T	B	M	E	O	P	R	F	G
I	N	V	R	N	O	B	O	F	S	M	H	X	E	R
A	G	J	O	A	J	P	E	T	O	E	O	H	T	Q
R	U	R	B	X	O	E	E	C	A	S	G	I	S	B
T	S	S	Y	I	M	O	Q	N	U	O	O	L	X	Q
H	J	I	E	A	B	P	U	N	Q	L	E	Q	K	S
R	I	S	I	L	U	C	I	L	A	N	A	C	X	R
O	I	N	A	M	A	S	Q	M	A	Q	K	E	C	T
S	T	S	A	L	C	O	E	T	S	O	U	I	D	G
E	T	S	Y	F	W	L	N	M	P	U	F	N	U	F
S	B	H	Q	H	L	O	U	S	A	R	X	I	T	V
R	P	M	P	A	F	M	G	X	K	D	S	L	G	A

Amphiarthroses	Fontanels	Osteoclasts
Articulation	Hemopoiesis	Periosteum
Axial	Lacunae	Sinus
Canaliculi	Lamella	Trabeculae
Compact	Osteoblasts	

DID YOU KNOW?

The bones of the hands and feet make up more than half of the total 206 bones of the body.

The size of your foot is approximately the size of your forearm.

The average person flexes their finger joints 25 million times during a lifetime.

Babies are born with 300 bones, but by adulthood we have only 206 in our bodies.

The bones of the middle ear are mature at birth.

SKELETAL SYSTEM

Fill in the crossword puzzle.

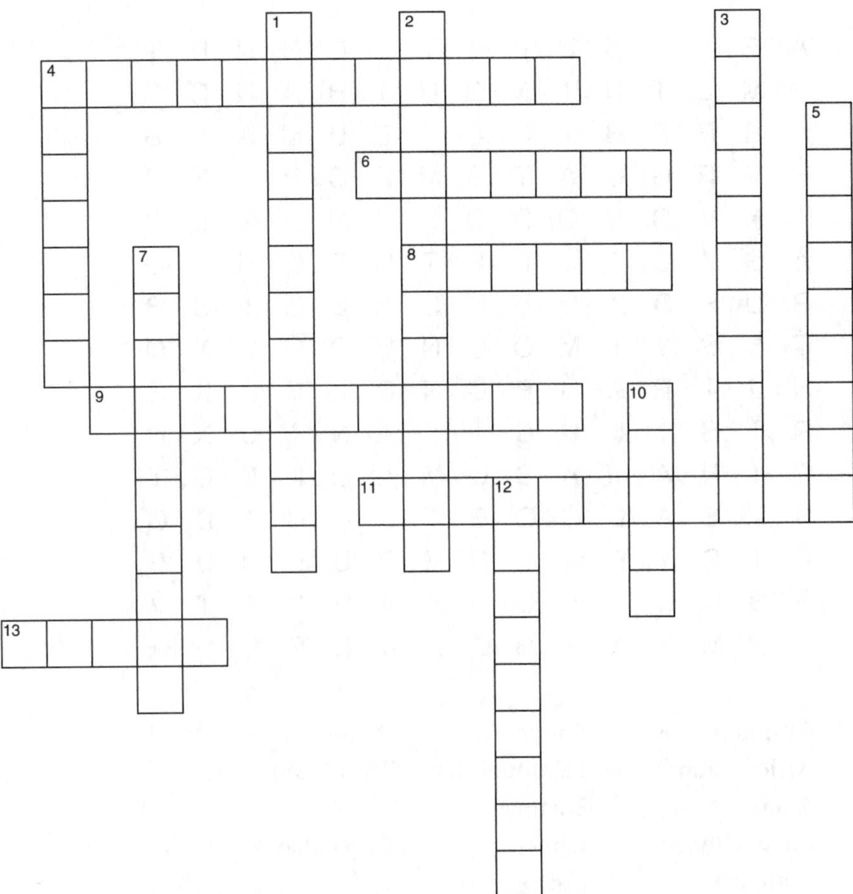

Across

4. Cartilage cells
6. Spaces in bones where osteocytes are found
8. Chest
9. Freely movable joints
11. Process of blood cell formation
13. Space inside cranial bone

Down

1. Joint
2. Suture joints
3. Bone absorbing cells
4. Type of bone
5. Ends of long bones
7. Covers long bone except at its joint surfaces
10. Division of skeleton
12. Bone cell

CHECK YOUR KNOWLEDGE

Multiple Choice

Select the best answer.

1. Which of the following is *not* a function of bones?
   A. Communication
   B. Storage
   C. Hematopoiesis
   D. Protection

2. The four types of bones are:
   A. Flat, irregular, short, and square
   B. Flat, cartilage, short, and long
   C. Flat, irregular, short, and long
   D. Small, long, flat, and heavy

3. Which of the following is *not* a main part of a long bone?
   A. Malleus
   B. Epiphyses
   C. Periosteum
   D. Diaphysis

4. All of the following bones are part of the appendicular skeleton *except*:
   A. Shoulder
   B. Hip
   C. Chest
   D. Feet

5. There are a total of __________ phalanges in the skeletal system.
   A. 28
   B. 60
   C. 56
   D. 72

6. Cartilage differs from bone because it:
   A. Is embedded in a firm gel rather than in a calcified cement substance
   B. Has the flexibility of a firm plastic rather than being rigid
   C. Rebuilds itself very slowly after injury
   D. All of the above

7. Which of the following is *not* a paranasal sinus?
   A. Frontal
   B. Ethmoid
   C. Lambdoidal
   D. Sphenoid

8. The last two ribs:
   A. Attach directly to the sternum
   B. Are attached to costal cartilage
   C. Are referred to as "floating ribs"
   D. None of the above

9. In an infant, each coxal bone consists of three separate bones. These bones are the:
   A. Ilium, ischium, and coccyx
   B. Ischium, pubis, and tuberosity
   C. Pubis, tuberosity, and coccyx
   D. Ilium, ischium, and pubis

10. An example of a synarthrotic joint is:
   A. A cranial suture
   B. The hip joint
   C. The shoulder joint
   D. The spine

Matching

Select the most correct answer from column B for each statement in column A. (Only one answer is correct.)

Column A	Column B
_____ 11. Articulation	A. "Funny bone"
_____ 12. Medullary cavity	B. Yellow bone marrow
_____ 13. Osteons	C. Immovable
_____ 14. Incus	D. Circumduct
_____ 15. Sternum	E. Manubrium
_____ 16. Zygomatic	F. Flexion
_____ 17. Olecranon process	G. Joint
_____ 18. Synarthroses	H. Cheekbone
_____ 19. Hinge joint	I. Haversian system
_____ 20. Thumb joint	J. Middle ear

LONGITUDINAL SECTION OF LONG BONE

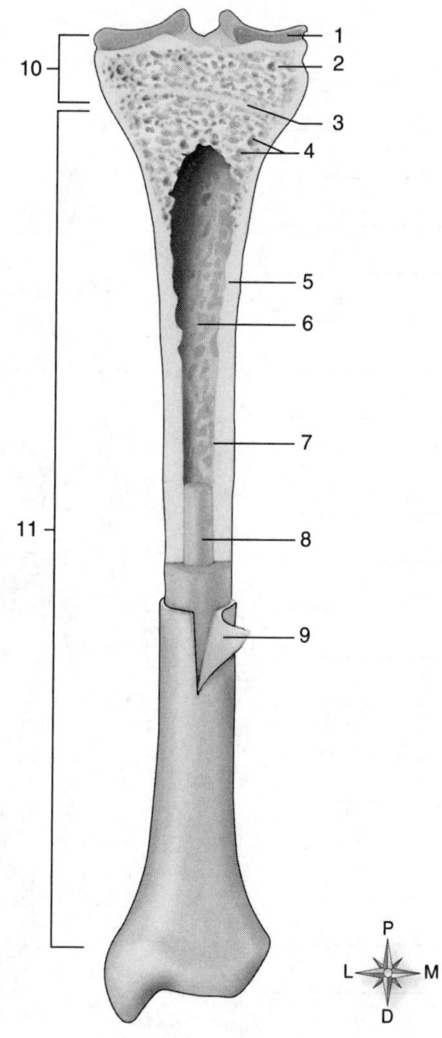

1. ______________________
2. ______________________
3. ______________________
4. ______________________
5. ______________________
6. ______________________
7. ______________________
8. ______________________
9. ______________________
10. ______________________
11. ______________________

ANTERIOR VIEW OF SKELETON

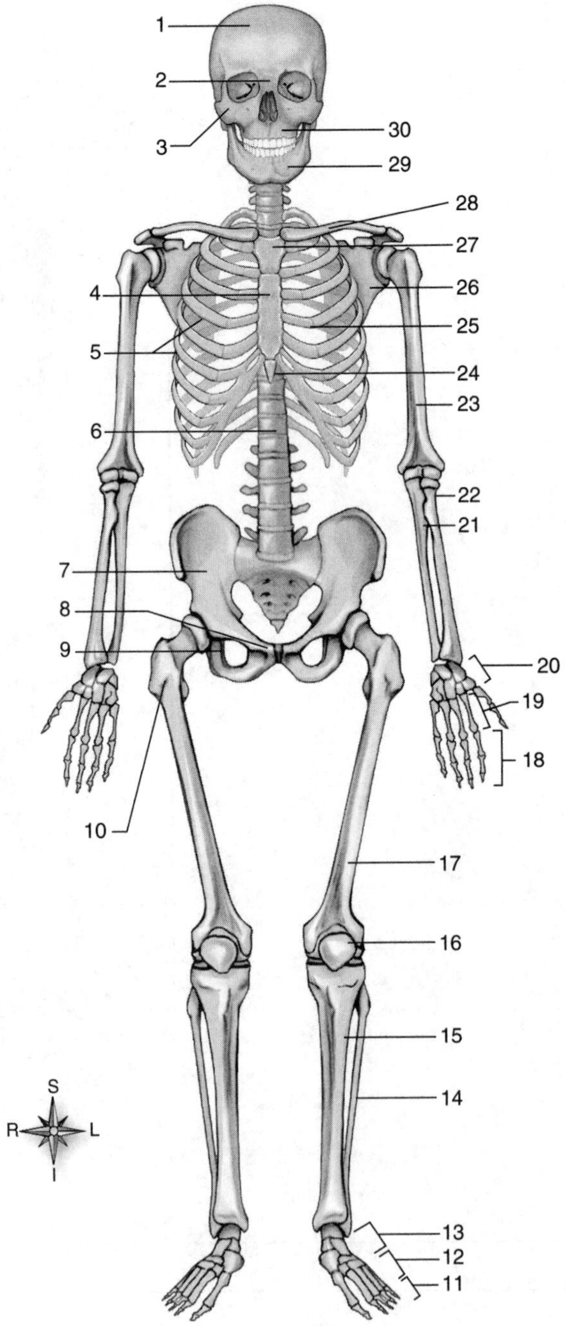

1. ____________________
2. ____________________
3. ____________________
4. ____________________
5. ____________________
6. ____________________
7. ____________________
8. ____________________
9. ____________________
10. ____________________
11. ____________________
12. ____________________
13. ____________________
14. ____________________
15. ____________________
16. ____________________
17. ____________________
18. ____________________
19. ____________________
20. ____________________
21. ____________________
22. ____________________
23. ____________________
24. ____________________
25. ____________________
26. ____________________
27. ____________________
28. ____________________
29. ____________________
30. ____________________

POSTERIOR VIEW OF SKELETON

1. ______________________
2. ______________________
3. ______________________
4. ______________________
5. ______________________
6. ______________________
7. ______________________
8. ______________________
9. ______________________
10. ______________________
11. ______________________
12. ______________________
13. ______________________
14. ______________________
15. ______________________
16. ______________________
17. ______________________
18. ______________________
19. ______________________
20. ______________________
21. ______________________
22. ______________________
23. ______________________
24. ______________________
25. ______________________
26. ______________________
27. ______________________

SKULL VIEWED FROM THE RIGHT SIDE

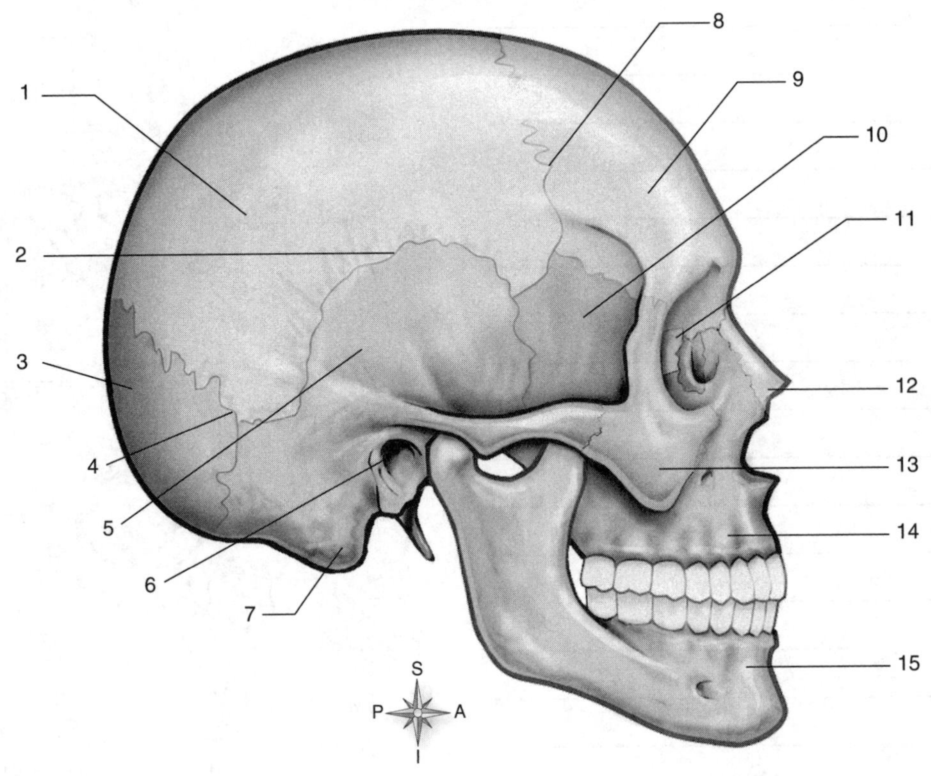

1. ______________________
2. ______________________
3. ______________________
4. ______________________
5. ______________________
6. ______________________
7. ______________________
8. ______________________
9. ______________________
10. ______________________
11. ______________________
12. ______________________
13. ______________________
14. ______________________
15. ______________________

SKULL VIEWED FROM THE FRONT

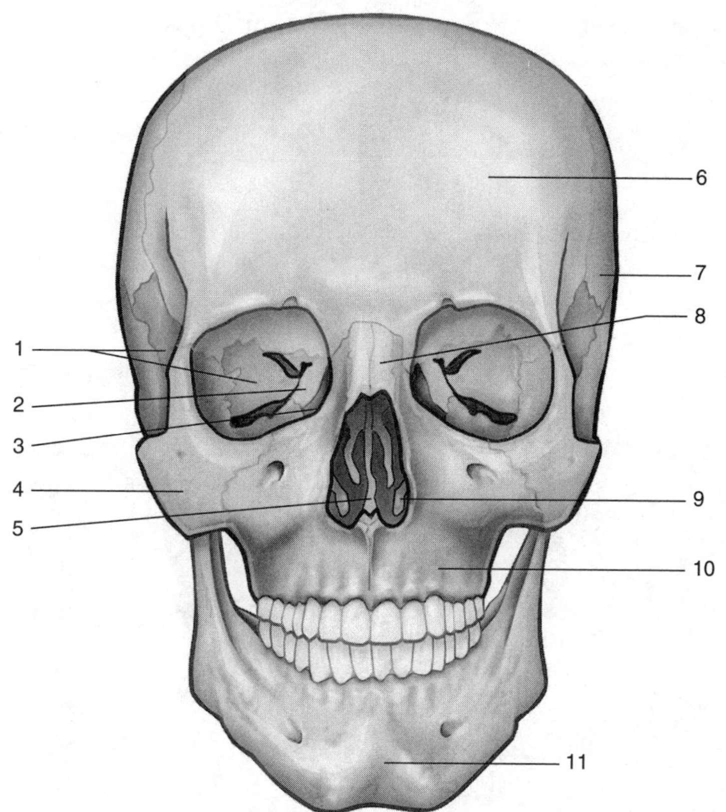

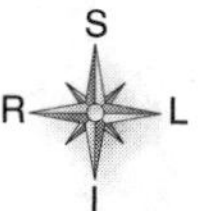

1. ______________________
2. ______________________
3. ______________________
4. ______________________
5. ______________________
6. ______________________
7. ______________________
8. ______________________
9. ______________________
10. ______________________
11. ______________________

STRUCTURE OF A DIARTHROTIC JOINT

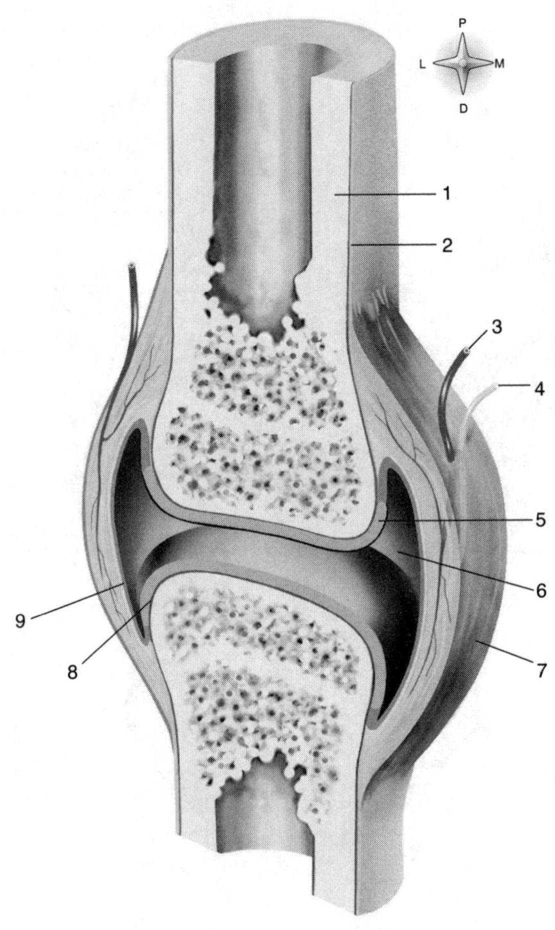

1. ______________________
2. ______________________
3. ______________________
4. ______________________
5. ______________________
6. ______________________
7. ______________________
8. ______________________
9. ______________________

CHAPTER 7

The Muscular System

The muscular system is often referred to as the *power system*; and rightfully so, because it is this system that provides the force necessary to move the body and perform organic functions. Just as an automobile relies on the engine to provide motion, the body depends on the muscular system to perform both voluntary and involuntary types of movement. Walking, breathing, and the digestion of food are but a few examples of body functions that require the healthy performance of the muscular system.

Although this system has several functions, the primary purpose is to provide movement or power. Muscles produce power by contracting. The ability of a large muscle or muscle group to contract depends upon the ability of microscopic muscle fibers that contract within the larger muscle. An understanding of these microscopic muscle fibers will assist you as your study progresses to the larger muscles and muscle groups.

Muscle contractions may be one of several types: isotonic, isometric, twitch, or tetanic. When skeletal or voluntary muscles contract, they provide us with a variety of motions. Flexion, extension, abduction, adduction, and rotation are examples of these movements that provide us with both strength and agility.

Muscles must be used to keep the body healthy and in good condition. Scientific evidence keeps pointing to the fact that the proper use and exercise of muscles may extend longevity. An understanding of the structure and function of the muscular system may, therefore, add quality and quantity to our lives.

TOPICS FOR REVIEW

Before progressing to Chapter 8, you should familiarize yourself with the structure and function of the three major types of muscle tissue. Your review should include the microscopic structure of skeletal muscle tissue, the mechanism by which a muscle is stimulated, the major types of skeletal muscle contractions, and the skeletal muscle groups. Your study should conclude with an understanding of the types of movements produced by skeletal muscle contractions.

MUSCLE TISSUE

Select the correct term(s) from the choices given and write the letter in the answer blank.

(A) Skeletal muscle (B) Cardiac muscle (C) Smooth muscle

_____ 1. Striated

_____ 2. Cells branch frequently

_____ 3. Moves food into stomach

_____ 4. Nonstriated

_____ 5. Voluntary

_____ 6. Increases efficiency of heart muscle in pumping blood.

_____ 7. Involuntary

_____ 8. Attaches to bone

_____ 9. Found in hollow internal organs

_____ 10. Also called *visceral muscle.*

If you have had difficulty with this section, review pages 140-143.

STRUCTURE OF SKELETAL MUSCLE

Match the term on the left with the proper selection on the right.

Group A

_____ 11. Origin — A. The muscle unit, excluding the ends

_____ 12. Insertion — B. Attachment to the more movable bone

_____ 13. Body — C. Fluid-filled sacs

_____ 14. Tendons — D. Attachment to more stationary bone

_____ 15. Bursae — E. Attach muscle to bones

MICROSCOPIC STRUCTURE AND FUNCTION

Group B

_____ 16. Muscle fibers — A. Protein that forms thick myofilaments

_____ 17. Actin — B. Basic functional unit of skeletal muscle

_____ 18. Sarcomere — C. Protein that forms thin myofilaments

_____ 19. Myosin — D. Microscopic threadlike structures found in skeletal muscle fibers

_____ 20. Myofilament — E. Elongated contractile cells of muscle tissue

If you have had difficulty with this section, review pages 143-145.

FUNCTIONS OF SKELETAL MUSCLE

Fill in the blanks.

21. Muscles move bones by _________________________ on them.

22. As a rule, only the _______________ bone moves.

23. The __________________ bone moves toward the ____________ bone.

24. Of all the muscles contracting simultaneously, the one mainly responsible for producing a particular movement is called the __________ __________ for that movement.

25. As prime movers contract, muscles called ________________ relax.

26. The biceps brachii is the prime mover during bending, and the brachialis is its helper or __________ muscle.

27. We are able to maintain our body position because of a specialized type of skeletal muscle contraction called ______________ ______________.

28. __________ _____________ maintains body posture by counteracting the pull of gravity.

29. A decrease in temperature, a condition known as __________________, will drastically affect cellular activity and normal body function.

30. Energy required to produce a muscle contraction is obtained from ________________.

If you have had difficulty with this section, review pages 145-147.

FATIGUE—ROLE OF BODY SYSTEMS MOTOR UNIT—MUSCLE STIMULUS

If the statement is true, write "T" on the answer blank. If the statement is false, correct the statement by circling the incorrect term and writing the correct term in the answer blank.

______________________ 31. The point of contact between the nerve ending and the muscle fiber is called a motor neuron.

______________________ 32. A motor neuron together with the cells it innervates is called a motor unit.

______________________ 33. If muscle cells are stimulated repeatedly without adequate periods of rest, the strength of the muscle contraction will decrease, resulting in fatigue.

______________________ 34. The depletion of oxygen in muscle cells during vigorous and prolonged exercise is known as fatigue.

______________________ 35. An adequate stimulus will contract a muscle cell completely because of the "must" theory.

______________________ 36. When oxygen supplies run low, muscle cells produce ATP and other waste products during contraction.

______________________ 37. In a laboratory setting, a single muscle fiber can be isolated and subjected to stimuli of varying intensities so that it can be studied.

______________________ 38. The minimal level of stimulation required to cause a fiber to contract is called the threshold stimulus.

______________________ 39. Smooth muscles bring about movements by pulling on bones across movable joints.

______________________ 40. A nervous system disorder that shuts off impulses to certain skeletal muscles may result in paralysis.

TYPES OF SKELETAL MUSCLE CONTRACTION EFFECTS OF EXERCISE ON SKELETAL MUSCLES

Select the best answer.

41. When a muscle does not shorten and no movement results, the contraction is:
    A. Isometric
    B. Isotonic
    C. Twitch
    D. Tetanic

42. Walking is an example of which type of contraction?
    A. Isometric
    B. Isotonic
    C. Twitch
    D. Tetanic

43. Pushing against a wall is an example of which type of contraction?
    A. Isotonic
    B. Isometric
    C. Twitch
    D. Tetanic

44. Endurance training is also known as:
    A. Isometrics
    B. Hypertrophy
    C. Aerobic training
    D. Strength training

45. Benefits of regular exercise include all of the following *except*:
    A. Improved lung function
    B. More efficient heart
    C. Less fatigue
    D. Atrophy

46. Twitch contractions can be easily seen in:
    A. Isolated muscles prepared for research
    B. A great deal of normal muscle activity
    C. During resting periods
    D. None of the above

47. Contractions that "melt" together to produce a sustained contraction are called:
    A. Twitch
    B. Tetanus
    C. Isotonic response
    D. Isometric response

48. In most cases, isotonic contraction of muscle produces movement at a(n):
    A. Insertion
    B. Origin
    C. Joint
    D. Bursa

49. Prolonged inactivity causes muscles to shrink in mass, producing a condition called:
    A. Hypertrophy
    B. Disuse atrophy
    C. Paralysis
    D. Muscle fatigue

50. Muscle hypertrophy can be best enhanced by a program of:
    A. Isotonic exercise
    B. Better posture
    C. High-protein diet
    D. Strength training

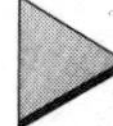
If you have had difficulty with this section, review pages 147-151.

MOVEMENTS PRODUCED BY SKELETAL MUSCLE CONTRACTIONS

Select the best answer.

51. A movement that makes the angle between two bones smaller is:
    A. Flexion
    B. Extension
    C. Abduction
    D. Adduction

52. Moving a part toward the midline is:
    A. Flexion
    B. Extension
    C. Abduction
    D. Adduction

53. Moving a part away from the midline is:
    A. Flexion
    B. Extension
    C. Abduction
    D. Adduction

54. When you move your head from side to side as in shaking your head "no," you are _______________ a muscle group.
    A. Rotating
    B. Pronating
    C. Supinating
    D. Abducting

55. _______________ occurs when you turn the palm of your hand from an anterior to posterior position.
    A. Dorsiflexion
    B. Plantar flexion
    C. Supination
    D. Pronation

56. *Dorsiflexion* refers to:
    A. Hand movements
    B. Eye movements
    C. Foot movements
    D. Head movements

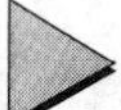
If you have had difficulty with this section, review pages 151-154.

SKELETAL MUSCLE GROUPS

Choose the proper function or functions for the muscles listed below and write the appropriate letter or letters in the answer blank.

(A) Flexor (B) Extensor (C) Abductor (D) Adductor (E) Rotator (F) Dorsiflexor or plantar flexor

_____ 57. Deltoid

_____ 58. Tibialis anterior

_____ 59. Gastrocnemius

_____ 60. Biceps brachii

_____ 61. Gluteus medius

_____ 62. Soleus

_____ 63. Iliopsoas

_____ 64. Pectoralis major

_____ 65. Gluteus maximus

_____ 66. Triceps brachii

_____ 67. Sternocleidomastoid

_____ 68. Trapezius

_____ 69. Gracilis

If you have had difficulty with this section, review pages 154-159.

UNSCRAMBLE THE WORDS

Take the circled letters, unscramble them, and fill in the statement.

70. **NFOXLIE**

71. **TNICA**

72. **VRSNEIOE**

73. **IORNIG**

74. **SEARRECMO**

What Kevin requested for his IOU.

75.

APPLYING WHAT YOU KNOW

76. Casey noticed pain whenever she reached for anything in her cupboards. Her doctor told her that the small fluid-filled sacs in her shoulder were inflamed. What condition did Casey have?

77. The nurse was preparing an injection for Mrs. Henry. The amount to be given was 2 ml. What area of the body will the nurse most likely select for this injection?

78. Chris was playing football and pulled a band of fibrous connective tissue that attached a muscle to a bone. What is the common term for this tissue?

79. WORD FIND

Can you find the 25 muscle terms in the box of letters? Words may be spelled top to bottom, bottom to top, right to left, left to right, or diagonally.

```
G A S T R O C N E M I U S D U
M S G I O N O I S N E T X E U
U R N N T O M S R B S F D T T
S U I S C I B O N T P N E A R
C B R E U X V T O O E C L I A
L Q T R D E C O D A C M T R P
E T S T B L M N N V I E O T E
X F M I A F Y I E Y B N I S Z
S I A O V I E C T L S S D I I
S Y H N S S R O T A T O R G U
U A M G A R H P A I D J N R S
E H A T R O P H Y L N J T E B
L N O H T D E U G I T A F N T
O R I G I N O S N V S B Z Y L
S B V T O J C T R I C E P S S
```

Abductor	Extension	Isometric	Striated
Atrophy	Fatigue	Isotonic	Synergist
Biceps	Flexion	Muscle	Tendon
Bursa	Gastrocnemius	Origin	Tenosynovitis
Deltoid	Hamstrings	Rotator	Trapezius
Diaphragm	Insertion	Soleus	Triceps
Dorsiflexion			

DID YOU KNOW?

If all of your muscles pulled in one direction, you would have the power to move 25 tons.

The simple act of walking requires the use of 200 muscles in the human body.

A cat has 32 muscles in each ear.

THE MUSCULAR SYSTEM

Fill in the crossword puzzle.

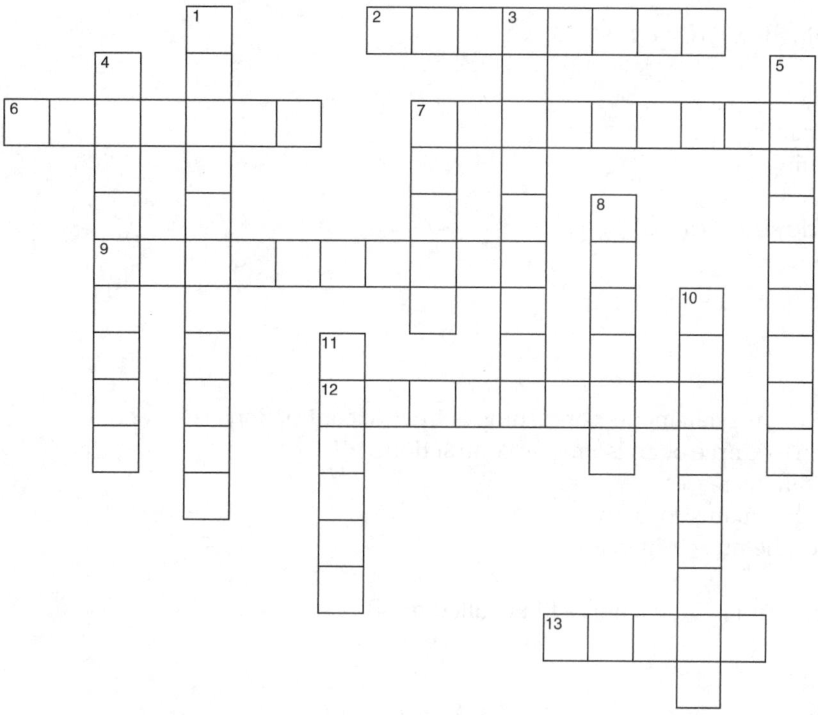

Across

2. Shaking your head "no"
6. Muscle shrinkage
7. Toward the body's midline
9. Produces movement opposite to prime movers
12. Movement that makes joint angles larger
13. Small fluid-filled sac between tendons and bones

Down

1. Increase in size
3. Away from the body's midline
4. Turning your palm from an anterior to posterior position
5. Attachment to the more movable bone
7. Protein that composes myofilaments
8. Attachment to the more stationary bone
10. Assists prime movers with movement
11. Anchors muscles to bones

CHECK YOUR KNOWLEDGE

Multiple Choice

Select the best answer.

1. Endurance training is also called:
   A. Isometrics
   B. Hypertrophy
   C. Anaerobic training
   D. Aerobic training

2. Increase in muscle size is called:
   A. Hypertrophy
   B. Atrophy
   C. Hyperplasia
   D. Treppe

3. Which of the following statements concerning isometric contractions is true?
   A. Walking is an example of an isometric contraction.
   B. Muscle tension decreases.
   C. Muscle length remains constant.
   D. Movement of the muscle increases.

4. Muscle cells are stimulated by a nerve fiber called a:
   A. Sarcomere
   B. Motor neuron
   C. Myofilament
   D. Prime mover

5. Muscles that help other muscles produce movement are called:
   A. Synergists
   B. Prime movers
   C. Antagonists
   D. None of the above

6. The connecting bridges between myofilaments form properly only if ________ is present.
   A. Potassium
   B. Calcium
   C. Sodium
   D. Chloride

7. Physiological muscle fatigue is caused by:
   A. Oxygen debt
   B. Inadequate periods of rest for muscles
   C. Lactic acid buildup in the muscles
   D. All of the above

8. The muscle's attachment to the more stationary bone is called its:
   A. Origin
   B. Body
   C. Insertion
   D. None of the above

9. Skeletal muscle:
   A. Is voluntary
   B. Is smooth
   C. Is also known as *visceral muscle*
   D. All of the above

10. Which of the following is *not* a hamstring muscle?
    A. Semimembranosus
    B. Semitendinosus
    C. Rectus femoris
    D. Biceps femoris

True or False

Indicate whether the following statements are true (T) or false (F).

_____ 11. The "all or none" principle states that when a muscle fiber is subjected to a threshold stimulus, it contracts completely.

_____ 12. Muscle tone maintains posture.

_____ 13. Thick myofilaments are formed from a protein called *actin*.

_____ 14. The triceps brachii is on the anterior surface of the upper arm.

_____ 15. Tendons anchor muscles firmly to bones.

_____ 16. Energy required to produce a muscle contraction is obtained from ATP.

_____ 17. Rotation is movement around a longitudinal axis.

_____ 18. Extension movements are the opposite of abduction.

_____ 19. The gastrocnemius is responsible for plantar flexion of the foot and is sometimes referred to as the *toe dancer's muscle*.

_____ 20. The zygomaticus is sometimes called the *kissing muscle*.

MUSCLES—ANTERIOR VIEW

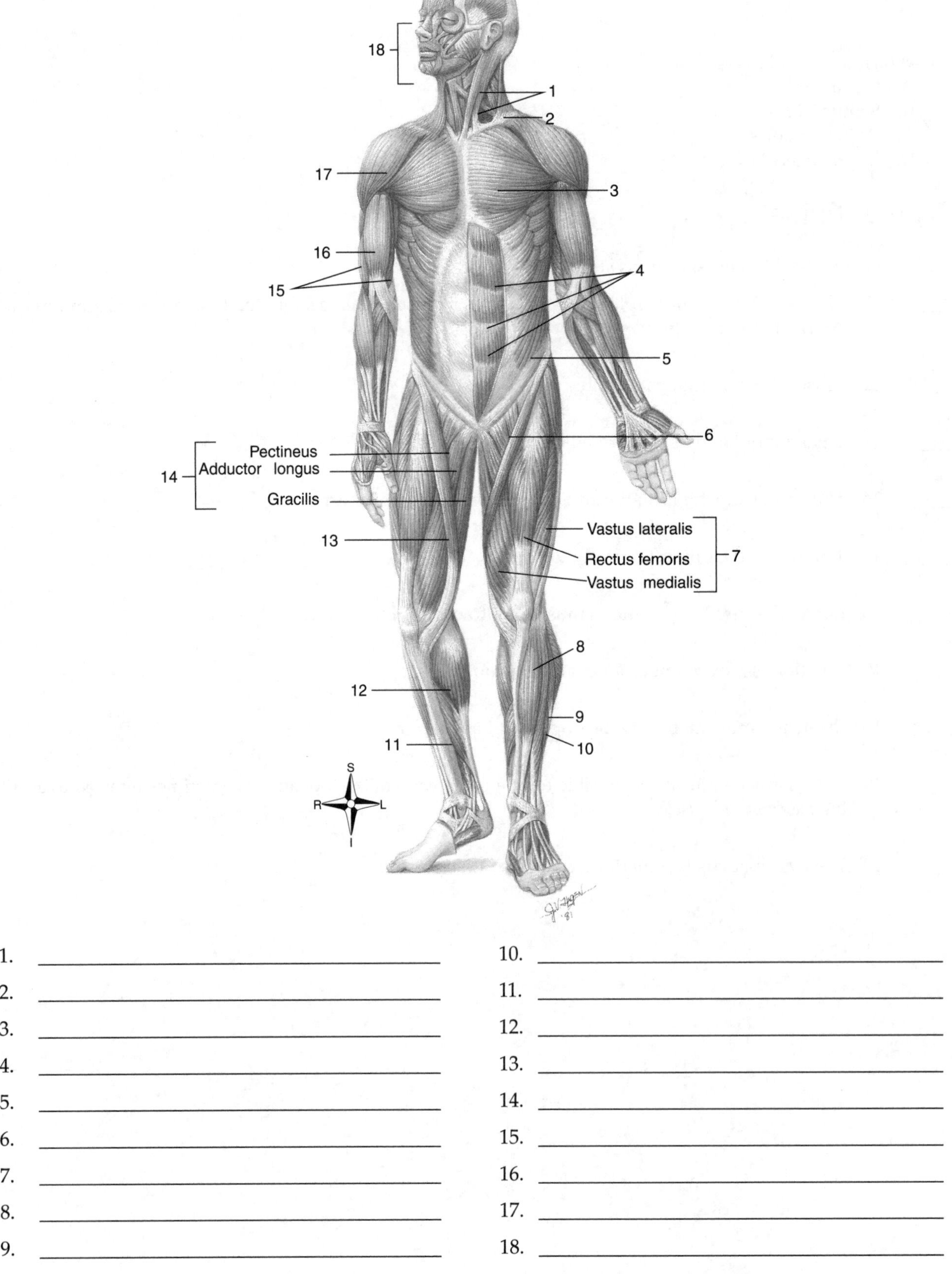

1. ______________________
2. ______________________
3. ______________________
4. ______________________
5. ______________________
6. ______________________
7. ______________________
8. ______________________
9. ______________________
10. ______________________
11. ______________________
12. ______________________
13. ______________________
14. ______________________
15. ______________________
16. ______________________
17. ______________________
18. ______________________

MUSCLES—POSTERIOR VIEW

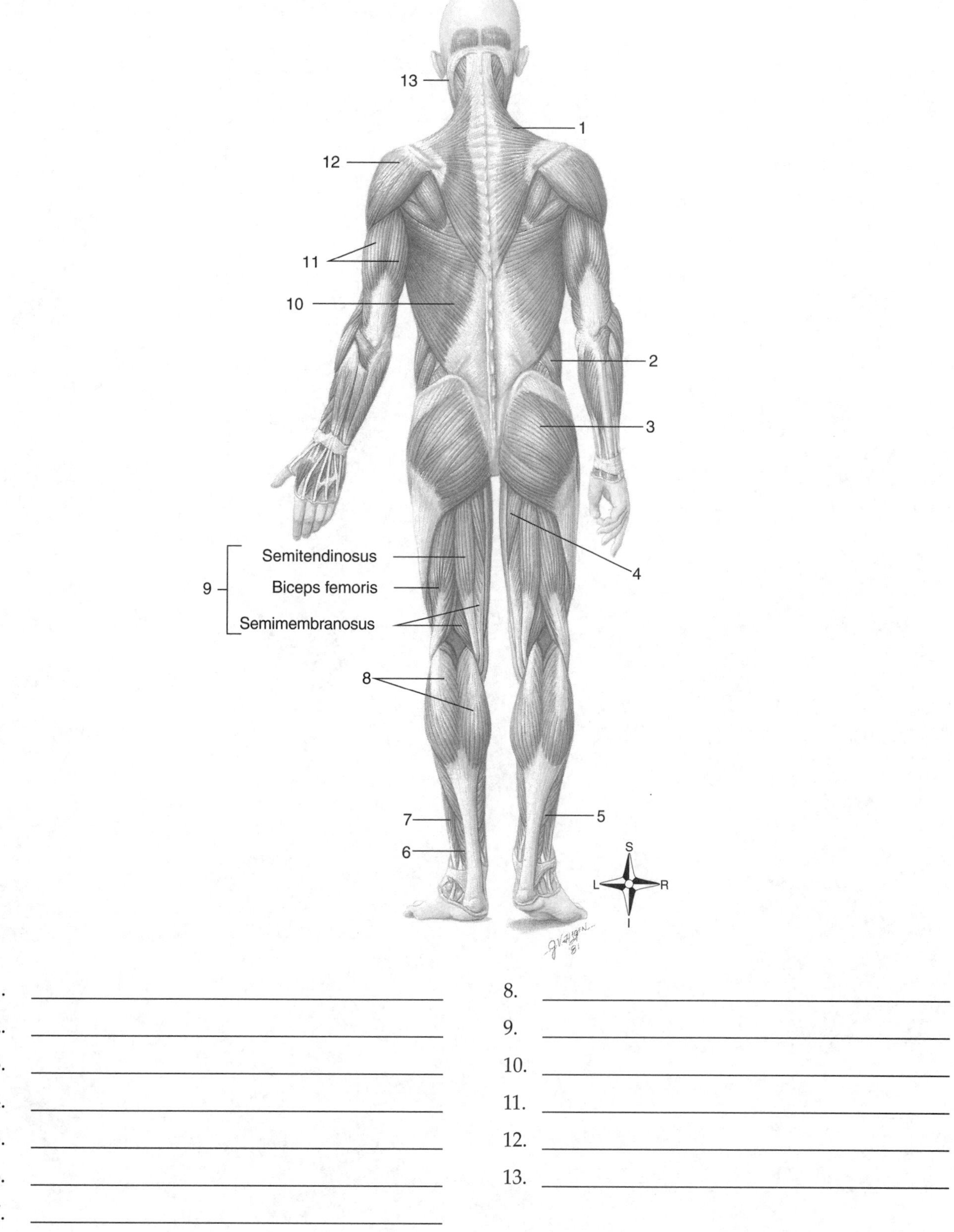

1. ______________________
2. ______________________
3. ______________________
4. ______________________
5. ______________________
6. ______________________
7. ______________________
8. ______________________
9. ______________________
10. ______________________
11. ______________________
12. ______________________
13. ______________________

CHAPTER 8

The Nervous System

The nervous system organizes and coordinates the millions of impulses received each day to make communication with and enjoyment of our environment possible. The functioning unit of the nervous system is the neuron. Three types of neurons—sensory neurons, motor neurons, and interneurons—exist, and are classified according to the direction in which they transmit impulses. Nerve impulses travel over routes made up of neurons and provide the rapid communication necessary for maintaining life. The central nervous system is made up of the spinal cord and brain. The spinal cord provides access to and from the brain by means of ascending and descending tracts. In addition, the spinal cord functions as the primary reflex center of the body. The brain can be subdivided for easier learning into the brain stem, cerebellum, diencephalon, and cerebrum. These areas provide the extraordinary network necessary to receive, interpret, and respond to the simplest or most complex impulses.

The peripheral nervous system is the system of nerves connecting the brain and spinal cord to other parts of the body. These nerves, known as the *cranial* and *spinal nerves*, may be further divided into the autonomic (involuntary) nervous system and the somatic (voluntary) nervous system. Sensory nerves are also considered part of the peripheral nervous system. The sensory nerves form the link between receptors and the central nervous system (CNS). They carry nerve impulses from stimulated receptors to the CNS and are considered part of the peripheral nervous system.

While you concentrate on this chapter, your body is performing a multitude of functions. Fortunately for us, breathing, beating of the heart, digestion of food, and most of our other day-to-day processes do not require our supervision or thought. They function automatically, and the division of the nervous system that regulates these functions is known as the *autonomic nervous system*.

The autonomic nervous system may be further subdivided into two divisions called the *sympathetic system* and the *parasympathetic system*. The sympathetic system functions as an emergency system and prepares us for "fight or flight." The parasympathetic system dominates control of many visceral effectors under normal everyday conditions. Together, these two divisions regulate the body's automatic functions in an effort to assist with the maintenance of homeostasis. Your understanding of this chapter will alert you to the complexity and functions of the nervous system and the "automatic pilot" of your body—the autonomic system.

TOPICS FOR REVIEW

Before progressing to Chapter 9, you should review the organs and divisions of the nervous system, the structure and function of the major types of cells in this system, the structure and function of a reflex arc, and the transmission of nerve impulses. Your study should include the anatomy and physiology of the brain and spinal cord and the nerves that extend from these two areas.

Finally, an understanding of the autonomic nervous system and the specific functions of the subdivisions of this system are necessary to complete the review of this chapter.

ORGANS AND DIVISIONS OF THE NERVOUS SYSTEM
CELLS OF THE NERVOUS SYSTEM
NERVES

Match the term on the left with the proper selection on the right.

Group A

Answer	Term		Selection
B	1. Sense organ	A.	Subdivision of peripheral nervous system
C	2. Central nervous system	B.	Ear
D	3. Peripheral nervous system	C.	Brain and spinal cord
A	4. Autonomic nervous system	D.	Nerves that extend to the outlying parts of the body

Group B

Answer	Term		Selection
B	5. Dendrite	A.	Indentations between adjacent Schwann cells
D	6. Schwann cell	B.	Branching projection of neuron
C	7. Motor neuron	C.	Also known as *efferent*
A	8. Nodes of Ranvier	D.	Forms myelin outside the central nervous system
F	9. Fascicles	E.	Tough sheath that covers the whole nerve
E	10. Epineurium	F.	Groups of wrapped axons

CELLS OF NERVOUS SYSTEM

Select the correct term from the choices given and write the letter in the answer blank.

(A) Neurons (B) Neuroglia

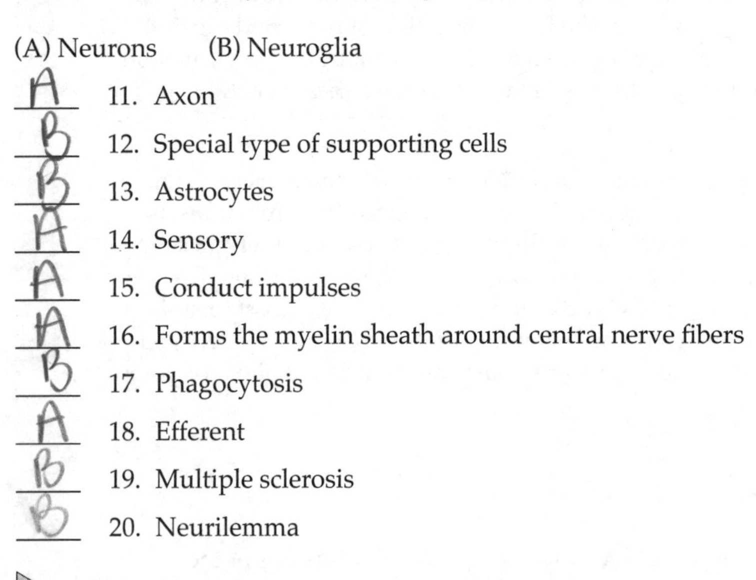

A 11. Axon

B 12. Special type of supporting cells

B 13. Astrocytes

A 14. Sensory

A 15. Conduct impulses

A 16. Forms the myelin sheath around central nerve fibers

B 17. Phagocytosis

A 18. Efferent

B 19. Multiple sclerosis

B 20. Neurilemma

If you have had difficulty with this section, review pages 166-171.

REFLEX ARCS

Fill in the blanks.

21. The simplest kind of reflex arc is a(n) ____________ ____________ ____________.

22. Three-neuron arcs consist of all three kinds of neurons, ____________, ____________, and ____________ ____________.

23. Impulse conduction in a reflex arc normally starts in ____________.

24. A(n) ____________ is the microscopic space that separates the axon of one neuron from the dendrites of another neuron.

25. A(n) ____________ is the response to impulse conduction over reflex arcs.

26. Contraction of a muscle that causes it to pull away from an irritating stimulus is known as the ____________ ____________.

27. A(n) ____________ is a group of nerve cell bodies located in the peripheral nervous system.

28. All ____________ lie entirely within the gray matter of the central nervous system.

29. In a patellar reflex, the nerve impulses that reach the quadriceps muscle (the effector) result in the classic "____________ ____________" response.

30. ____________ ____________ forms the H-shaped inner core of the spinal cord.

If you have had difficulty with this section, review pages 171-174.

NERVE IMPULSES THE SYNAPSE

Circle the correct answer.

31. Nerve impulses (do or do not) continually race along every nerve cell's surface.

32. When a stimulus acts on a neuron, it (increases or decreases) the permeability of the stimulated point of its membrane to sodium ions.

33. An inward movement of positive ions leaves (a lack or an excess) of negative ions outside.

34. The plasma membrane of the (presynaptic or postsynaptic) neuron makes up a portion of the synapse.

35. A synaptic knob is a tiny bulge at the end of the (presynaptic or postsynaptic) neuron's axon.

36. Acetylcholine is an example of a (neurotransmitter or protein molecule receptor).

37. Neurotransmitters are chemicals that allow neurons to (communicate or reproduce) with one another.

38. Neurotransmitters are distributed (randomly or specifically) into groups of neurons.

39. Catecholamines may play a role in (sleep or reproduction).

40. Endorphins and enkephalins are neurotransmitters that inhibit conduction of (fear or pain) impulses.

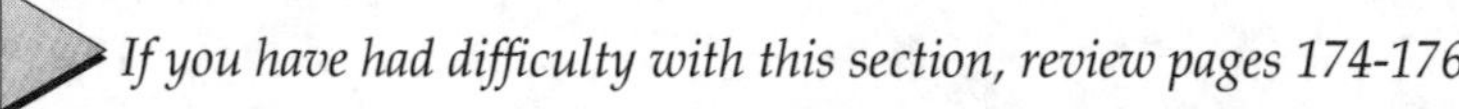

If you have had difficulty with this section, review pages 174-176.

CENTRAL NERVOUS SYSTEM
DIVISIONS OF THE BRAIN

Select the best answer.

41. Which one of the following is a part of the brainstem?
   A. Thalamus
   B. Cerebellum
   C. Cerebrum
   D. Hypothalamus
   E. Medulla

42. Which one of the following is *not* a function of the brainstem?
   A. Conduction of sensory impulses from the spinal cord to the higher centers of the brain
   B. Conduction of motor impulses from the cerebrum to the spinal cord
   C. Control of heartbeat, respiration, and blood vessel diameter
   D. Containment of centers for speech and memory

43. Which one of the following is *not* part of the diencephalon?
   A. Cerebrum
   B. Thalamus
   C. Hypothalamus
   D. All of the above are correct

44. ADH is produced by the:
   A. Pituitary gland
   B. Medulla
   C. Mammillary bodies
   D. Third ventricle
   E. Hypothalamus

45. Which one of the following is *not* true about the hypothalamus?
   A. It helps control the rate of heartbeat.
   B. It helps control the constriction and dilation of blood vessels.
   C. It helps control the contraction of the stomach and intestines.
   D. It produces releasing hormones that control the release of certain anterior pituitary hormones.
   E. All of the above are true.

46. Which one of the following parts of the brain helps in the association of sensations with emotions and also aids in the arousal or alerting mechanism?
   A. Pons
   B. Hypothalamus
   C. Cerebellum
   D. Thalamus
   E. None of the above

47. Which of the following is *not* true of the cerebrum?
   A. Its lobes correspond to the bones that lie over them.
   B. Its grooves are called *gyri*.
   C. Most of its gray matter lies on the surface of the cerebrum.
   D. Its outer region is called the *cerebral cortex*.
   E. Its two hemispheres are connected by a structure called the *corpus callosum*.

48. Which one of the following is *not* a function of the cerebrum?
    A. Willed movement
    B. Consciousness
    C. Memory
    D. Conscious awareness of sensations
    E. All of the above are functions of the cerebrum

49. The area of the cerebrum responsible for the perception of sound lies in the ___________ lobe.
    A. Frontal
    B. Temporal
    C. Occipital
    D. Parietal

50. Visual perception is located in the ___________ lobe.
    A. Frontal
    B. Temporal
    C. Parietal
    D. Occipital
    E. None of the above

51. Which one of the following is *not* a function of the cerebellum?
    A. Maintains equilibrium
    B. Helps with production of smooth, coordinated movements
    C. Helps maintain normal posture
    D. Associates sensations with emotions

52. Within the interior of the cerebrum are a few islands of gray matter known as:
    A. Fissures
    B. Basal ganglia
    C. Gyri
    D. Myelin

53. A cerebrovascular accident is commonly referred to as:
    A. A stroke
    B. Parkinson's disease
    C. A tumor
    D. Multiple sclerosis

54. Parkinson's disease is a disease of the:
    A. Myelin
    B. Axons
    C. Neuroglia
    D. Cerebral nuclei

55. The largest section of the brain is the:
    A. Cerebellum
    B. Pons
    C. Cerebrum
    D. Midbrain

If you have had difficulty with this section, review pages 176-183.

SPINAL CORD

If the statement is true, write "T" in the answer blank. If the statement is false, correct the statement by circling the incorrect term and writing the correct term in the answer blank.

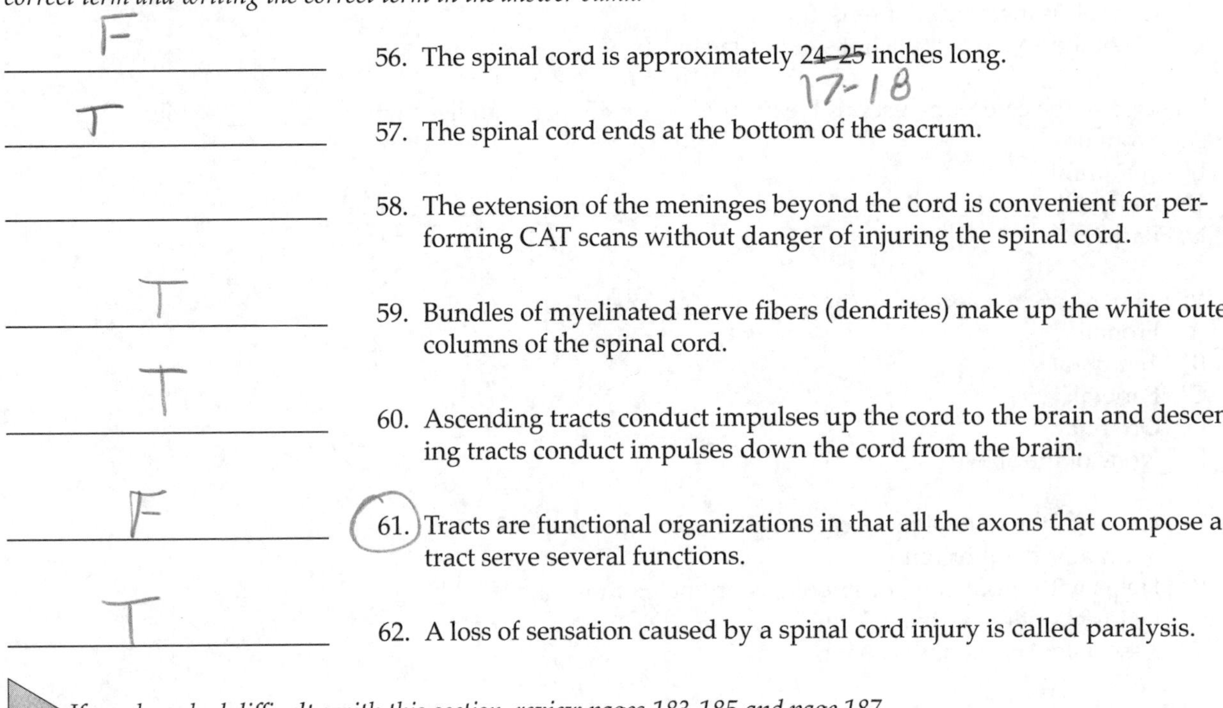

F ______ 56. The spinal cord is approximately 24–25 inches long. 17-18

T ______ 57. The spinal cord ends at the bottom of the sacrum.

______ 58. The extension of the meninges beyond the cord is convenient for performing CAT scans without danger of injuring the spinal cord.

T ______ 59. Bundles of myelinated nerve fibers (dendrites) make up the white outer columns of the spinal cord.

T ______ 60. Ascending tracts conduct impulses up the cord to the brain and descending tracts conduct impulses down the cord from the brain.

F ______ 61. Tracts are functional organizations in that all the axons that compose a tract serve several functions.

T ______ 62. A loss of sensation caused by a spinal cord injury is called paralysis.

If you have had difficulty with this section, review pages 183-185 and page 187.

COVERINGS AND FLUID SPACES OF BRAIN AND SPINAL CORD

Circle the one that does not *belong.*

63. Meninges	Pia mater	Ventricles	Dura mater
64. Arachnoid	Middle layer	CSF	Cobweb-like
65. CSF	Ventricles	Subarachnoid space	Pia mater
66. Tough	Outer layer	Dura mater	Choroid plexus
67. Brain tumor	Subarachnoid space	CSF	Fourth lumbar vertebra

If you have had difficulty with this section, review pages 185-187.

PERIPHERAL NERVOUS SYSTEM—CRANIAL NERVES

68. *Fill in the missing areas on the chart below.*

NERVE		CONDUCT IMPULSES	FUNCTION
I		From nose to brain	Sense of smell
II	Optic		From eye to brain
III	Oculomotor		Eye movements
IV		From brain to external eye muscles	Eye movements
V	Trigeminal	From skin and mucous membrane of head and from teeth to brain; also from brain to chewing muscles	
VI	Abducens		Eye movements
VII	Facial	From taste buds of tongue to brain; from brain to face muscles	
VIII		From ear to brain	Hearing; sense of balance
IX	Glossopharyngeal		Sensations of throat, taste, swallowing movements, secretion of saliva
X		From throat, larynx, and organs in thoracic and abdominal cavities to brain; also from brain to muscles of throat and to organs in thoracic and abdominal cavities	Sensations of throat, larynx, and of thoracic and abdominal organs; swallowing, voice production, slowing of heartbeat, acceleration of peristalsis (gut movements)
XI	Accessory	From brain to certain shoulder and neck muscles	
XII		From brain to muscles of tongue	Tongue movements

If you have had difficulty with this section, review page 189, Table 8-2.

CRANIAL NERVES
SPINAL NERVES

Select the correct term from the choices given and write its letter in the answer blank.

(A) Cranial nerves (B) Spinal nerves

_____ 69. 12 pairs

_____ 70. Dermatome

_____ 71. Vagus

_____ 72. Shingles

_____ 73. 31 pairs

_____ 74. Optic

_____ 75. C1

_____ 76. Plexus

If you have had difficulty with this section, review pages 187-189.

AUTONOMIC NERVOUS SYSTEM

Match the term on the left with the proper selection on the right.

_____ 77. Autonomic nervous system A. Division of ANS

_____ 78. Autonomic neurons B. Tissues to which autonomic neurons conduct impulses

_____ 79. Preganglionic neurons C. Voluntary actions

_____ 80. Visceral effectors D. Regulates body's involuntary functions

_____ 81. Sympathetic system E. Motor neurons that make up the ANS

_____ 82. Somatic nervous system F. Conduct impulses between the spinal cord and a ganglion

SYMPATHETIC NERVOUS SYSTEM
PARASYMPATHETIC NERVOUS SYSTEM

Select the best answer.

83. Dendrites and cell bodies of sympathetic preganglionic neurons are located in the:
    A. Brainstem and sacral portion of the spinal cord
    B. Sympathetic ganglia
    C. Gray matter of the thoracic and upper lumbar segments of the spinal cord
    D. Ganglia close to effectors

84. Which of the following statements is *not* correct?
    A. Sympathetic preganglionic neurons have their cell bodies located in the lateral gray column of certain parts of the spinal cord.
    B. Sympathetic preganglionic axons pass along the dorsal root of certain spinal nerves.
    C. There are synapses within sympathetic ganglia.
    D. Sympathetic responses are usually widespread, involving many organs.

85. Another name for the parasympathetic nervous system is:
    A. Thoracolumbar
    B. Craniosacral
    C. Visceral
    D. ANS
    E. Cholinergic

86. Which of the following statements is *not* correct?
    A. Sympathetic postganglionic neurons have their dendrites and cell bodies in sympathetic ganglia or collateral ganglia.
    B. Sympathetic ganglions are located in front of and at each side of the spinal column.
    C. Separate autonomic nerves distribute many sympathetic postganglionic axons to various internal organs.
    D. Very few sympathetic preganglionic axons synapse with postganglionic neurons.

87. Sympathetic stimulation usually results in:
    A. Response by numerous organs
    B. Response by only one organ
    C. Increased peristalsis
    D. Constriction of pupils

88. Parasympathetic stimulation frequently results in:
    A. Response by only one organ
    B. Responses by numerous organs
    C. The "fight-or-flight" response
    D. Increased heartbeat

Select the correct term from the choices given and write the letter in the answer blank.

(A) Sympathetic control (B) Parasympathetic control

_____ 89. Constricts pupils

_____ 90. Produces "goose pimples"

_____ 91. Increases sweat secretion

_____ 92. Increases secretion of digestive juices

_____ 93. Constricts blood vessels

_____ 94. Slows heartbeat

_____ 95. Relaxes bladder

_____ 96. Increases epinephrine secretion

_____ 97. Increases peristalsis

_____ 98. Stimulates lens for near vision

If you have had difficulty with this section, review pages 189-194.

AUTONOMIC NEUROTRANSMITTERS
AUTONOMIC NERVOUS SYSTEM AS A WHOLE

Fill in the blanks.

99. Sympathetic preganglionic axons release the neurotransmitter ____________________.

100. Axons that release norepinephrine are classified as ____________ ____________.

101. Axons that release acetylcholine are classified as ____________ ____________.

102. The function of the autonomic nervous system is to regulate the body's involuntary functions in ways that maintain or restore ____________.

103. Your ____________ ________________ is determined by the combined forces of the sympathetic and parasympathetic nervous system.

104. According to some physiologists, meditation leads to ________________ sympathetic activity and changes opposite to those of the "fight-or-flight" response.

If you have had difficulty with this section, review pages 194-196.

UNSCRAMBLE THE WORDS

Take the circled letters, unscramble them, and fill in the statement.

105. **RONNESU**

106. **APSYENS**

107. **CIATUNOMO**

108. **SHTOMO ULMSEC**

What the man hoped the IRS agent would be during his audit.

109.

APPLYING WHAT YOU KNOW

110. Mr. Hemstreet suffered a cerebrovascular accident and it was determined that the damage affected the left side of his cerebrum. On which side of his body will he most likely notice any paralysis?

111. Baby Dania was born with an excessive accumulation of cerebrospinal fluid in the ventricles. A catheter was placed in the ventricle and the fluid was drained by means of a shunt into the circulatory bloodstream. What condition does this medical history describe?

112. Mrs. Muhlenkamp looked out her window to see a man trapped under the wheel of a car. Although slightly built, Mrs. Muhlenkamp rushed to the car, lifted it, and saved the man underneath the wheel. What division of the autonomic nervous system made this seemingly impossible task possible?

113. Madison's heart raced and her palms became clammy as she watched the monster movie at the local theater. When the movie was over, however, she told her friends that she was not afraid at all. She appeared to be as calm as before the movie. What division of the autonomic nervous system made this possible?

114. Bill is going to his boss for his annual evaluation. He is planning to ask for a raise and hopes the evaluation will be good. Which subdivision of the autonomic nervous system will be active during this conference? Should he have a large meal before his appointment? Support your answer with facts from the chapter.

115. WORD FIND

Can you find the 14 terms from this chapter in the box of letters? Words may be spelled top to bottom, bottom to top, right to left, left to right, or diagonally.

```
M C C D Q S Y N A P S E Q G O
E N A Q D W H N W E J N A L W
S R O T P E C E R Y Z N I S M
I D S X E K N O K X G G C Y Y
J O T R A C T D F L O N E N A
R P W E K O H X I D A L H A M
F A L O N A Y O E I I I X P C
C M Z I F D N N L N G Z U T Z
S I N V C G D G Z A N A K I P
G N A T Z R O W V A M Y T C O
K E N D O R P H I N S I L C X
C P Q G C J X F J D Q S N L F
X U L I H I G Q A N S W O E U
A I M H Q E X K D B W Y T F S
A A D A X O C K G B F H B T K
```

Axon	Glia	Serotonin
Catecholamines	Microglia	Synapse
Dopamine	Myelin	Synaptic cleft
Endorphins	Oligodendroglia	Tract
Ganglion	Receptors	

DID YOU KNOW?

Although all pain is felt and interpreted in the brain, it has no pain sensation itself—even when cut!

In the adult human body, there are 46 miles of nerves.

The areas of the brain that track emotion and memory are larger and more sensitive in the female brain.

"Rejection" actually hurts like physical pain because it triggers the same circuits in the brain.

THE NERVOUS SYSTEM

Fill in the crossword puzzle.

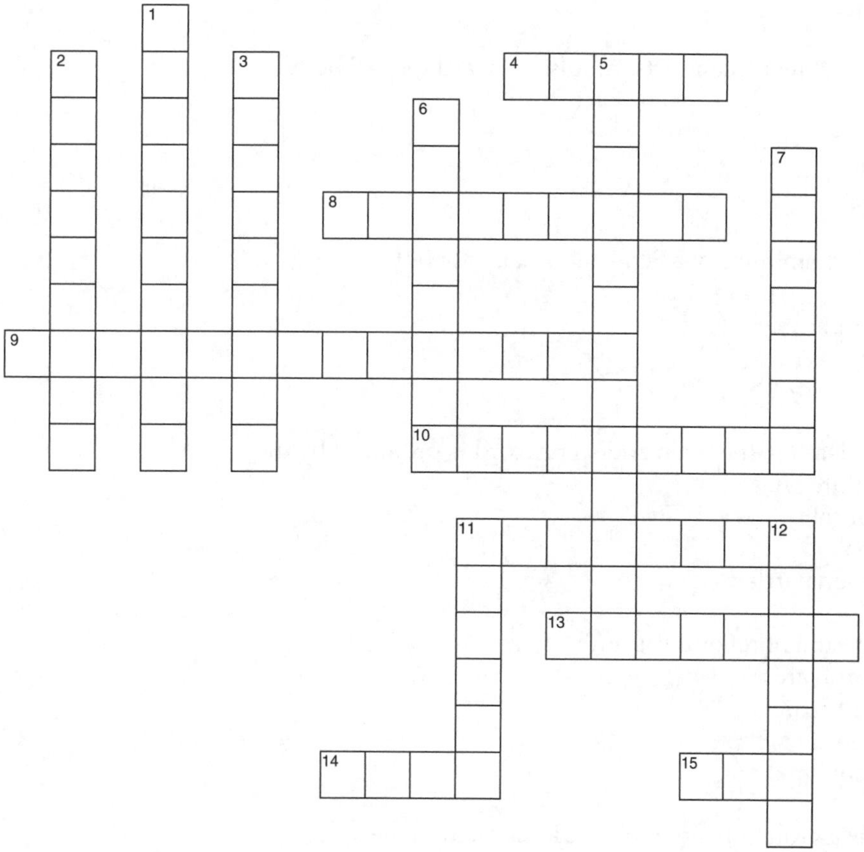

Across

4. Bundle of axons located within the CNS
8. Transmits impulses toward the cell body
9. Neurons that conduct impulses from a ganglion
10. Astrocytes
11. Pia mater
13. Nerve cells
14. Transmits impulses away from the cell body
15. Peripheral nervous system (abbreviation)

Down

1. Neuroglia
2. Peripheral beginning of a sensory neuron's dendrite
3. Two neuron arc (two words)
5. Neurotransmitter
6. Cluster of nerve cell bodies outside the central nervous system
7. Area of brain stem
11. Fatty substance found around some nerve fibers
12. Where impulses are transmitted from one neuron to another

CHECK YOUR KNOWLEDGE

Multiple Choice

Select the best answer.

1. Which of the following conducts impulses toward the cell body?
   A. Axons
   B. Astrocytes
   C. Microglia
   D. Dendrites

2. The outer cell membrane of a Schwann cell is called the:
   A. Glioma
   B. Neurilemma
   C. Cell body
   D. Dendrite

3. The myelin sheath in the brain and spinal cord is produced by the:
   A. Oligodendrocytes
   B. Schwann cells
   C. Microglia
   D. Blood-brain barrier

4. The simplest kind of reflex arc is a(n):
   A. One-neuron arc
   B. Two-neuron arc
   C. Three-neuron arc
   D. Action potential

5. A ganglion is a group of nerve cell bodies located in the:
   A. PNS
   B. CNS
   C. Brain and spinal cord
   D. All of the above

6. Each synaptic knob vesicle contains a very small quantity of a chemical compound called a:
   A. Synapse
   B. ADH
   C. Releasing hormone
   D. Neurotransmitter

7. Which of the following is located in the brainstem?
   A. Medulla oblongata
   B. Pons
   C. Midbrain
   D. All of the above

8. Which of the following is a function of the hypothalamus?
   A. Muscle coordination
   B. Willed movements
   C. Regulation of body temperature
   D. Relay for visual impulses

9. Which of the following is *not* true regarding the meninges?
   A. The tough outer layer is the dura mater.
   B. The arachnoid mater is the membrane between the dura mater and the pia mater.
   C. The pia mater resembles a "cobweb" and the name comes from the Greek word for spider.
   D. All of the above statements are true.

10. The autonomic nervous system consists of certain motor neurons that conduct impulses from the spinal cord or brainstem to the:
    A. Cardiac muscle tissue
    B. Smooth muscle tissue
    C. Glandular epithelial tissue
    D. All of the above

Matching

Select the most correct answer from column B for each statement in column A. (Only one answer is correct.)

Column A		Column B
_____	11. Multiple sclerosis	A. Corpus callosum
_____	12. Cerebrum	B. Abducens
_____	13. CVA	C. Myelin disorder
_____	14. Cerebrospinal fluid	D. Slows heartbeat
_____	15. Cranial nerves	E. "Fight or flight"
_____	16. Spinal nerves	F. Visceral effectors
_____	17. Autonomic neurons	G. Parkinson's disease
_____	18. Sympathetic nervous system	H. Ventricles
_____	19. Parasympathetic nervous system	I. Thirty-one pairs
_____	20. Dopamine	J. Stroke

NEURON

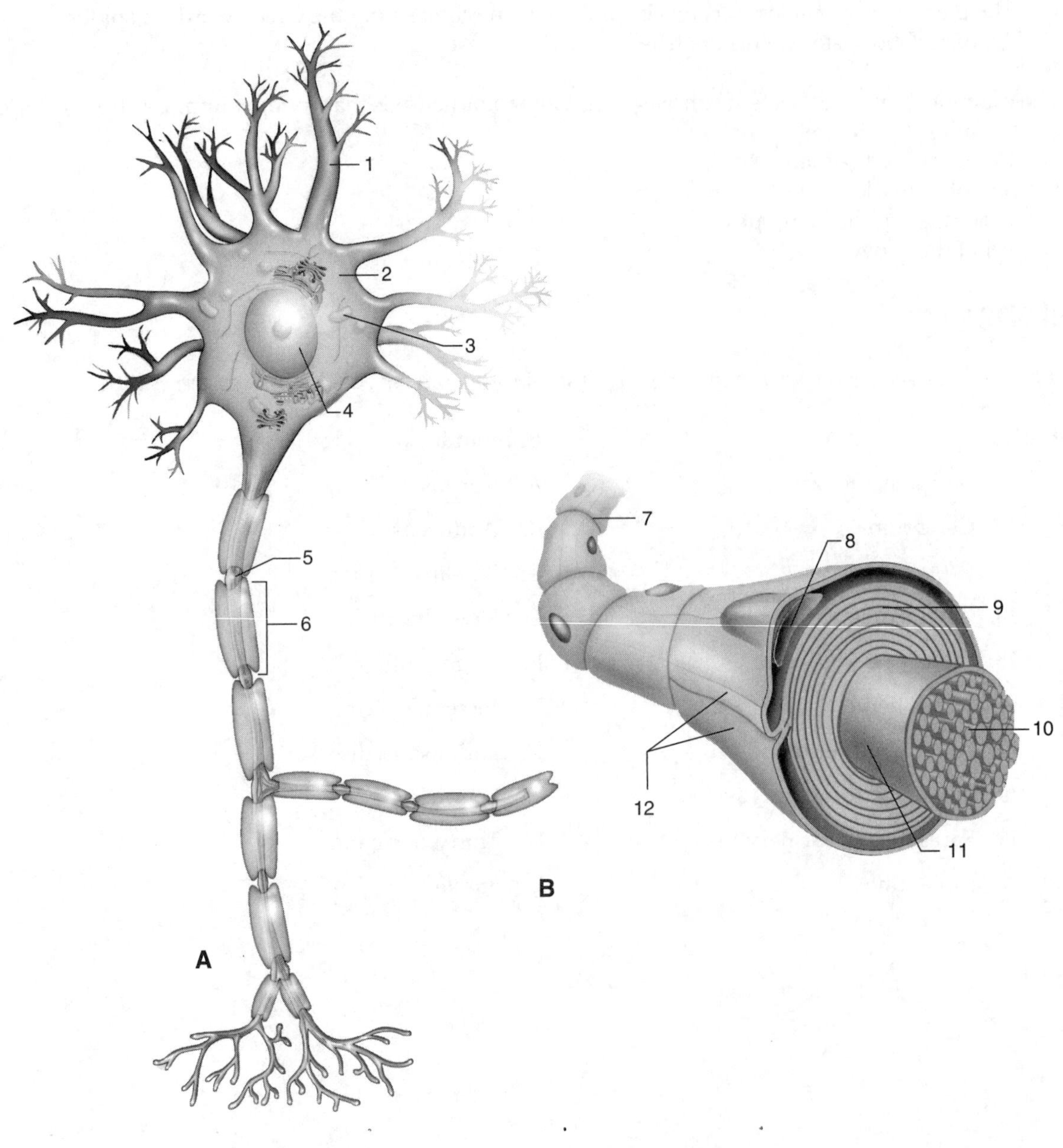

1. ______________________
2. ______________________
3. ______________________
4. ______________________
5. ______________________
6. ______________________
7. ______________________
8. ______________________
9. ______________________
10. ______________________
11. ______________________
12. ______________________

CRANIAL NERVES

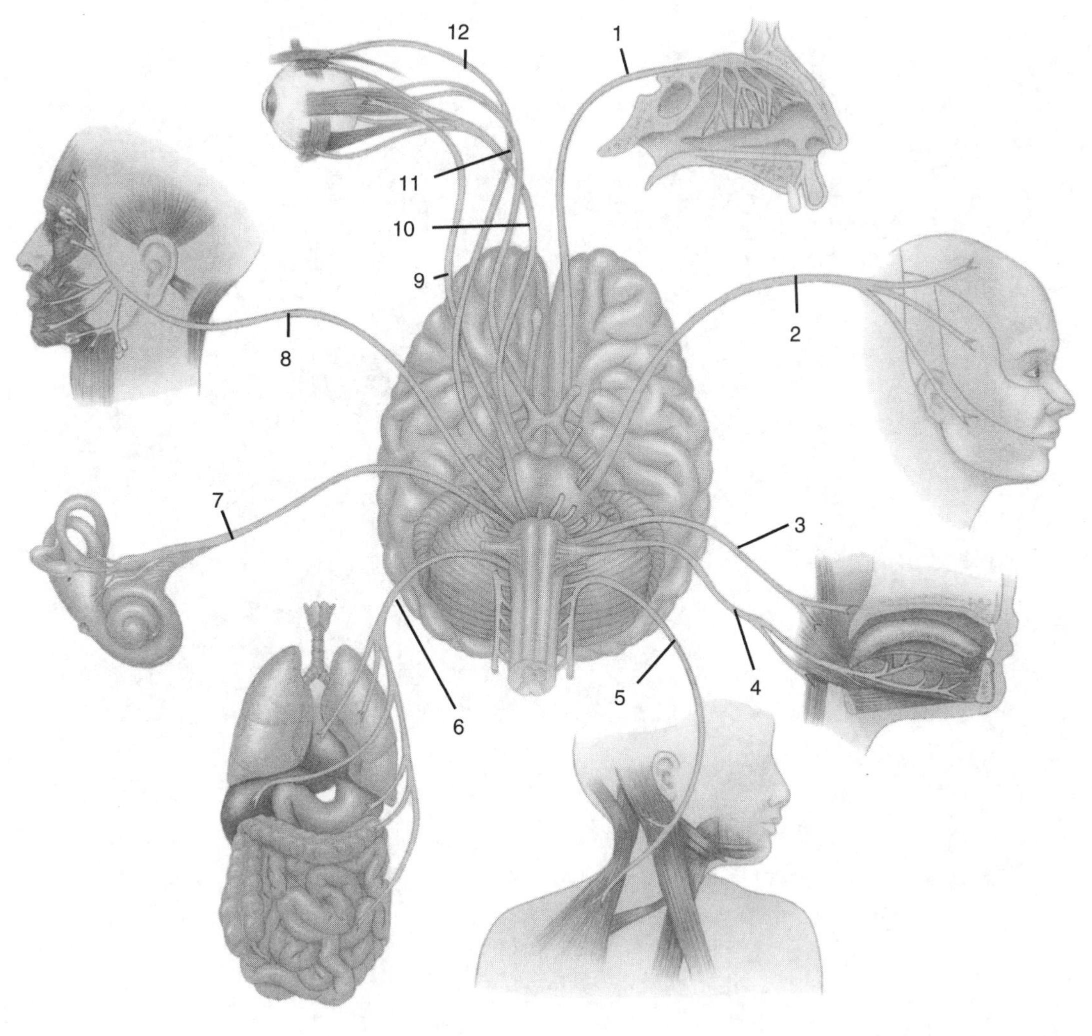

1. ____________________
2. ____________________
3. ____________________
4. ____________________
5. ____________________
6. ____________________
7. ____________________
8. ____________________
9. ____________________
10. ____________________
11. ____________________
12. ____________________

NEURAL PATHWAY INVOLVED IN THE PATELLAR REFLEX

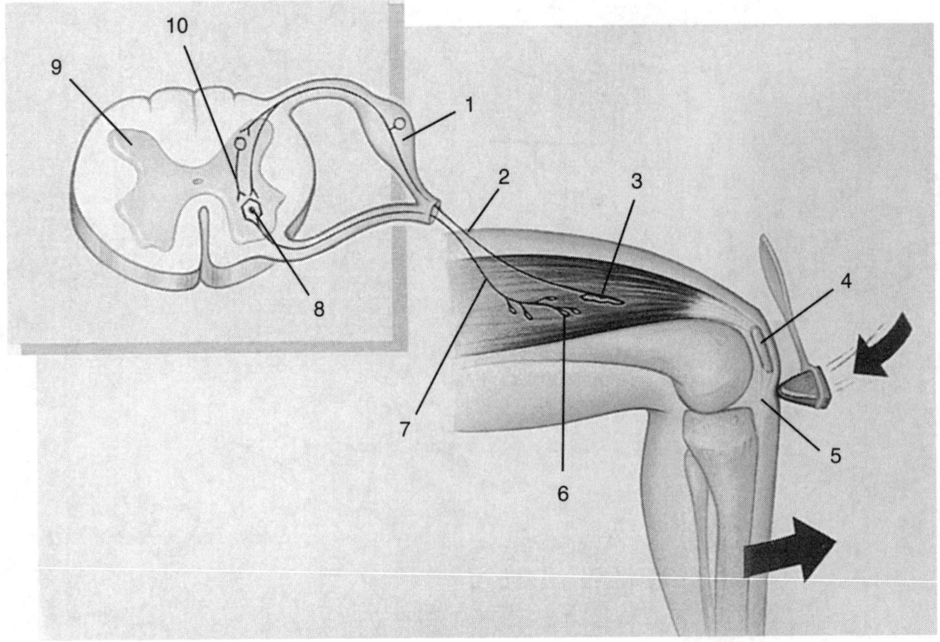

1. ______________________
2. ______________________
3. ______________________
4. ______________________
5. ______________________
6. ______________________
7. ______________________
8. ______________________
9. ______________________
10. ______________________

AUTONOMIC CONDUCTION PATHS

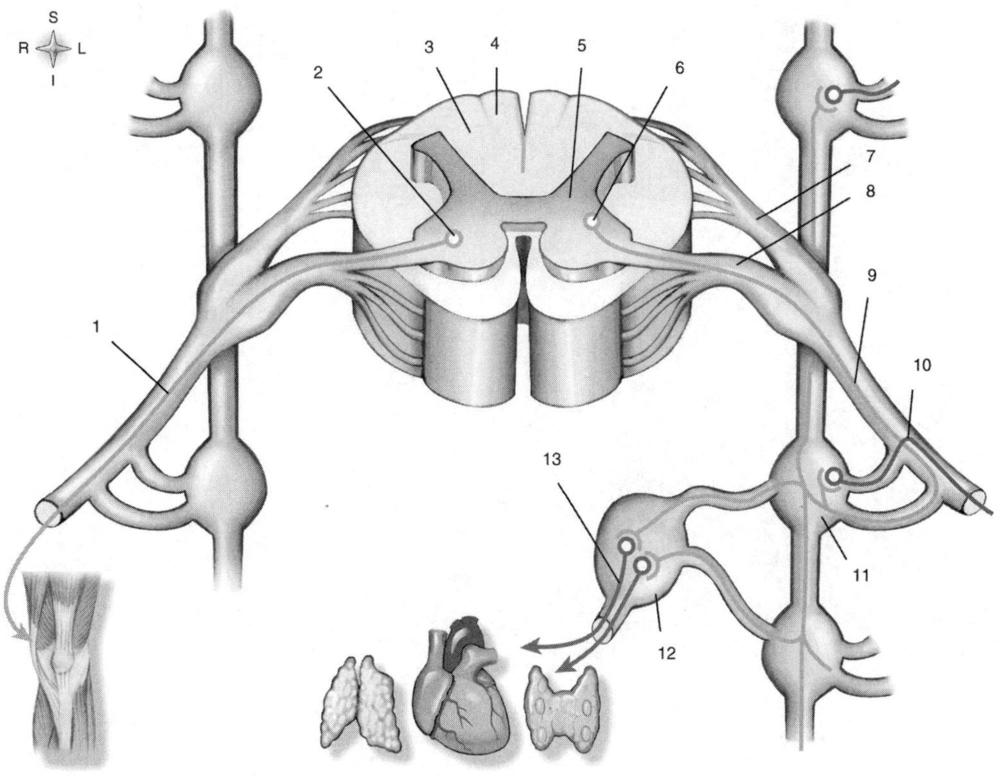

1. ______________________
2. ______________________
3. ______________________
4. ______________________
5. ______________________
6. ______________________
7. ______________________
8. ______________________
9. ______________________
10. ______________________
11. ______________________
12. ______________________
13. ______________________

CHAPTER 9

The Senses

Consider this scene for a moment. You are walking along a beautiful beach watching the sunset. You notice the various hues and are amazed at the multitude of shades that cover the sky. The waves are indeed melodious as they splash along the shore, and you wiggle your feet with delight as you sense the warm, soft sand trickling between your toes. You sip on a soda and then inhale the fresh salt air as you continue your stroll along the shore. It is a memorable scene, but one that would not be possible without the assistance of your sense organs. The sense organs pick up messages that are sent over nerve pathways to specialized areas in the brain for interpretation. They make communication with and enjoyment of the environment possible. The visual, auditory, tactile, olfactory, and gustatory sense organs not only protect us from danger but also add an important dimension to our daily pleasures of life.

Your study of this chapter will give you an understanding of another of the systems necessary for homeostasis and survival.

TOPICS FOR REVIEW

Before progressing to Chapter 10, you should review the classification of sense organs and the process for converting a stimulus into a sensation. Your study should also include an understanding of the special sense organs and the general sense organs.

CLASSIFICATION OF SENSE ORGANS
CONVERTING A STIMULUS INTO A SENSATION
GENERAL SENSE ORGANS

Match the term on the left with the proper selection on the right.

_____	1. Special sense organ	A. Olfactory cells
_____	2. General sense organ	B. Meissner's corpuscles
_____	3. Nose	C. Chemoreceptor
_____	4. Krause's end-bulbs	D. Eye
_____	5. Taste buds	E. Touch

If you have had difficulty with this section, review pages 205-208.

SPECIAL SENSE ORGANS

Eye

Select the best answer.

6. The "white" of the eye is more commonly called the:
   A. Choroid
   B. Cornea
   C. Sclera
   D. Retina
   E. None of the above

7. The "colored" part of the eye is known as the:
   A. Retina
   B. Cornea
   C. Pupil
   D. Sclera
   E. Iris

8. The transparent portion of the sclera, referred to as the *window* of the eye, is the:
   A. Retina
   B. Cornea
   C. Pupil
   D. Iris

9. The mucous membrane that covers the front of the eye is called the:
   A. Cornea
   B. Choroid
   C. Conjunctiva
   D. Ciliary body
   E. None of the above

10. The structure that can contract or dilate to allow more or less light to enter the eye is the:
    A. Lens
    B. Choroid
    C. Retina
    D. Cornea
    E. Iris

11. When the eye is looking at objects far in the distance, the lens is ____________________ and the ciliary muscle is ____________________.
    A. Rounded; contracted
    B. Rounded; relaxed
    C. Slightly rounded; contracted
    D. Slightly curved; relaxed
    E. None of the above

12. The lens of the eye is held in place by the:
    A. Ciliary muscle
    B. Aqueous humor
    C. Vitreous humor
    D. Cornea

13. When the lens loses its elasticity and can no longer bring near objects into focus, the condition is known as:
    A. Glaucoma
    B. Presbyopia
    C. Astigmatism
    D. Strabismus

14. The fluid in front of the lens that is constantly being formed, drained, and replaced in the anterior chamber is the:
    A. Vitreous humor
    B. Protoplasm
    C. Aqueous humor
    D. Conjunctiva

15. If drainage of the aqueous humor is blocked, the internal pressure within the eye will increase and a condition known as ________________ could occur.
    A. Presbyopia
    B. Glaucoma
    C. Color blindness
    D. Cataracts

16. The rods and cones are the photoreceptor cells and are located on the:
    A. Sclera
    B. Cornea
    C. Choroid
    D. Retina

17. The area which contains the greatest concentration of cones on the retina is the:
    A. Fovea centralis
    B. Retinal artery
    C. Ciliary body
    D. Optic disc

18. If our eyes are abnormally elongated, the image focuses in front of the retina and a condition known as ________________ occurs.
    A. Hyperopia
    B. Cataracts
    C. Night blindness
    D. Myopia

If you have had difficulty with this section, review pages 208-213.

Ear

Select the correct term from the choices given and write the letter in the answer blank.

(A) External ear (B) Middle ear (C) Inner ear

_____ 19. Malleus

_____ 20. Perilymph

_____ 21. Incus

_____ 22. Ceruminous glands

_____ 23. Cochlea

_____ 24. Auditory canal

_____ 25. Semicircular canals

_____ 26. Stapes

_____ 27. Eustachian tube

_____ 28. Organ of Corti

Fill in the blanks.

29. The external ear has two parts: the ______________________________ and the ____________ ____________ ______________.

30. Another name for the tympanic membrane is the ____________________.

31. The bones of the middle ear are collectively referred to as ______________.

32. The stapes presses against a membrane that covers a small opening called the ______________ ______________.

33. A middle ear infection is called ________________ ______________.

34. The ____________________ is located adjacent to the oval window between the semicircular canals and the cochlea.

35. Located within the semicircular canals and the vestibule are ____________ for balance and equilibrium.

36. The sensory cells in the ______________ ________________ are stimulated when movement of the head causes the endolymph to move.

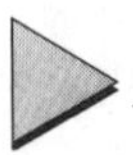
If you have had difficulty with this section, review pages 213-216.

TASTE RECEPTORS SMELL RECEPTORS

Circle the correct answer.

37. Structures known as (papillae or olfactory cells) are found on the tongue.

38. Nerve impulses generated by stimulation of taste buds travel primarily through two (cranial or spinal) nerves.

39. To be detected by olfactory receptors, chemicals must be dissolved in the watery (mucus or plasma) that lines the nasal cavity.

40. The pathways taken by olfactory nerve impulses and the areas where these impulses are interpreted are closely associated with areas of the brain important in (hearing or memory).

41. (Chemoreceptor or mechanoreceptor) is the term used to describe the type of receptors that generate nervous impulses resulting in the sense of taste or smell.

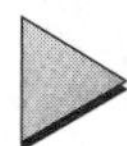
If you have had difficulty with this section, review pages 216-219.

UNSCRAMBLE THE WORDS

Take the circled letters, unscramble them, and fill in the statement.

42. C A L R I E U

43. R A E C L S

44. L A P I L A E P

45. C T V N U C N O I A J

What Mr. Tuttle liked best about his classroom.

46.

APPLYING WHAT YOU KNOW

47. Mr. Nay was an avid swimmer and competed regularly in his age group. He had to withdraw from the last competition due to an infection of his ear. Antibiotics and analgesics were prescribed by the doctor. What is the medical term for his condition?

48. Mrs. Metheny loved the outdoors and spent a great deal of her spare time basking in the sun on the beach. Her physician suggested that she begin wearing sunglasses regularly when he noticed milky spots beginning to appear on Mrs. Metheny's lenses. What condition was Mrs. Metheny's physician trying to prevent?

49. Shelley repeatedly became ill with throat infections during her first few years of school. Lately, however, she has noticed that whenever she has a throat infection, her ears become very sore also. What might be the cause of this additional problem?

50. Julius was hit in the nose with a baseball during practice. His sense of smell was temporarily gone. What nerve receptors were damaged during the injury?

51. WORD FIND

Can you find the 19 terms from this chapter in the box of letters? Words may be spelled top to bottom, bottom to top, right to left, left to right, or diagonally.

```
M E C H A N O R E C E P T O R
H R A T B Q I R T B N H M A E
P F T Y R O T C A F L O X R C
G U A Y I N A I H C A T S U E
G P R A C E R U M E N O P X P
I E A I P O Y B S E R P K D T
W L C P L Y N E Y K E I T O O
C Q T O I B R J B S F G L M R
Z U S R C L E O U J R M N N S
F D M E O H L Q T N A E Y I S
H I D P N D L A M A C N X S Z
A M L Y E S S E E D T T M Z H
D D M H S F E X A Y I S I I A
J C G N J T I S L P O G U V J
P H G Y A K H S U C N I S G A
```

Cataracts
Cerumen
Cochlea
Cones
Conjunctiva
Eustachian
Eye
Gustatory
Hyperopia
Incus
Mechanoreceptor
Olfactory
Papillae
Photopigment
Presbyopia
Receptors
Refraction
Rods
Senses

DID YOU KNOW?

The human eye blinks an average of 4,200,000 times a year.

Our eyes are always the same size from birth, but our nose and ears never stop growing.

If your mouth was completely dry, you would not be able to distinguish the taste of anything.

Tongue prints are as unique as fingerprints.

THE SENSES

Fill in the crossword puzzle.

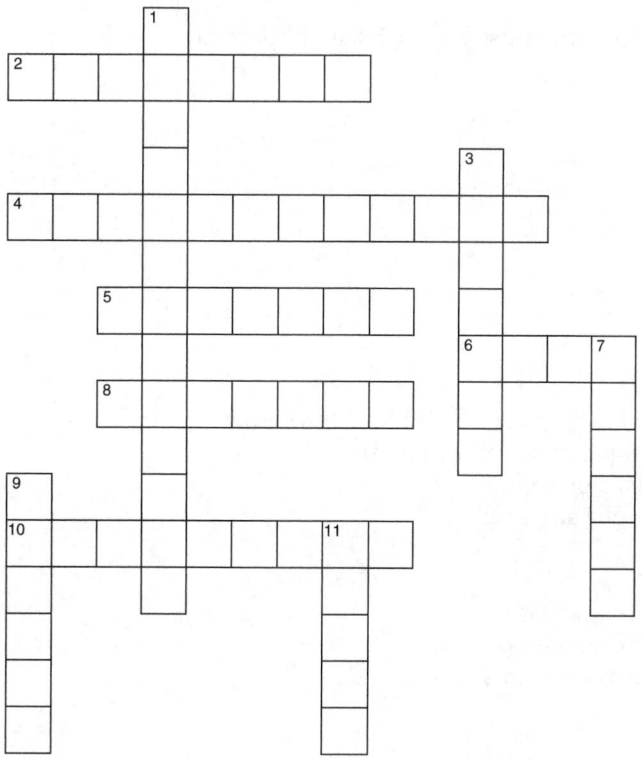

Across

2. Bones of the middle ear
4. Located in anterior cavity in front of lens (two words)
5. External ear
6. Transparent body behind pupil
8. Front part of this coat is the ciliary muscle and iris
10. Membranous labyrinth filled with this fluid

Down

1. Located in posterior cavity (two words)
3. Organ of Corti located here
7. White of the eye
9. Innermost layer of the eye
11. Hole in center of the iris

CHECK YOUR KNOWLEDGE

Multiple Choice

Select the best answer.

1. The Golgi tendon receptors and muscle spindles are important:
   A. Proprioceptors
   B. Photoreceptors
   C. Chemoreceptors
   D. None of the above

2. Another name for *farsightedness* is:
   A. Myopia
   B. Hyperopia
   C. Astigmatism
   D. None of the above

3. In addition to its role in hearing, the ear also functions as:
   A. The sense organ of equilibrium and balance
   B. A sense organ for chemoreceptors
   C. The sense organ for gustatory cells
   D. None of the above

4. The occipital lobe is responsible for:
   A. Interpretation of mechanoreceptors
   B. Interpretation of chemoreceptors
   C. Visual interpretation
   D. None of the above

5. Another name for the tympanic membrane is the:
   A. Ossicle
   B. Eardrum
   C. External auditory canal
   D. Oval window

6. The inner ear consists of three spaces in the temporal bone, assembled in a complex maze called the:
   A. Crista ampullaris
   B. Bony labyrinth
   C. Organ of Corti
   D. Ossicles

7. Three layers of tissue form the eyeball. They are the:
   A. Iris, conjunctiva, and cornea
   B. Choroid, iris, and pupil
   C. Retina, rods, and cones
   D. Sclera, choroid, and retina

8. The jellylike fluid behind the lens in the posterior chamber is the:
   A. Aqueous humor
   B. Vitreous humor
   C. Endolymph
   D. Perilymph

9. The Eustachian tube connects the throat with the:
   A. Tympanic membrane
   B. External ear
   C. Inner ear
   D. Middle ear

10. The receptors for night vision are the:
    A. Rods
    B. Cones
    C. Fovea centralis
    D. Chemoreceptors

True or False

Indicate whether the following statements are true (T) or false (F).

_____ 11. The sense organs are often classified as either general sense organs or special sense organs.

_____ 12. The cornea is sometimes spoken of as the *white of the eye*.

_____ 13. Two involuntary muscles make up the front part of the choroid: the iris and the ciliary muscle.

_____ 14. When the lens becomes hard and loses its transparency, a condition called *glaucoma* occurs.

_____ 15. A laser surgery approved by the USFDA for hyperopia is laser thermal keratoplasty.

_____ 16. The optic disc is also known as the *blind spot*.

_____ 17. The malleus, incus, and stapes are also known as the *ossicles*.

_____ 18. A middle ear infection may also be referred to as *otitis media*.

_____ 19. The chemoreceptors of the taste buds are called *gustatory cells*.

_____ 20. Tears are formed in the lacrimal gland.

EYE

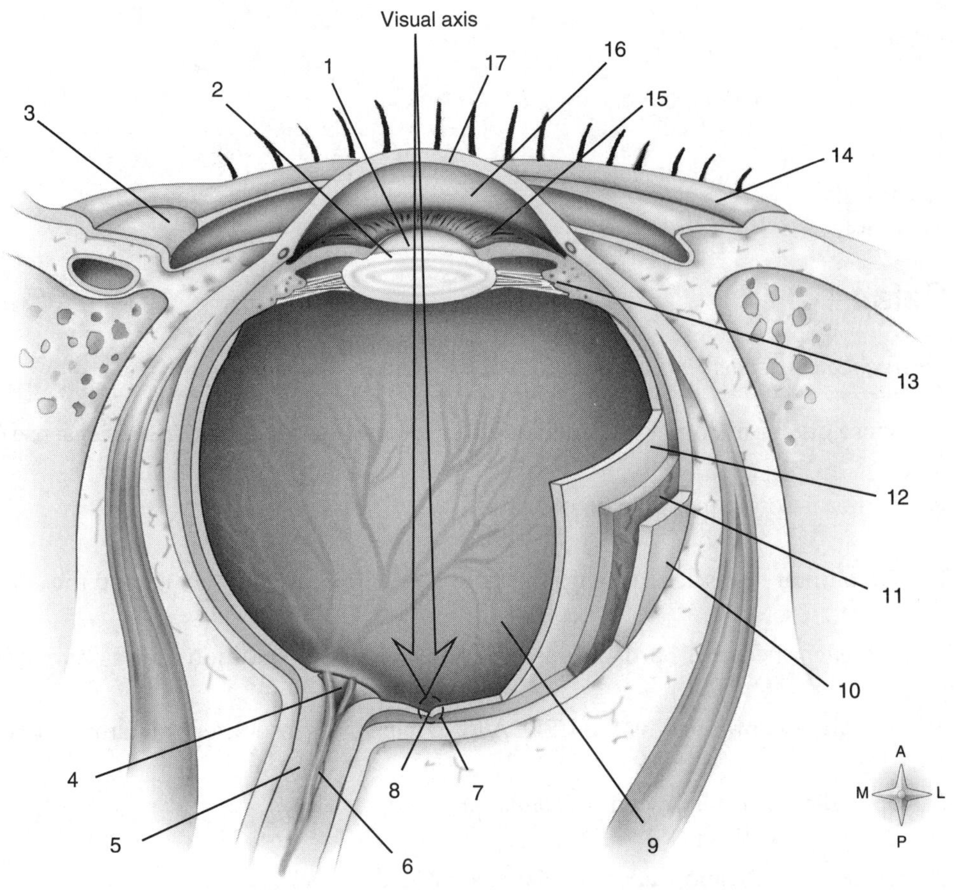

1. ______________________
2. ______________________
3. ______________________
4. ______________________
5. ______________________
6. ______________________
7. ______________________
8. ______________________
9. ______________________
10. ______________________
11. ______________________
12. ______________________
13. ______________________
14. ______________________
15. ______________________
16. ______________________
17. ______________________

EAR

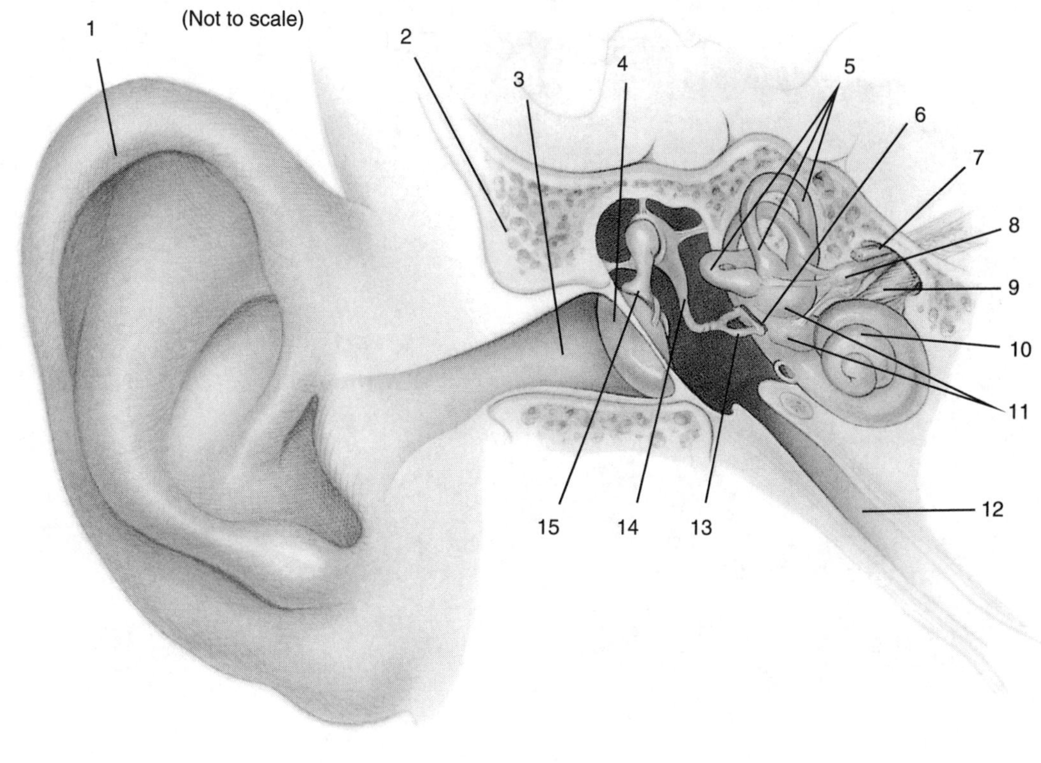

1. ______________________
2. ______________________
3. ______________________
4. ______________________
5. ______________________
6. ______________________
7. ______________________
8. ______________________
9. ______________________
10. ______________________
11. ______________________
12. ______________________
13. ______________________
14. ______________________
15. ______________________

CHAPTER 10

The Endocrine System

The endocrine system has often been compared to a fine symphony concert. When all instruments are playing properly, the sound is melodious. If one instrument plays too loudly or too softly, however, it affects the overall quality of the performance.

The endocrine system is a ductless system that releases hormones into the bloodstream to help regulate body functions. The pituitary gland may be considered the conductor of the orchestra, as it stimulates many of the endocrine glands to secrete their powerful hormones. All hormones, whether stimulated in this manner or by other control mechanisms, are interdependent. A change in the level of one hormone may affect the level and performance of many other hormones.

In addition to the endocrine glands, prostaglandins ("tissue hormones") are powerful substances similar to hormones that have been found in a variety of body tissues. These hormones are often produced in a tissue and diffuse only a short distance to act on cells within that area. Prostaglandins influence respiration, blood pressure, gastrointestinal secretions, and the reproductive system, and they may someday play an important role in the treatment of diseases such as hypertension, asthma, and ulcers.

The endocrine system is a system of communication and control. It differs from the nervous system in that hormones provide a slower, longer-lasting effect than do nerve stimuli and responses. Your understanding of the "system of hormones" will alert you to the mechanism of our emotions, responses to stress, growth, chemical balances, and many other body functions.

TOPICS FOR REVIEW

Before progressing to Chapter 11, you should be able to identify and locate the primary endocrine glands of the body. Your understanding should include the hormones that are produced by these glands and the method by which these secretions are regulated. Your study will conclude with the pathological conditions that result from the malfunctioning of this system.

MECHANISMS OF HORMONE ACTION REGULATION OF HORMONE SECRETION PROSTAGLANDINS

Match the term on the left with the proper selection on the right.

Group A

_____ 1. Pituitary
_____ 2. Parathyroids
_____ 3. Adrenals
_____ 4. Ovaries
_____ 5. Thymus

A. Pelvic cavity
B. Mediastinum
C. Neck
D. Cranial cavity
E. Abdominal cavity

Group B

_____ 6. Negative feedback
_____ 7. Tissue hormones
_____ 8. Second messenger
_____ 9. Exocrine glands
_____ 10. Target organ cells

A. Cyclic AMP is an example of one
B. Respond to a particular hormone
C. Prostaglandins
D. Discharge secretions into ducts
E. Specialized homeostatic mechanism that regulates release of hormones

Fill in the blanks.

Nonsteroid hormones serve as (11) __________ ______________ providing communication between (12) ____________ and (13) _________ _________. Another molecule such as (14) ________ ___________ then acts as the (15) __________ __________ providing (16) __________________ within a hormone's (17) ______________ ____________.

If you have had difficulty with this section, review pages 224-231.

PITUITARY GLAND HYPOTHALAMUS

Select the best answer.

18. The pituitary gland lies in the ________________ bone.
    A. Ethmoid
    B. Sphenoid
    C. Temporal
    D. Frontal
    E. Occipital

19. Which one of the following structures would *not* be stimulated by a tropic hormone from the anterior pituitary?
    A. Ovaries
    B. Testes
    C. Thyroid
    D. Adrenals
    E. Uterus

20. Which one of the following is *not* a function of FSH?
    A. Stimulates the growth of follicles
    B. Stimulates the production of estrogens
    C. Stimulates the growth of seminiferous tubules
    D. Stimulates the interstitial cells of the testes

21. Which one of the following is *not* a function of LH?
    A. Stimulates maturation of a developing follicle
    B. Stimulates the production of estrogens
    C. Stimulates the formation of a corpus luteum
    D. Stimulates sperm cells to mature in the male
    E. Causes ovulation

22. Which one of the following is *not* a function of GH?
    A. Increases glucose catabolism
    B. Increases fat catabolism
    C. Speeds up the movement of amino acids into cells from the bloodstream
    D. All of the above are functions of GH

23. Which one of the following hormones is *not* released by the anterior pituitary gland?
    A. ACTH
    B. TSH
    C. ADH
    D. FSH
    E. LH

24. Which one of the following is *not* a function of prolactin?
    A. Stimulates breast development during pregnancy
    B. Stimulates milk secretion after delivery
    C. Causes the release of milk from glandular cells of the breast
    D. All of the above are functions of prolactin

25. The anterior pituitary gland secretes:
    A. Eight major hormones
    B. Tropic hormones that stimulate other endocrine glands to grow and secrete
    C. ADH
    D. Oxytocin

26. TSH acts on the:
    A. Thyroid
    B. Thymus
    C. Pineal
    D. Testes

27. ACTH stimulates the:
    A. Adrenal cortex
    B. Adrenal medulla
    C. Hypothalamus
    D. Ovaries

28. Which hormone is secreted by the posterior pituitary gland?
    A. MSH
    B. LH
    C. GH
    D. ADH

29. ADH serves the body by:
    A. Initiating labor
    B. Accelerating water reabsorption from urine into the blood
    C. Stimulating the pineal gland
    D. Regulating the calcium/phosphorus levels in the blood

30. What disease is caused by hyposecretion of ADH?
    A. Diabetes insipidus
    B. Diabetes mellitus
    C. Acromegaly
    D. Myxedema

31. The actual production of ADH and oxytocin takes place in which area?
    A. Anterior pituitary
    B. Posterior pituitary
    C. Hypothalamus
    D. Pineal

32. Inhibiting hormones are produced by the:
    A. Anterior pituitary
    B. Posterior pituitary
    C. Hypothalamus
    D. Pineal

Select the correct term from the choices given and write the letter in the answer blank.

(A) Anterior pituitary (B) Posterior pituitary (C) Hypothalamus

_____ 33. Adenohypophysis

_____ 34. Neurohypophysis

_____ 35. Induced labor

_____ 36. Appetite

_____ 37. Acromegaly

_____ 38. Body temperature

_____ 39. Sex hormones

_____ 40. Tropic hormones

_____ 41. Gigantism

_____ 42. Releasing hormones

If you have had difficulty with this section, review pages 231-234.

THYROID GLAND
PARATHYROID GLANDS

Circle the correct answer.

43. The thyroid gland lies (above or below) the larynx.
44. The thyroid gland secretes (calcitonin or glucagon).
45. For thyroxine to be produced in adequate amounts, the diet must contain sufficient (calcium or iodine).
46. Most endocrine glands (do or do not) store their hormones.
47. Colloid is a storage medium for the (thyroid or parathyroid) hormone.
48. Calcitonin (increases or decreases) the concentration of calcium in the blood.
49. Simple goiter results from (hyperthyroidism or hypothyroidism).
50. Hyposecretion of thyroid hormones during the formative years leads to (cretinism or myxedema).
51. The parathyroid glands secrete the hormone (PTH or PTA).
52. Parathyroid hormone tends to (increase or decrease) the concentration of calcium in the blood.

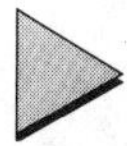

If you have had difficulty with this section, review pages 234-236.

ADRENAL GLANDS

Fill in the blanks.

53. The adrenal gland is actually two separate endocrine glands, the ____________ ____________ and the ____________ ____________.
54. Hormones secreted by the adrenal cortex are known as ________________.
55. The outer zone of the adrenal cortex secretes ____________________.
56. The middle zone secretes __________________.
57. The innermost zone secretes ________________ ____________________.
58. Glucocorticoids act in several ways to increase ____________________.
59. Glucocorticoids also play an essential part in maintaining ____________ ________________.
60. The adrenal medulla secretes the hormones ____________________ and __________________.
61. The adrenal medulla may help the body resist __________________.
62. Deficiency or hyposecretion of adrenal cortex hormones results in a condition called __________ ________.

Select the correct term from the choices given and write the letter in the answer blank.

(A) Adrenal cortex (B) Adrenal medulla

_____ 63. Mineralocorticoids

_____ 64. Anti-immunity

_____ 65. Adrenaline

_____ 66. Cushing syndrome

_____ 67. "Fight-or-flight" response

_____ 68. Aldosterone

_____ 69. Androgens

If you have had difficulty with this section, review pages 236-240.

PANCREATIC ISLETS, SEX GLANDS, THYMUS, PLACENTA, PINEAL GLAND

Circle the term that does not *belong.*

70. Alpha cells	Glucagon	Beta cells	Glycogenolysis
71. Insulin	Glucagon	Beta cells	Diabetes mellitus
72. Estrogens	Progesterone	Corpus luteum	Thymosin
73. Chorion	Interstitial cells	Testosterone	Semen
74. Immune system	Mediastinum	Aldosterone	Thymosin
75. Pregnancy	ACTH	Estrogen	Chorion
76. Melatonin	Menstruation	"Third eye"	Semen

Match the term on the left with the proper selection on the right.

Group A

_____ 77. Alpha cells	A. Estrogen
_____ 78. Beta cells	B. Progesterone
_____ 79. Corpus luteum	C. Insulin
_____ 80. Interstitial cells	D. Testosterone
_____ 81. Ovarian follicles	E. Glucagon

Group B

_____ 82. Placenta	A. Melatonin
_____ 83. Pineal	B. ANH
_____ 84. Heart atria	C. Testosterone
_____ 85. Testes	D. Thymosin
_____ 86. Thymus	E. Chorionic gonadotropins

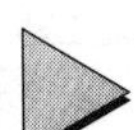

If you have had difficulty with this section, review pages 240-244.

UNSCRAMBLE THE WORDS

Take the circled letters, unscramble them, and fill in the statement.

87. ROODIITSCC

88. SIUISERD

89. UOOOTDCSIILRCCG

90. RIODSTES

Why Billy didn't like to take exams.

91.

APPLYING WHAT YOU KNOW

92. Mrs. Langston made a routine visit to her physician last week. When the laboratory results came back, the report indicated a high level of chorionic gonadotropin in her urine. What did this mean to Mrs. Langston?

93. Mrs. Wilcox noticed that her daughter was beginning to take on some of the secondary sex characteristics of a male. The pediatrician diagnosed the condition as a tumor of an endocrine gland. Where specifically was the tumor located?

94. Mrs. Florez was pregnant and was 2 weeks past her due date. Her doctor suggested that she enter the hospital and said he would induce labor. What hormone will he give Mrs. Florez?

95. WORD FIND

Can you find the 16 terms from the chapter in the box of letters? Words may be spelled top to bottom, bottom to top, right to left, left to right, or diagonally.

```
S S I S E R U I D M E S I T W
N D N X E B A M E D E X Y M I
I I G O N R S G X T I I Y V B
D O M S I N I T E R C C U Q D
N C X S R T N B O T V M Y O M
A I M E C L A C R E P Y H I X
L T Y R O I E Z Q R T J V K F
G R E T D P S N I L D J M X N
A O O S N I D K I N K S P P O
T C P R E T I O G R I F M X G
S L M H Y P O G L Y C E M I A
O A J L H O R M O N E O T G C
R C E L T S E L C N P N X U U
P I O S W R T X C G U L O E L
G G V Y H M S H Y K A K N Q G
```

Corticoids	Glucagon	Myxedema
Cretinism	Goiter	Prostaglandins
Diabetes	Hormone	Steroids
Diuresis	Hypercalcemia	Stress
Endocrine	Hypoglycemia	
Exocrine	Luteinization	

DID YOU KNOW?

The pituitary weighs little more than a small paper clip.

The total daily output of the pituitary gland is less than 1/1,000,000 of a gram, yet this small amount is responsible for stimulating the majority of all endocrine functions.

There are almost 30 hormones that are continuously being produced for us by various glands of the endocrine system.

THE ENDOCRINE SYSTEM

Fill in the crossword puzzle.

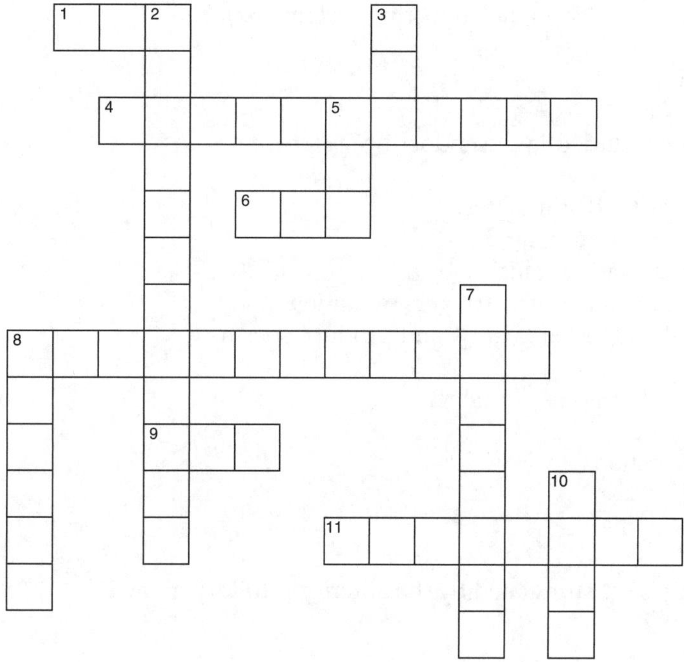

Across

1. Secreted by cells in the walls of the heart's atria
4. Adrenal medulla
6. Estrogens
8. Converts amino acids to glucose
9. Melanin
11. Labor

Down

2. Hypersecretion of insulin
3. Antagonist to diuresis
5. Increases calcium concentration
7. Hyposecretion of islets of Langerhans (one word)
8. Hyposecretion of thyroid
10. Adrenal cortex

CHECK YOUR KNOWLEDGE

Multiple Choice

Select the best answer.

1. All of the following are included in the endocrine system *except*:
   A. Exocrine glands
   B. Steroid hormones
   C. Nonsteroid hormones
   D. All of the above are included in the endocrine system

2. The luteinizing hormone (LH) stimulates:
   A. Breast development during pregnancy
   B. The development of ovarian follicles
   C. Maturation of ovarian follicle and triggers ovulation
   D. Seminiferous tubules of testes to grow and produce sperm

3. Prostaglandins or tissue hormones influence:
   A. Respiration
   B. Gastrointestinal secretions
   C. Blood pressure
   D. All of the above

4. Which of the following is *not* stimulated by the anterior pituitary gland?
   A. TSH
   B. ACTH
   C. ADH
   D. FSH

5. Too much insulin in the blood:
   A. Has the same effect on blood glucose as the growth hormone
   B. Increases blood glucose concentration
   C. Stimulates retention of water by the kidneys
   D. Produces hypoglycemia

6. The posterior pituitary gland and hypothalamus:
   A. Release two hormones
   B. Produce substances called *releasing* and *inhibiting* hormones
   C. Cause the glandular cells of the breast to release milk into ducts for nursing a baby
   D. All of the above

7. In addition to producing thyroid hormones, the thyroid gland also secretes:
   A. Hydrocortisone
   B. Calcitonin
   C. Aldosterone
   D. Glucagon

8. The adrenal medulla produces hormones that are:
   A. Not essential for life
   B. Helpful in responding to stress
   C. Responsible for the "fight-or-flight" response
   D. All of the above

9. The pineal gland produces several hormones in small quantities, with the most significant being:
   A. ANH
   B. Leptin
   C. Chorionic gonadotropins
   D. Melatonin

10. What plays a critical role in the body's defenses against infections?
    A. Pancreas
    B. Thymus
    C. Pineal body
    D. Thyroid

Matching

Select the most correct answer from column B for each statement in column A. (Only one answer is correct.)

Column A	Column B
_____ 11. Steroid hormones	A. Pancreas
_____ 12. Positive feedback	B. Adrenal cortex
_____ 13. Tropic hormones	C. Progesterone
_____ 14. Myxedema	D. Diabetes mellitus
_____ 15. Glucocorticoids	E. "Third eye"
_____ 16. Aldosterone	F. Mineralocorticoid
_____ 17. Islets of Langerhans	G. Occurs during labor
_____ 18. Glycosuria	H. Anterior pituitary
_____ 19. Pineal gland	I. Thyroid gland
_____ 20. Corpus luteum	J. Lipid soluble

ENDOCRINE GLANDS

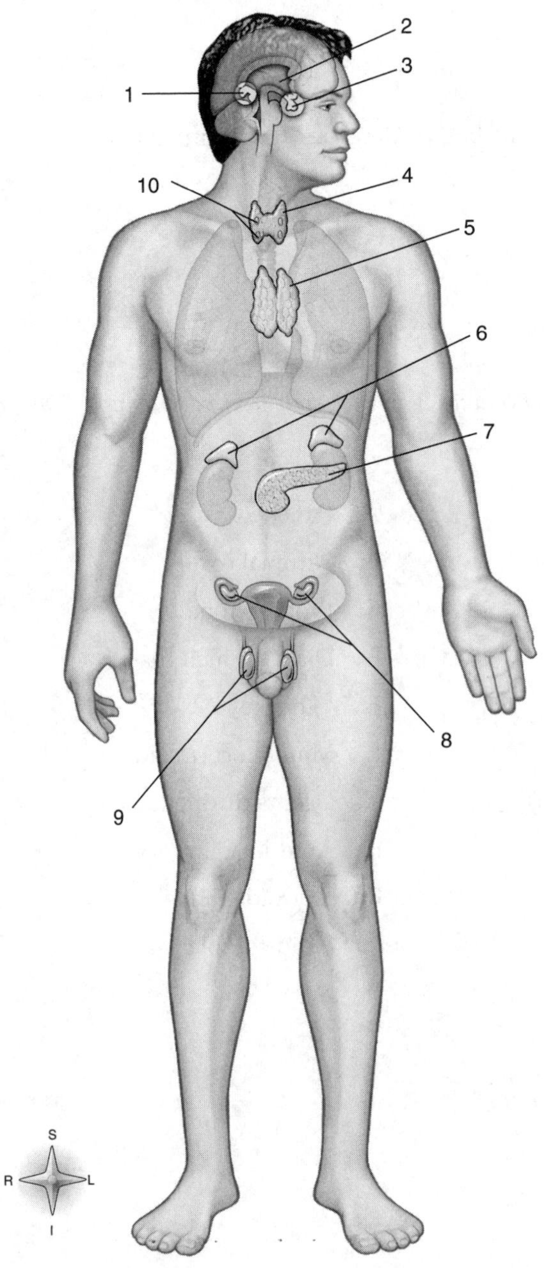

1. ______________________
2. ______________________
3. ______________________
4. ______________________
5. ______________________
6. ______________________
7. ______________________
8. ______________________
9. ______________________
10. ______________________

CHAPTER 11

Blood

Blood, the river of life, is the body's primary means of transportation. Although it is the respiratory system that provides oxygen for the body, the digestive system that provides nutrients, and the urinary system that eliminates wastes, none of these functions could be provided for the individual cells without the blood. In less than one minute, a drop of blood will complete a trip through the entire body, distributing nutrients and collecting the wastes of metabolism.

Blood is divided into plasma (the liquid portion of blood) and the formed elements (the blood cells). There are three types of blood cells: red blood cells, white blood cells, and platelets. Together these cells and plasma provide a means of transportation that delivers the body's daily necessities.

Although the red blood cells in all of us are of a similar shape, we have different blood types. Blood types are identified by the presence of certain antigens in the red blood cells. Every person's blood belongs to one of four main blood groups: Type A, B, AB, or O. Any one of the four groups or "types" may or may not have the specific antigen called the *Rh factor* present in the red blood cells. If an individual has the Rh factor present in his or her blood, the blood is Rh positive. If this factor is missing, the blood is Rh negative. Approximately 85% of the population has the Rh factor (Rh positive), and 15% do not have the Rh factor (Rh negative).

Your understanding of this chapter will be necessary to prepare a proper foundation for the circulatory system.

TOPICS FOR REVIEW

Before progressing to Chapter 12, you should have an understanding of the structure and function of blood plasma and cells. Your review should also include knowledge of blood types and Rh factors.

BLOOD COMPOSITION

Select the best answer.

1. Which one of the following substances is *not* a part of the plasma?
   A. Hormones
   B. Salts
   C. Nutrients
   D. Wastes
   E. All of the above are part of the plasma

2. The normal volume of blood in an adult is about:
   A. 2–3 pints
   B. 2–3 quarts
   C. 2–3 gallons
   D. 4–6 liters

3. Another name for red blood cells is:
   A. Leukocytes
   B. Thrombocytes
   C. Platelets
   D. Erythrocytes

4. Another name for white blood cells is:
   A. Erythrocytes
   B. Leukocytes
   C. Thrombocytes
   D. Platelets

5. Another name for platelets is:
   A. Neutrophils
   B. Eosinophils
   C. Thrombocytes
   D. Erythrocytes

6. Pernicious anemia is caused by:
   A. A lack of vitamin B_{12}
   B. Hemorrhage
   C. Radiation
   D. Bleeding ulcers

7. The laboratory test called *hematocrit* tells the physician the volume of:
   A. White cells in a blood sample
   B. Red cells in a blood sample
   C. Platelets in a blood sample
   D. Plasma in a blood sample

8. An example of a nongranular leukocyte is a(n):
   A. Platelet
   B. Erythrocyte
   C. Eosinophil
   D. Monocyte

9. An abnormally high white blood cell count is known as:
   A. AIDS
   B. Leukopenia
   C. Leukocytosis
   D. Anemia

10. A critical component of hemoglobin is:
    A. Potassium
    B. Calcium
    C. Vitamin K
    D. Iron

11. Sickle cell anemia is caused by the production of:
    A. An abnormal type of hemoglobin
    B. Excessive neutrophils
    C. Excessive platelets
    D. Abnormal leukocytes

12. The practice of using blood transfusions to increase oxygen delivery to muscles during athletic events is called blood:
    A. Antigen
    B. Doping
    C. Agglutination
    D. Proofing

13. The term used to describe the condition of a circulating blood clot is:
    A. Thrombosis
    B. Embolism
    C. Hemoglobin
    D. Platelet

14. Which one of the following types of cells is *not* a granular leukocyte?
    A. Neutrophil
    B. Lymphocyte
    C. Basophil
    D. Eosinophil

15. If a blood cell has no nucleus and is shaped like a biconcave disc, then the cell most likely is a(n):
    A. Platelet
    B. Lymphocyte
    C. Basophil
    D. Eosinophil
    E. Red blood cell

16. Red bone marrow forms all kinds of blood cells *except*:
    A. Platelets
    B. Lymphocytes
    C. Red blood cells
    D. Neutrophils

17. Myeloid tissue is found in all of the following locations *except*:
    A. Sternum
    B. Ribs
    C. Wrist bones
    D. Hip bones
    E. Cranial bones

18. Lymphatic tissue is found in all of the following locations *except*:
    A. Lymph nodes
    B. Thymus
    C. Spleen
    D. All of the above contain lymphatic tissue

19. The "buffy coat" layer in a hematocrit tube contains:
    A. Red blood cells and platelets
    B. Plasma only
    C. Platelets only
    D. White blood cells and platelets
    E. None of the above

20. The hematocrit value for red blood cells should be:
    A. 75%
    B. 60%
    C. 50%
    D. 45%
    E. 35%

21. An unusually low white blood cell count would be termed:
    A. Leukemia
    B. Leukopenia
    C. Leukocytosis
    D. Anemia
    E. None of the above

22. Most of the oxygen transported in the blood is carried by:
    A. Platelets
    B. Plasma
    C. Basophils
    D. Red blood cells
    E. None of the above

23. The most numerous of the phagocytes are the ________________.
    A. Lymphocytes
    B. Neutrophils
    C. Basophils
    D. Eosinophils
    E. Monocytes

24. Which one of the following types of cells is *not* phagocytic?
    A. Neutrophils
    B. Eosinophils
    C. Lymphocytes
    D. Monocytes
    E. All of the above are phagocytic cells

25. Which of the following cell types functions in the immune process?
    A. Neutrophils
    B. Lymphocytes
    C. Monocytes
    D. Basophils
    E. Reticuloendothelial cells

26. The organ that manufactures prothrombin is the:
    A. Liver
    B. Pancreas
    C. Thymus
    D. Kidney
    E. Spleen

27. Which one of the following vitamins acts to accelerate blood clotting?
    A. A
    B. B
    C. C
    D. D
    E. K

If you have had difficulty with this section, review pages 250-260.

BLOOD TYPES—RH FACTOR

28. *Fill in the missing areas of the chart.*

Blood Type	Antigen Present in RBCs	Antibody Present in Plasma
A		Anti-B
B	B	
AB		None
O	None	

Fill in the blanks.

29. A(n) ________________ is a substance that can activate the immune system to make antibodies.

30. A(n) ________________ is a substance made by the body in response to stimulation by an antigen.

31. Many antibodies react with their antigens to clump or ________________ them.

32. If a baby is born to an Rh-negative mother and Rh-positive father, it may develop the disease ________________ ________________.

33. The term *Rh* is used because the antigen was first discovered in the blood of a(n) ________________ ________________.

34. ________________ stops an Rh-negative mother from forming anti-Rh antibodies and thus prevents the possibility of harm to the next Rh-positive baby.

35. Blood type __________ has been called the *universal recipient*.

If you have had difficulty with this section, review pages 260-264.

UNSCRAMBLE THE WORDS

Take the circled letters, unscramble them, and fill in the statement.

36. **HGAPOYCET**

37. **NTHIRBMO**

38. **ATNIGNE**

39. **BRNIFI**

What Shelley thought was the most difficult task to learn on her new computer.

40.

APPLYING WHAT YOU KNOW

41. Mrs. Lassiter's blood type is O positive. Her husband's type is O negative. Her newborn baby's blood type is O negative. Is there any need for concern with this combination?

42. After Mrs. Freund's baby was born, the doctor applied a gauze dressing for a short time on the umbilical cord. He also gave the baby a dose of vitamin K. Why did the doctor perform these two procedures?

43. WORD FIND

Can you find 24 terms from this chapter in the box of letters? Words may be spelled top to bottom, bottom to top, right to left, left to right, or diagonally.

```
H S H K L S U L O B M E A E S
K E E V M Z H E P A R I N D N
D T M F A C T O R Y E T I Q P
O Y A O H N B A T Q Y A R A R
N C T J G W E H N P N L B U D
O O O S Q L R M E T I S I P M
R K C E M O O N I H I Q F W W
H U R T C N I B P A S G Z T G
E E I Y O B O O I V E W E T X
S L T C M D S E C N R T U N R
U E Y O Y A I M E K U E L Y S
S T R G B S T H R O M B U S Q
E H Z A M S A L P N D Z P O N
T E N H F P D A P M E E I B W
E W B P H K B O N C K W X V J
```

AIDS	Factor	Phagocytes
Anemia	Fibrin	Plasma
Antibody	Hematocrit	Recipient
Antigen	Hemoglobin	Rhesus
Basophil	Heparin	Serum
Donor	Leukemia	Thrombin
Embolus	Leukocytes	Thrombus
Erythrocytes	Monocyte	Type

DID YOU KNOW?

In the second it takes to turn the page of a book, you will lose about 3 million red blood cells. During that same second, your bone marrow will have produced the same number of new ones.

There is enough iron in a human to make a small nail.

Each whole blood donation can help as many as three people. One unit is divided into three parts: red blood cells, platelets, and plasma.

Statistics show that 25% or more of us will require blood at least once in our lifetime.

BLOOD

Fill in the crossword puzzle.

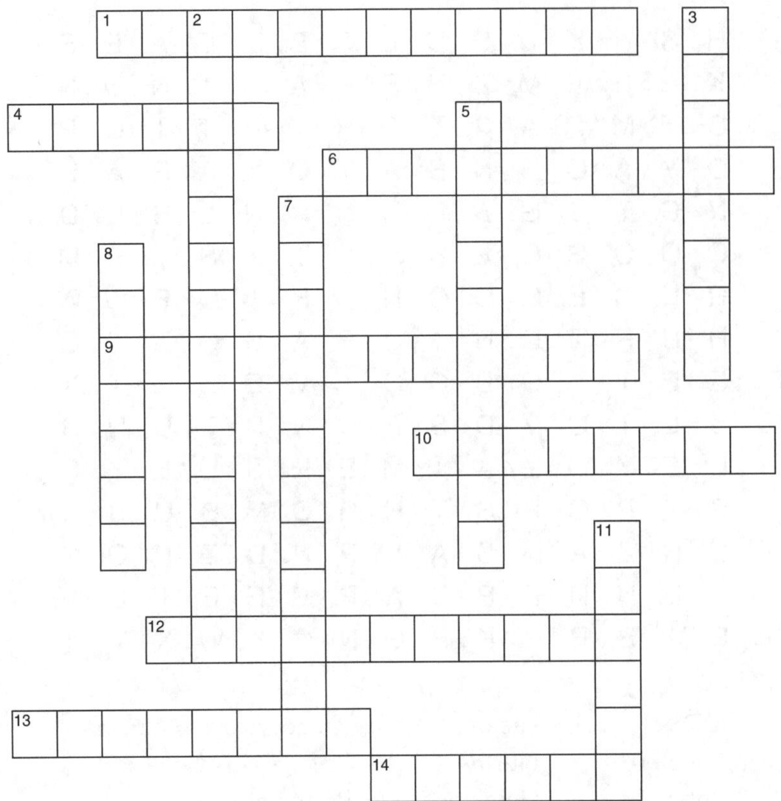

Across

1. Abnormally high WBC count
4. Final stage of clotting process
6. Oxygen-carrying mechanism of blood
9. To engulf and digest microbes
10. Stationary blood clot
12. RBC
13. Circulating blood clot
14. Liquid portion of blood

Down

2. Type O (two words)
3. Substances that stimulate the body to make antibodies
5. Type of leukocyte
7. Platelets
8. Prevents clotting of blood
11. Inability of the blood to carry sufficient oxygen

CHECK YOUR KNOWLEDGE

Multiple Choice

Select the best answer.

1. The two primary functions of blood are:
   A. Communication and integration of body functions
   B. Transportation and protection
   C. Elimination of wastes and regulation of body temperature
   D. Synthesis of chemicals and regulation of acid-base balance

2. Which of the following is *not* a formed element?
   A. Neutrophils
   B. Blood serum
   C. Platelets
   D. Erythrocytes

3. Which of the following is an agranulocyte?
   A. Macrophage
   B. Neutrophil
   C. Eosinophil
   D. Basophil

4. Without adequate __________ in the diet, the body cannot manufacture enough hemoglobin.
   A. Iron
   B. Calcium
   C. Sodium
   D. Vitamin C

5. All of the following are necessary for successful blood clotting *except*:
   A. Platelets
   B. Prothrombin
   C. Fibrin
   D. Heparin

6. The function of white blood cells is to:
   A. Defend the body from microorganisms invading the body
   B. Transport oxygen to the cells
   C. Play an essential part in blood clotting
   D. None of the above

7. A blood clot that is stationary and stays in the place where it formed is called a(n):
   A. Thrombus
   B. Embolus
   C. Anticoagulant
   D. Coumadin

8. An *antibody* may be defined as:
   A. A substance made by the body in response to stimulation by an antigen
   B. A substance that reacts with the antigen that stimulated its formation
   C. A substance that causes antigens to agglutinate
   D. All of the above

9. Which blood type is considered the *universal recipient*?
   A. A-negative
   B. B-positive
   C. AB-positive
   D. O-negative

10. Erythroblastosis fetalis is now avoidable by treating all Rh-negative mothers who carry an Rh-positive baby with a protein marketed as:
   A. Rhesus immune treatment
   B. RhoGAM
   C. PolyHeme
   D. None of the above

Matching

Select the most correct answer from column B for each statement in column A. (Only one answer is correct.)

Column A	Column B
_____ 11. Plasma	A. RBC volume
_____ 12. Erythrocytes	B. Abnormally high WBC count
_____ 13. Myeloid tissue	C. Allergy protection
_____ 14. Hematocrit	D. Liquid portion of blood
_____ 15. Buffy coat	E. Abnormally high RBC count
_____ 16. Eosinophils	F. No nuclei
_____ 17. Leukocytosis	G. WBCs and platelets
_____ 18. Polycythemia	H. Hematopoiesis
_____ 19. Leukopenia	I. Abnormally low WBC count
_____ 20. Agglutinate	J. Clump

HUMAN BLOOD CELLS

BODY CELL		FUNCTION

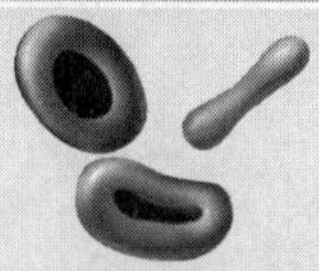

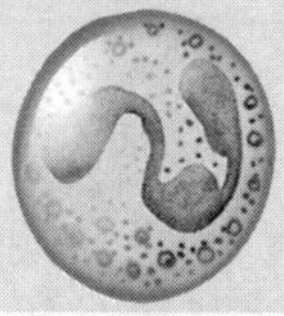

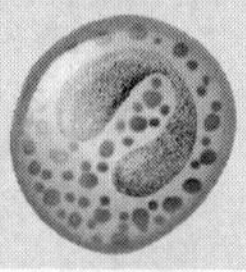

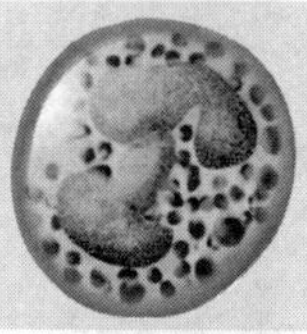

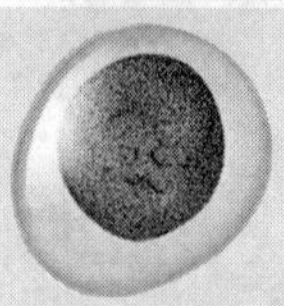

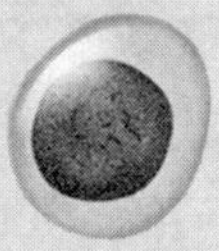

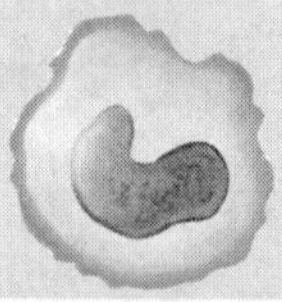

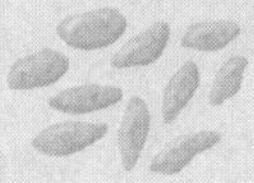

BLOOD TYPING

Using the key below, draw the appropriate reaction with the donor's blood in the circles.

Recipient's blood		*Reactions with donor's blood*			
RBC antigens	Plasma antibodies	Donor type O	Donor type A	Donor type B	Donor type AB
None (Type O)	Anti-A Anti-B				
A (Type A)	Anti-B				
B (Type B)	Anti-A				
AB (Type AB)	(none)				

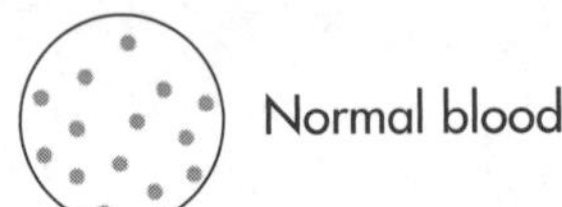

Normal blood

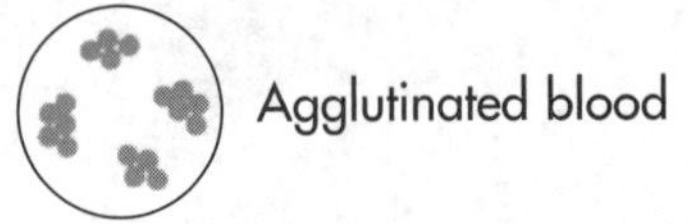

Agglutinated blood

CHAPTER 12

The Cardiovascular System

The heart is actually two pumps: one to move blood to the lungs, the other to push it out into the body. These two functions seem rather elementary in comparison to the complex and numerous functions performed by most of the other body organs, and yet, if either of these pumps stop, within a few short minutes all life ceases.

The heart is divided into two upper compartments, called *atria,* that serve as receiving chambers, and two lower compartments, called *ventricles,* that serve as discharging chambers. By the time a person reaches age 45, approximately 300,000 tons of blood will have passed through these chambers to be circulated to the blood vessels. These vessels—arteries, veins, and capillaries—serve different functions. Arteries carry blood from the heart, veins carry blood to the heart, and capillaries are exchange vessels or connecting links between the arteries and veins. This closed system of circulation provides distribution of blood to the whole body (systemic circulation) and to specific regions, such as pulmonary circulation or hepatic portal circulation.

Blood pressure is the force of blood in the vessels. This force is highest in arteries and lowest in veins. Normal blood pressure varies among individuals and depends on the volume of blood in the arteries. The larger the volume of blood in the arteries, the more pressure is exerted on the walls of the arteries, and the higher the arterial pressure. Conversely, the less blood in the arteries, the lower the blood pressure.

A functional cardiovascular system is vital for survival because, without circulation, tissues would lack a supply of oxygen and nutrients. Waste products would begin to accumulate and could become toxic. Your review of this system will provide you with an understanding of the complex transportation mechanism of the body that is necessary for survival.

TOPICS FOR REVIEW

Before progressing to Chapter 13 you should have an understanding of the structure and function of the heart and blood vessels. Your review should include a study of systemic, pulmonary, hepatic portal, and fetal circulations, and should conclude with a thorough understanding of blood pressure and pulse.

HEART

Fill in the blanks.

1. Rhythmic compression of the heart combined with effective artificial respiration is known as ____________________.

2. The ______________ ______________ divides the heart into right and left sides between the atria.
3. The ______________ are the two upper chambers of the heart.
4. The ______________ are the two lower chambers of the heart.
5. The cardiac muscle tissue is referred to as the ______________.
6. Inflammation of the heart lining is ______________.
7. The two AV valves are ______________ and ______________.
8. ______________ ______________ involves the movement of blood from the right ventricle to the lungs.
9. An occlusion of a coronary artery is known as a(n) ______________.
10. ______________ ______________ occurs when heart muscle cells are deprived of oxygen and become damaged or die.
11. The pacemaker of the heart is the ______________ node.
12. A normal ECG tracing has three characteristic waves. They are ______________, ______________, and ______________ waves.
13. ______________ begins just before the relaxation phase of cardiac muscle activity noted on an ECG.

Choose the correct term and write the letter in the space next to the appropriate definition below.

A. Pericardium
B. Severe chest pain
C. Thrombus
D. Pulmonary
E. Heart block
F. Ventricles
G. Systemic
H. Coronary arteries
I. Systole
J. Depolarization
K. Atria
L. Apex
M. Epicardium

_____ 14. Covering of heart
_____ 15. Receiving chambers
_____ 16. Circulation from left ventricle throughout body
_____ 17. Blood clot
_____ 18. Semilunar valve
_____ 19. Discharging chambers
_____ 20. Supplies oxygen to heart muscle
_____ 21. Angina pectoris
_____ 22. Slow heart rate caused by blocked impulses
_____ 23. Contraction of the heart
_____ 24. Electrical activity associated with ECG
_____ 25. Blunt-pointed lower edge of heart
_____ 26. Visceral pericardium

If you have had difficulty with this section, review pages 268-279.

BLOOD VESSELS—CIRCULATION

Matching

Match the term on the left with the proper selection on the right.

_____ 27. Arteries	A.	Smooth muscle cells that guard entrance to capillaries
_____ 28. Veins	B.	Carry blood to the heart
_____ 29. Capillaries	C.	Carry blood into venules
_____ 30. Tunica externa	D.	Carry blood away from the heart
_____ 31. Precapillary sphincters	E.	Largest vein
_____ 32. Superior vena cava	F.	Largest artery
_____ 33. Aorta	G.	Outermost layer of arteries and veins

Multiple Choice

Select the best answer.

34. The aorta carries blood out of the:
    A. Right atrium
    B. Left atrium
    C. Right ventricle
    D. Left ventricle
    E. None of the above

35. The superior vena cava returns blood to the:
    A. Left atrium
    B. Left ventricle
    C. Right atrium
    D. Right ventricle
    E. None of the above

36. Which one of the following vessel's walls are made up entirely of endothelial cells?
    A. Vein
    B. Capillary
    C. Artery
    D. Venule
    E. Arteriole

37. The _____________ is made up of smooth muscle.
    A. Tunica media
    B. Tunica adventitia
    C. Tunica intima
    D. Endothelium
    E. Myocardium

38. The _____________ function as exchange vessels.
    A. Venules
    B. Capillaries
    C. Arteries
    D. Arterioles
    E. Veins

39. Blood returns from the lungs during pulmonary circulation via the:
    A. Pulmonary artery
    B. Pulmonary veins
    C. Aorta
    D. Inferior vena cava

40. The hepatic portal circulation serves the body by:
    A. Removing excess glucose and storing it in the liver as glycogen
    B. Detoxifying blood
    C. Removing various poisonous substances present in blood
    D. All of the above

41. The structure used to bypass the liver in fetal circulation is the:
    A. Foramen ovale
    B. Ductus venosus
    C. Ductus arteriosus
    D. Umbilical vein

42. The foramen ovale serves the fetal circulation by:
    A. Connecting the aorta and the pulmonary artery
    B. Shunting blood from the right atrium directly into the left atrium
    C. Bypassing the liver
    D. Bypassing the lungs

43. The structure used to connect the aorta and pulmonary artery in fetal circulation is the:
    A. Ductus arteriosus
    B. Ductus venosus
    C. Aorta
    D. Foramen ovale

44. Which of the following is *not* an artery?
    A. Femoral
    B. Popliteal
    C. Coronary
    D. Inferior vena cava

45. Which of the following has valves to assist the blood flow?
    A. Veins
    B. Arteries
    C. Capillaries
    D. Arterioles

If you have had difficulty with this section, review pages 279-289.

BLOOD PRESSURE—PULSE

If the statement is true, write "T" in the answer blank. If the statement is false, correct the statement by circling the incorrect term and writing the correct term in the answer blank.

____________________ 46. Blood pressure is highest in the veins and lowest in the arteries.

____________________ 47. The difference between two blood pressures is referred to as blood pressure deficit.

____________________ 48. If the blood pressure in the arteries were to decrease so that it became equal to the average pressure in the arterioles, circulation would increase.

____________________ 49. A stroke is often the result of low blood pressure.

____________________ 50. Massive hemorrhage increases blood pressure.

____________________ 51. Blood pressure is the volume of blood in the vessels.

____________________ 52. Both the strength and the rate of heartbeat affect cardiac output and blood pressure.

____________________ 53. The diameter of the arterioles helps to determine how much blood drains out of arteries into arterioles.

____________________ 54. A stronger heartbeat tends to decrease blood pressure and a weaker heartbeat tends to increase it.

____________________ 55. The systolic pressure is the pressure while the ventricles relax.

____________________ 56. The diastolic pressure is the pressure while the ventricles contract.

____________________ 57. The pulse is a vein expanding and then recoiling.

____________________ 58. The radial artery is located at the wrist.

____________________ 59. The common carotid artery is located in the neck along the front edge of the sternocleidomastoid muscle.

____________________ 60. The artery located at the bend of the elbow and used for locating the pulse is the dorsalis pedis.

If you have had difficulty with this section, review pages 289-294.

UNSCRAMBLE THE WORDS

Take the circled letters, unscramble them, and fill in the statement.

61. **S T M E S Y C I**

62. **N U L V E E**

63. **R Y T R E A**

64. **U S L E P**

How Noah survived the flood.

65.

APPLYING WHAT YOU KNOW

66. Mr. Rainey was experiencing angina pectoris. His doctor suggested a surgical procedure that would require the removal of a vein from another region of his body. This vein would then be used to bypass a partial blockage in his coronary arteries. What is this procedure called?

67. Phil has heart block. His electrical impulses are being blocked from reaching the ventricles. An electrical device that causes ventricular contractions at a rate necessary to maintain circulation is being considered as possible treatment for his condition. What is this device called?

68. Mrs. Haygood was diagnosed with an acute case of endocarditis. What is the real danger of this diagnosis?

69. Dan returned from surgery in stable condition. The nurse noted that each time she took Dan's pulse and blood pressure, the pulse became higher and the blood pressure lower than the last time. What might be the cause?

70. WORD FIND

Can you find 15 terms from this chapter in the box of letters? Words may be spelled top to bottom, bottom to top, right to left, left to right, or diagonally.

```
Y H Y S I S O B M O R H T A R
L A C I L I B M U O A Y N I Y
E E S Y S T E M I C C G D E U
M V E N U L E D D C I X M D I
E Y M U I R T A R N L E C G Y
N O I T A Z I R A L O P E D N
U D L A T R O P C I T A P E H
S I U K M U E T O E S L U P U
R P N F Y C B E D R A L Z P J
D S A H T I T V N L I I B D W
Q U R O I V A Q E O D A K R K
K C R M P G A I G N D D Z Y J
Y I Y R I N E A F Z L Q S P X
S R M I C C Q O A W U N H O K
P T A V H H Z L H I J J X K Z
```

Angina pectoris	ECG	Systemic
Apex	Endocardium	Thrombosis
Atrium	Hepatic portal	Tricuspid
Depolarization	Pulse	Umbilical
Diastolic	Semilunar	Venule

DID YOU KNOW?

Your heart pumps more than 5 quarts of blood every minute or 2,000 gallons a day.

Every pound of excess fat contains some 200 miles of additional capillaries to push blood through each minute.

If laid out in a straight line, the average adult's circulatory system would be nearly 60,000 miles long—enough to circle the earth 2.5 times!

People who have an optimistic attitude as opposed to a pessimistic attitude suffer fewer strokes and heart attacks and have a 55% less chance of suffering cardiovascular diseases.

CARDIOVASCULAR SYSTEM

Fill in the crossword puzzle.

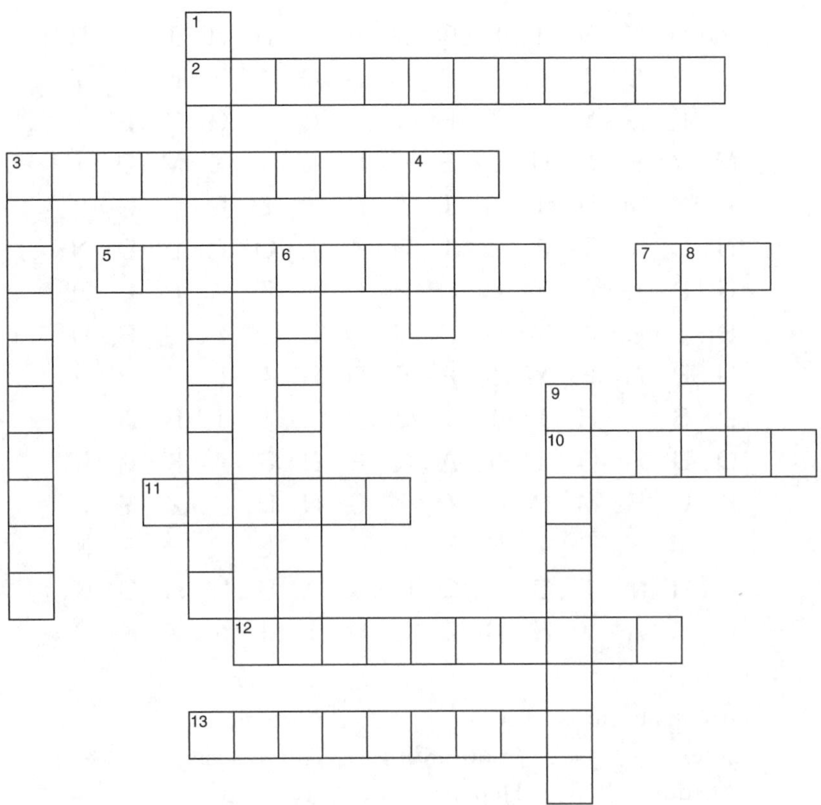

Across

2. Inflammation of the lining of the heart
3. Bicuspid valve (2 words)
5. Inner layer of pericardium
7. Cardiopulmonary resuscitation (abbreviation)
10. Carries blood away from the heart
11. Upper chamber of heart
12. Lower chambers of the heart
13. SA node

Down

1. Unique blood circulation through the liver (2 words)
3. Muscular layer of the heart
4. Carries blood to the heart
6. Tiny artery
8. Heart rate
9. Carries blood from arterioles into venules

CHECK YOUR KNOWLEDGE

Multiple Choice

Select the best answer.

1. Heart sounds are most easily heard by placing a stethoscope:
   A. Directly over the apex of the heart
   B. Over the space between the first and second ribs
   C. Over the upper portion of the mediastinum
   D. None of the above

2. The valve located between the right atrium and ventricle is the:
   A. Bicuspid
   B. Aortic semilunar valve
   C. Tricuspid
   D. Pulmonary semilunar valve

3. Blood rich in oxygen returns from the lungs and enters the left atrium of the heart through the:
   A. Aorta
   B. Pulmonary veins
   C. Superior vena cava
   D. Pulmonary artery

4. Heart block is often successfully treated by:
   A. Implanting an artificial pacemaker
   B. Coronary bypass surgery
   C. Angioplasty
   D. None of the above

5. The outermost layer of the arteries and veins is the:
   A. Tunica externa
   B. Tunica media
   C. Tunica intima
   D. Endothelium

6. An electrocardiogram or ECG:
   A. Is a graphic record of the heart's electrical activity
   B. Records damage to cardiac muscle tissue that affects the heart's conduction system
   C. Has three deflections known as the *P wave,* the *QRS complex,* and the *T wave*
   D. All of the above

7. The blood pressure gradient is:
   A. The pressure against the arteries during contraction
   B. The pressure against the arteries at rest
   C. Vitally involved in keeping the blood flowing
   D. The artery expanding and then recoiling alternately

8. A structure unique to fetal circulation is the:
   A. Ductus venosus
   B. Ductus arteriosus
   C. Foramen ovale
   D. All of the above

9. *Stroke volume* refers to the:
   A. Volume of blood pumped by one ventricle per minute
   B. Flow of blood into the cardiac veins
   C. Volume of blood ejected from the ventricles during each beat
   D. Flow of blood into the coronary sinus

10. A structural feature *not* present in arteries and unique to veins is:
    A. Tunica intima
    B. Tunica media
    C. One-way valves
    D. Tunica adventitia

Matching

Select the most correct answer from column B for each statement in column A. (Only one answer is correct.)

Column A	Column B
_____ 11. Atria	A. Right atrium
_____ 12. Endocardium	B. AV bundle
_____ 13. Pericardium	C. Discharging chambers
_____ 14. Superior vena cava	D. Radial artery
_____ 15. Aorta	E. Ventricles relaxed
_____ 16. Bundle of His	F. Receiving chambers
_____ 17. Ventricles	G. Lining of heart
_____ 18. Central venous pressure	H. Covering of heart
_____ 19. Pulse	I. Vein
_____ 20. Diastole	J. Artery

THE HEART

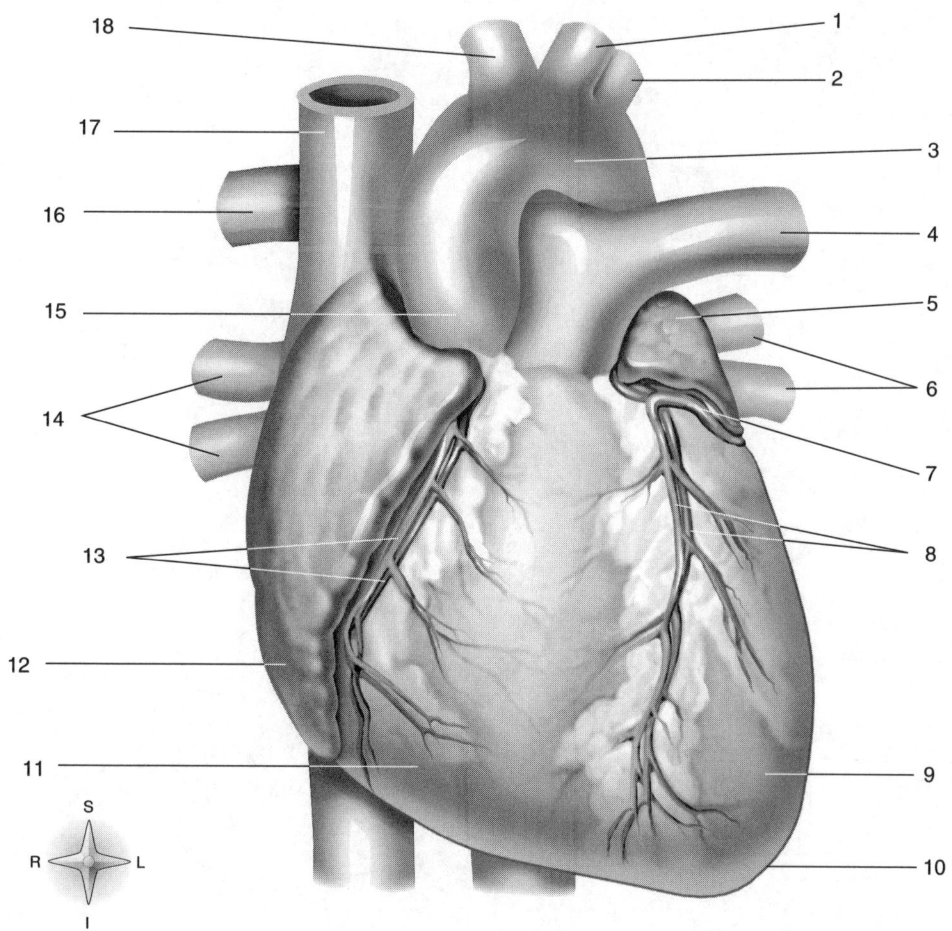

1. ______________________
2. ______________________
3. ______________________
4. ______________________
5. ______________________
6. ______________________
7. ______________________
8. ______________________
9. ______________________
10. ______________________
11. ______________________
12. ______________________
13. ______________________
14. ______________________
15. ______________________
16. ______________________
17. ______________________
18. ______________________

CONDUCTION SYSTEM OF THE HEART

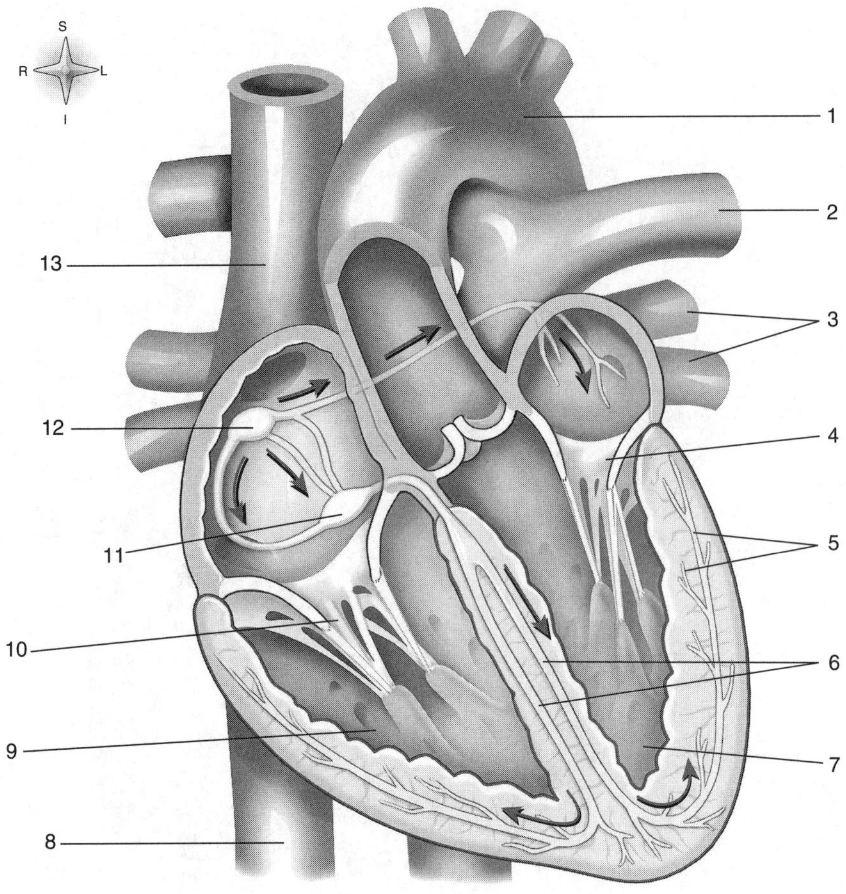

1. ______________________
2. ______________________
3. ______________________
4. ______________________
5. ______________________
6. ______________________
7. ______________________
8. ______________________
9. ______________________
10. ______________________
11. ______________________
12. ______________________
13. ______________________

FETAL CIRCULATION

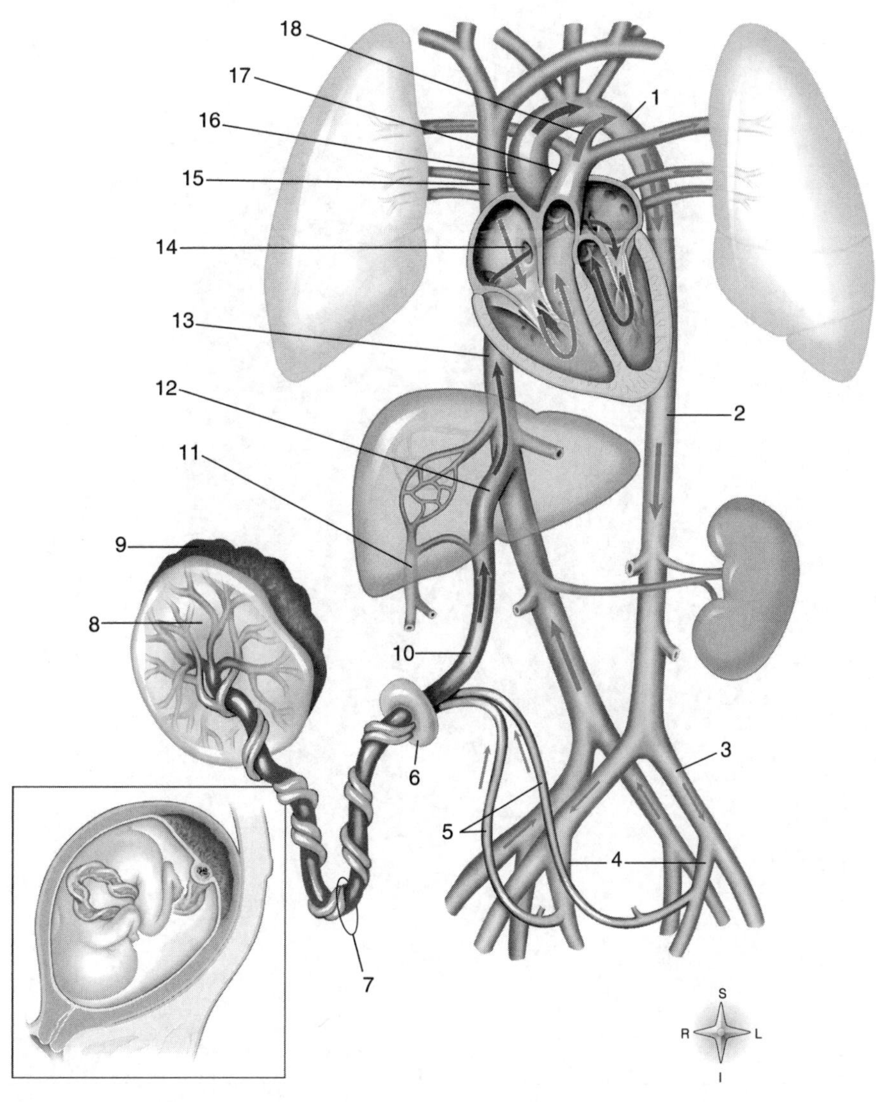

1. ______________________
2. ______________________
3. ______________________
4. ______________________
5. ______________________
6. ______________________
7. ______________________
8. ______________________
9. ______________________
10. ______________________
11. ______________________
12. ______________________
13. ______________________
14. ______________________
15. ______________________
16. ______________________
17. ______________________
18. ______________________

HEPATIC PORTAL CIRCULATION

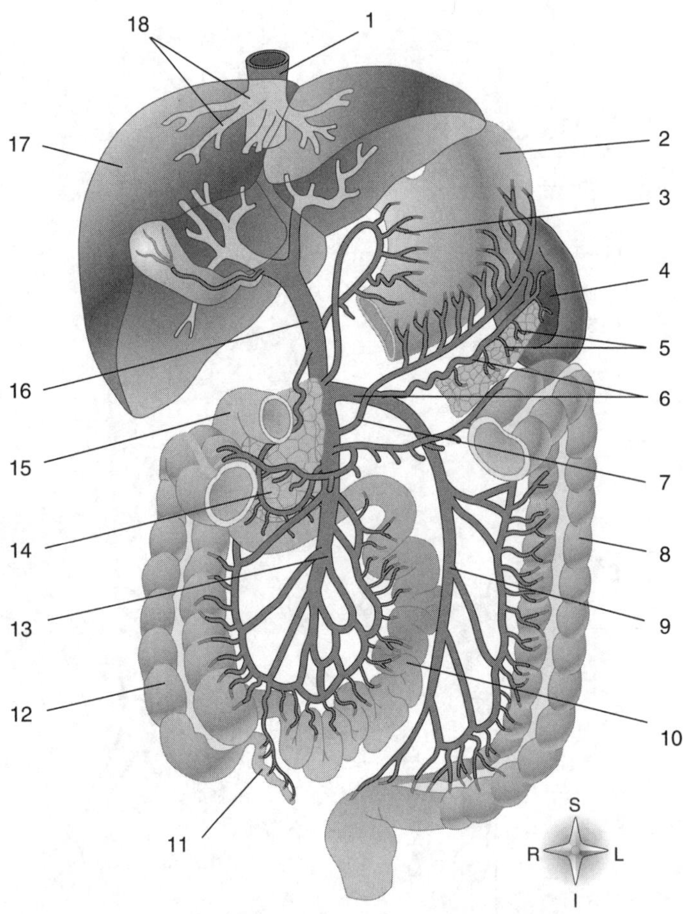

1. ______________________
2. ______________________
3. ______________________
4. ______________________
5. ______________________
6. ______________________
7. ______________________
8. ______________________
9. ______________________
10. ______________________
11. ______________________
12. ______________________
13. ______________________
14. ______________________
15. ______________________
16. ______________________
17. ______________________
18. ______________________

PRINCIPAL ARTERIES OF THE BODY

1. ______________________
2. ______________________
3. ______________________
4. ______________________
5. ______________________
6. ______________________
7. ______________________
8. ______________________
9. ______________________
10. ______________________
11. ______________________
12. ______________________
13. ______________________
14. ______________________
15. ______________________
16. ______________________
17. ______________________
18. ______________________
19. ______________________
20. ______________________
21. ______________________
22. ______________________
23. ______________________
24. ______________________
25. ______________________
26. ______________________
27. ______________________
28. ______________________
29. ______________________
30. ______________________

PRINCIPAL VEINS OF THE BODY

1. ______________________
2. ______________________
3. ______________________
4. ______________________
5. ______________________
6. ______________________
7. ______________________
8. ______________________
9. ______________________
10. ______________________
11. ______________________
12. ______________________
13. ______________________
14. ______________________
15. ______________________
16. ______________________
17. ______________________
18. ______________________
19. ______________________
20. ______________________
21. ______________________
22. ______________________
23. ______________________
24. ______________________
25. ______________________
26. ______________________
27. ______________________
28. ______________________
29. ______________________
30. ______________________
31. ______________________
32. ______________________
33. ______________________
34. ______________________
35. ______________________
36. ______________________
37. ______________________
38. ______________________

NORMAL ECG DEFLECTIONS

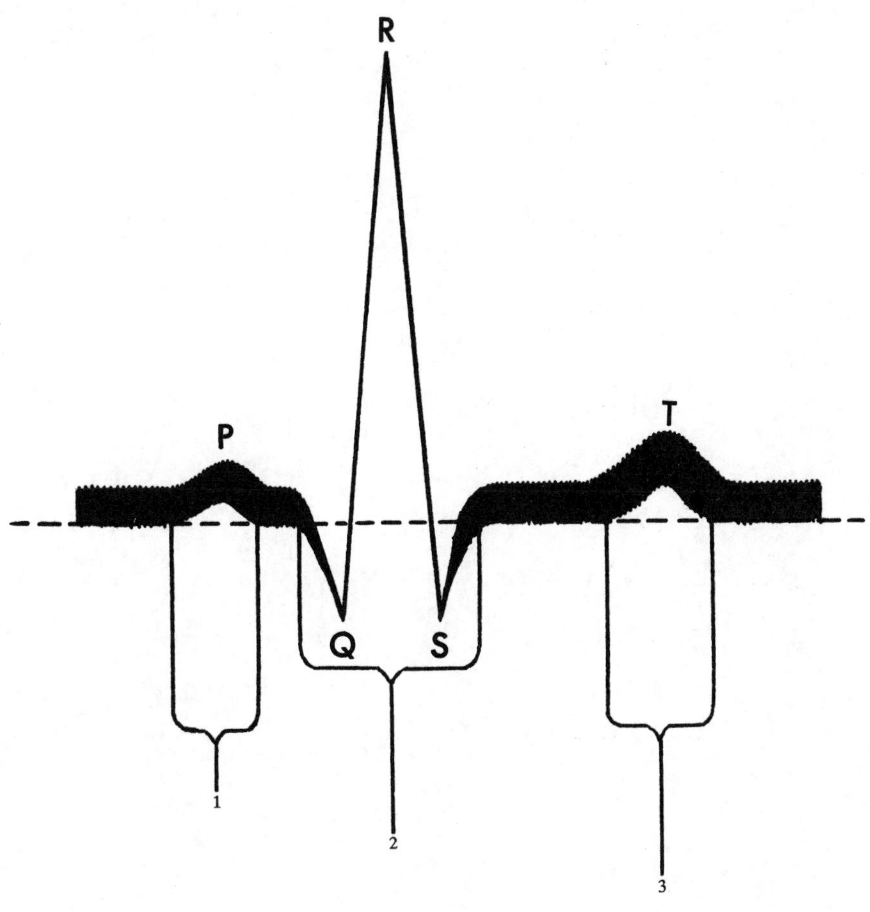

1. ______________________________
2. ______________________________
3. ______________________________

CHAPTER 13

The Lymphatic System and Immunity

The lymphatic system is similar to the circulatory system. Lymph, like blood, flows through an elaborate route of vessels. In addition to lymphatic vessels, the lymphatic system consists of lymph nodes, lymph, and the spleen. Unlike the circulatory system, the lymphatic vessels do not form a closed circuit. Lymph flows only once through the vessels before draining into the general blood circulation. This system is a filtering mechanism for microorganisms and serves as a protective device against foreign invaders, such as cancer.

The immune system is the armed forces division of the body. Ready to attack at a moment's notice, the immune system defends us against the major enemies of the body: microorganisms, foreign transplanted tissue cells, and our own cells that have turned malignant.

The most numerous cells of the immune system are the lymphocytes. These cells circulate in the body's fluids seeking invading organisms and destroying them with powerful lymphotoxins, lymphokines, or antibodies.

Phagocytes, another large group of immune system cells, assist with the destruction of foreign invaders by a process known as *phagocytosis*. Neutrophils, monocytes, and connective tissue cells called *macrophages* use this process to surround unwanted microorganisms, ingest and digest them, and render them harmless to the body.

Another weapon that the immune system possesses is complement. Normally a group of inactive enzymes present in the blood, complement can be activated to kill invading cells by drilling holes in their cytoplasmic membranes allowing fluid to enter the cell until it bursts.

Your review of this chapter will give you an understanding of how the body defends itself from the daily invasion of destructive substances.

TOPICS FOR REVIEW

Before progressing to Chapter 14 you should familiarize yourself with the functions of the lymphatic system, the immune system, and the major structures that make up these systems. Your review should include knowledge of lymphatic vessels, lymph nodes, lymph, antibodies, complement, and the development of B and T cells. Your study should conclude with an understanding of the differences in humoral and cell-mediated immunity.

THE LYMPHATIC SYSTEM

Fill in the blanks.

1. ____________________ is a fluid formed in the tissue spaces that will be transported by way of vessels to eventually reenter the circulatory system.

2. Blood plasma that has filtered out of capillaries into microscopic spaces between cells is called ______________ __________________.

3. The network of tiny blind-ended tubes distributed in the tissue spaces is called __________ __________.

4. Lymph eventually empties into two terminal vessels called the ___________ ____________ ______________ and the _____________ ________________.

5. The thoracic duct has an enlarged pouchlike structure called the ____________ ________________.

6. Lymph is filtered by moving through _____________ ________________, located in clusters along the pathway of lymphatic vessels.

7. Lymph enters the node through four ______________________ lymph vessels.

8. Lymph exits from the node through a single _______________ lymph vessel.

If you have had difficulty with this section, review pages 300-308.

THYMUS, TONSILS, SPLEEN

Select the correct term from the options given and write the letter in the answer blank.

(A) Thymus (B) Tonsils (C) Spleen

_____ 9. Palatine, pharyngeal, and lingual are examples
_____ 10. Largest lymphoid organ in the body
_____ 11. Destroys worn-out red blood cells
_____ 12. Located in the mediastinum
_____ 13. Serves as a reservoir for blood
_____ 14. T-lymphocytes
_____ 15. Largest at puberty

If you have had difficulty with this section, review pages 300-308.

THE IMMUNE SYSTEM

Match the term on the left with the proper selection on the right.

_____	16. Nonspecific immunity	A. Natural passive immunity
_____	17. Mother's milk	B. Injection of antibodies
_____	18. Specific immunity	C. General protection
_____	19. Artificial passive immunity	D. Artificial active exposure
_____	20. Immunization	E. Adaptive immunity

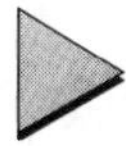
If you have had difficulty with this section, review pages 308-310.

IMMUNE SYSTEM MOLECULES

Choose the term that applies to each of the following descriptions. Write the letter for the term in the appropriate answer blank.

A. Antibodies	F. Complement cascade
B. Antigen	G. Complement
C. Allergy	H. Humoral immunity
D. Anaphylactic shock	I. Combining site
E. Monoclonal	J. hCG

_____ 21. Hypersensitivity of the immune system to harmless antigens

_____ 22. Life-threatening allergic reaction

_____ 23. Type of very specific antibodies produced from a population of identical cells

_____ 24. Protein compounds normally present in the body

_____ 25. Also known as *antibody-mediated immunity*

_____ 26. Combines with antibody to produce humoral immunity

_____ 27. Antibody

_____ 28. Process of changing molecule shape slightly to expose binding sites

_____ 29. Pregnancy test kits

_____ 30. Inactive proteins in blood

Circle the one that does not *belong.*

31. Antibody	Allergy	Protein compound	Combining site
32. Antigen	Invading cells	Foreign protein	Complement
33. Monoclonal	Antibodies	Antigen	Specific
34. Allergy	Complement	Anaphylactic shock	Antigen
35. Monoclonal	14	Complement	Proteins

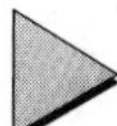
If you have had difficulty with this section, review pages 310-312.

IMMUNE SYSTEM CELLS

Multiple Choice

Select the best answer.

36. The most numerous cells of the immune system are the:
    A. Monocytes
    B. Eosinophils
    C. Neutrophils
    D. Lymphocytes
    E. Complement

37. Which of the terms listed below occurs third in the immune process?
    A. Plasma cells
    B. Stem cells
    C. Antibodies
    D. Activated B cells
    E. Inactive B cells

38. Which one of the terms listed below occurs last in the immune process?
    A. Plasma cells
    B. Stem cells
    C. Antibodies
    D. Activated B cells
    E. Inactive B cells

39. Moderate exercise has been found to:
    A. Decrease white blood cells
    B. Increase white blood cells
    C. Decrease platelets
    D. Decrease red blood cells

40. Which one of the following is part of the cell membrane of B cells?
    A. Complement
    B. Antigens
    C. Antibodies
    D. Epitopes
    E. None of the above

41. Immature B cells have:
    A. Four types of defense mechanisms on their cell membrane
    B. Several kinds of defense mechanisms on their cell membrane
    C. One specific kind of defense mechanism on their cell membrane
    D. No defense mechanisms on their cell membrane

42. Activation of a B cell depends on the B cell coming in contact with:
    A. Complement
    B. Antibodies
    C. Lymphotoxins
    D. Lymphokines
    E. Antigens

43. The kind of cell that produces large numbers of antibodies is the:
    A. B cell
    B. Stem cell
    C. T cell
    D. Memory cell
    E. Plasma cell

44. Just one of these short-lived cells that make antibodies can produce ______________ of them per second.
    A. 20
    B. 200
    C. 2,000
    D. 20,000

45. Which of the following statements is *not* true of memory cells?
    A. They produce large numbers of antibodies.
    B. They are found in lymph nodes.
    C. They develop into plasma cells.
    D. They can react with antigens.
    E. All of the above are true of memory cells.

46. T cell development begins in the:
    A. Lymph nodes
    B. Liver
    C. Pancreas
    D. Spleen
    E. Thymus

47. Human immunodeficiency virus (HIV) has its most obvious effects in:
    A. B cells
    B. Stem cells
    C. Plasma cells
    D. T cells

48. Interferon:
    A. Is produced by T cells within hours after infection by a virus
    B. Decreases the severity of many virus-related diseases
    C. Shows promise as an anticancer agent
    D. Has been shown to be effective in treating breast cancer
    E. All of the above

49. B cells function indirectly to produce:
    A. Humoral immunity
    B. Cell-mediated immunity
    C. Lymphotoxins
    D. Lymphokines

50. T cells function to produce:
    A. Humoral immunity
    B. Cell-mediated immunity
    C. Antibodies
    D. Memory cells

Fill in the blanks.

51. All lymphocytes that circulate in the tissues arise from primitive cells in the bone marrow called ____________ ____________.

52. The first stage of B cell development—transformation of stem cells into immature B cells—occurs in the ________ and the ________ ________ before birth but only in the ________ ________ in adults.

53. ____________ ____________ secrete copious amounts of antibody into the blood—nearly 2,000 antibody molecules for every second they live.

54. T cells are lymphocytes that have undergone their first stage of development in the ____________ ____________.

55. ________________ blocks HIV's ability to reproduce within infected cells.

56. ________________ is a disease caused by a retrovirus that enters the bloodstream and integrates into the DNA of T cell lymphocytes.

57. Like many viruses such as the common cold, HIV changes rapidly so the development of a ________________ may not occur for several years.

If you have had difficulty with this section, review pages 312-319.

UNSCRAMBLE THE WORDS

Take the circled letters, unscramble them, and fill in the statement.

58. **N T C M P E O L E M**

☐☐◯◯☐◯☐☐

59. **M T M Y I U N I**

☐◯☐☐☐☐◯

60. **O E N C L S**

◯◯☐☐☐◯

61. **F N R O E R T E N I**

☐☐☐☐◯☐◯☐◯

What the student was praying for the night before exams.

62.

☐☐☐☐☐☐ ☐☐☐☐☐

APPLYING WHAT YOU KNOW

63. Two-year old baby Metcalfe was exposed to chickenpox. He had been a particularly sickly child and so the doctor decided to give him a dose of interferon. What effect was the physician hoping for in baby Metcalfe's case?

64. Marcia was an intravenous drug user. She was recently diagnosed with Kaposi's sarcoma. What is another possible diagnosis?

65. Baby Phelps was born without a thymus gland. Immediate plans were made for a transplant to be performed. In the meantime, baby Phelps was placed in strict isolation. Why was this done?

66. WORD FIND

Can you find 14 terms from the chapter in the box of letters? Words may be spelled top to bottom, bottom to top, right to left, left to right, or diagonally.

```
I N F L A M M A T O R Y F C G
Q N L O Y Z O C C P A O F S X
M W T A A M N J X Q K R N P H
U R L E R M P X B R U I A L C
C M A C R O P H A G E I E D Z
X M N D K F M N O T U C R N M
A E O R E Z E U O C F B Y E B
Y P L E B G G R H T Y T S E D
Y S C R I S P J O E I T M L A
Z M O T J X E T O N A E E P X
T O N S I L S S U M Y H T S Y
W A O C J N I M W K O Z E N D
D W M K W R M O I P S H Y B G
F H W U J I Z F V D Z L Y T X
```

Acquired	Interferon	Proteins
Antigen	Lymph	Spleen
Humoral	Lymphocytes	Thymus
Immunity	Macrophage	Tonsils
Inflammatory	Monoclonal	

DID YOU KNOW?

There are more living organisms on the skin of a single human being than there are human beings on the surface of the earth.

According to the Centers for Disease Control (CDC), 18 million courses of antibiotics are prescribed for the common cold in the United States per year. Research shows that colds are caused by viruses. Fifty million unnecessary antibiotics are prescribed for viral respiratory infections.

The lymphatic system returns approximately 3.17 quarts (3 liters) of fluid each day from the tissues to the circulatory system.

LYMPH AND IMMUNITY

Fill in the crossword puzzle.

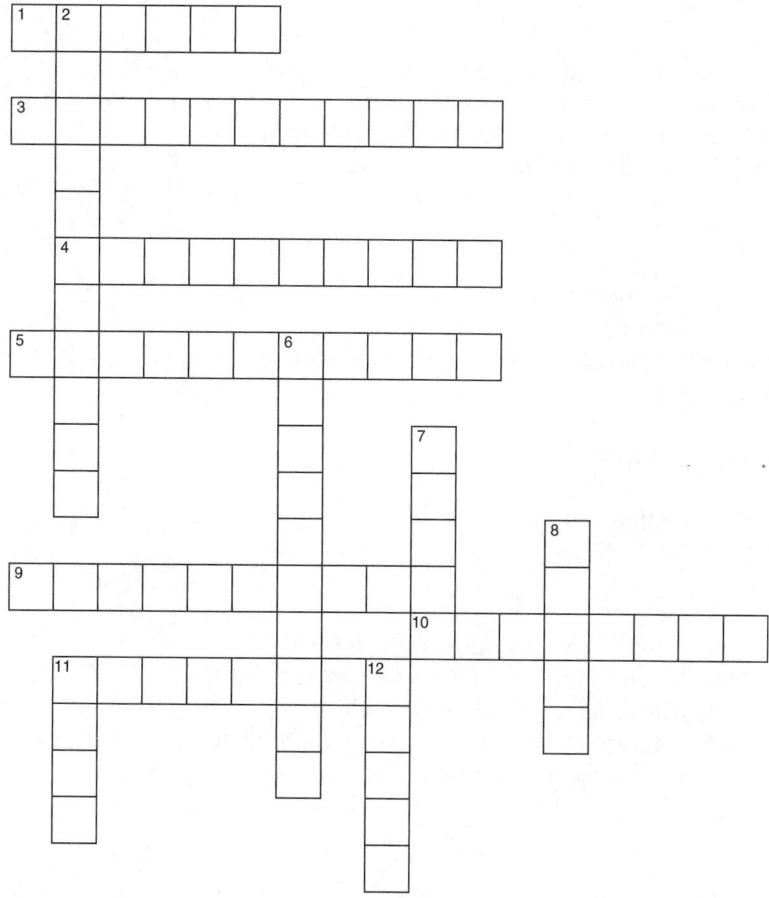

Across

1. Largest lymphoid organ in the body
3. Connective tissue cells that are phagocytes
4. Protein compounds normally present in the body
5. Remain in reserve then turn into plasma cells when needed (2 words)
9. Synthetically produced to fight certain diseases
10. Lymph exits the node through this lymph vessel
11. Lymph enters the node through these lymph vessels

Down

2. Secretes a copious amount of antibodies into the blood (2 words)
6. Inactive proteins
7. Family of identical cells descended from one cell
8. Type of lymphocyte (humoral immunity—2 words)
11. Immune deficiency disorder
12. Type of lymphocyte (cell-mediated immunity—2 words)

CHECK YOUR KNOWLEDGE

Multiple Choice

Select the best answer.

1. Which of the following is true about both lymphatic and blood capillaries?
   A. Both types of vessels are microscopic and are formed from sheets of endothelium.
   B. The movement and route of blood and lymph are identical.
   C. Both lymph and blood terminate into the same veins.
   D. All of the above are true.

2. The spleen
   A. Is the largest lymphoid organ in the body
   B. Has a limited blood supply
   C. Is located in the upper right quadrant of the abdomen lateral to the stomach
   D. All of the above

3. Lymph nodes are responsible for:
   A. Defense
   B. White blood cell formation
   C. Biological filtration
   D. All of the above

4. Which of the following is *not* true regarding lymph vessels?
   A. Lymph enters the node through four afferent lymph vessels.
   B. Lymph exits the node through four efferent vessels.
   C. Once lymph enters the node, it "percolates" slowly through spaces called *sinuses*.
   D. Lymph from the breast drains into many different and widely placed nodes.

5. The thymus is:
   A. Largest at puberty
   B. A source of lymphocytes before birth
   C. Replaced by a process called *involution*
   D. All of the above

6. Which of the following is *not* an example of tonsils?
   A. Palatine
   B. Humoral
   C. Pharyngeal
   D. Lingual

7. Active immunity occurs when:
   A. Immunity to a disease that has developed in another individual is transferred to someone not previously immune
   B. An infant receives antibodies in her mother's milk
   C. Immunity is inherited
   D. A vaccination confers immunity

8. The function of T cells is to:
   A. Produce cell-mediated immunity
   B. Kill infected cells by releasing a substance that poisons cells
   C. Release chemicals that attract and activate macrophages to kill cells by phagocytosis
   D. All of the above

9. Which of the following is an example of nonspecific immunity?
   A. Skin
   B. Tears and mucus
   C. Inflammation
   D. All of the above

10. In general, antibodies produce __________ immunity.
    A. Complement
    B. Phagocytic
    C. Humoral
    D. Inherited

Matching

Select the most correct answer from column B for each statement in column A. (Only one answer is correct.)

Column A	Column B
_____ 11. Lymph vessel	A. Humoral
_____ 12. Thymus	B. Allergy
_____ 13. Nonspecific immunity	C. Interferon
_____ 14. Specific immunity	D. T-cells
_____ 15. Protein compounds in the body	E. Efferent
_____ 16. Antigen hypersensitivity	F. Macrophages
_____ 17. Antibody-mediated immunity	G. Antibodies
_____ 18. Monoclonal antibodies	H. Adaptive immunity
_____ 19. Synthetic treatment for viral infections	I. Phagocytosis
_____ 20. Act as antigen-presenting cells (APCs)	J. Pregnancy test kits

PRINCIPAL ORGANS OF THE LYMPHATIC SYSTEM

1. ______________________________
2. ______________________________
3. ______________________________
4. ______________________________
5. ______________________________
6. ______________________________
7. ______________________________
8. ______________________________
9. ______________________________
10. ______________________________
11. ______________________________
12. ______________________________
13. ______________________________

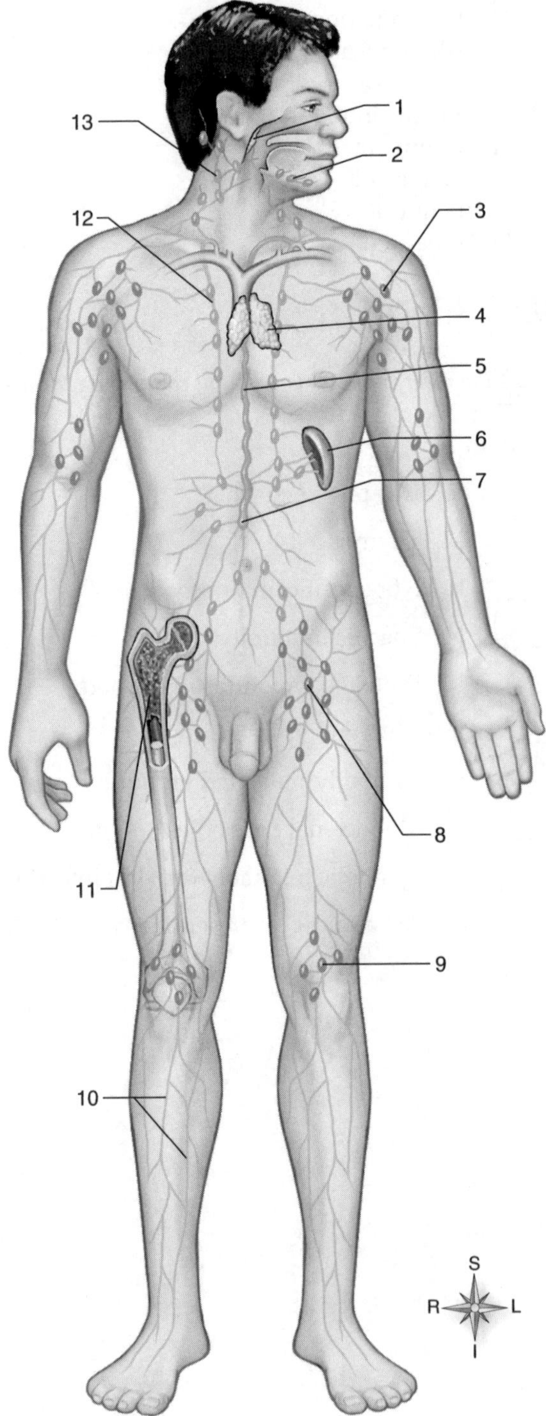

CHAPTER 14

The Respiratory System

As you sit reviewing this system, your body needs 16 quarts of air per minute. Walking requires 24 quarts of air per minute, and running requires 50 quarts per minute. The respiratory system provides the air necessary for you to perform your daily activities and eliminates the waste gases from the air that you breathe. Take a deep breath, and think of the air as entering some 250 million tiny air sacs similar in appearance to clusters of grapes. These microscopic air sacs expand to let air in and contract to force it out. These tiny sacs, alveoli, are the functioning units of the respiratory system. They provide the necessary volume of oxygen and eliminate carbon dioxide 24 hours a day.

Air enters either through the mouth or the nasal cavity. It next passes through the pharynx and past the epiglottis, then through the glottis and the rest of the larynx. It then continues down the trachea, into the bronchi to the bronchioles, and finally through the alveoli. The reverse occurs for expelled air.

The exchange of gases between air in the lungs and in the blood is known as *external respiration*. The exchange of gases that occurs between the blood and the cells of the body is known as *internal respiration*. By constantly supplying adequate oxygen and by removing carbon dioxide as it forms, the respiratory system helps to maintain an environment conducive to maximum cell efficiency.

Your review of this system is necessary to provide you with an understanding of this essential homeostatic mechanism.

TOPICS FOR REVIEW

Before progressing to Chapter 15, you should have an understanding of the structure and function of the organs of the respiratory system. Your review should include knowledge of the mechanisms responsible for both internal and external respiration. Your study should conclude with knowledge of the volumes of air exchanged in pulmonary ventilation and an understanding of how respiration is regulated.

STRUCTURAL PLAN
RESPIRATORY TRACTS
RESPIRATORY MUCOSA

Match the term with the definition.

A. Diffusion
B. Sinuses
C. Alveoli
D. URI
E. Respiration
F. Respiratory mucosa
G. Upper respiratory tract
H. Lower respiratory tract
I. Cilia
J. Air distributor

_____ 1. Function of respiratory system

_____ 2. Pharynx

_____ 3. Passive transport process responsible for actual exchange of gases

_____ 4. Assists with the movement of mucus towards the pharynx

_____ 5. Make olfaction possible

_____ 6. Lines the tubes of the respiratory tree

_____ 7. Terminal air sacs

_____ 8. Trachea

_____ 9. Head cold

_____ 10. Homeostatic mechanism

Fill in the blanks.

The organs of the respiratory system are designed to perform two basic functions. They serve as a(n): (11)__________ __________ and as a(n) (12) __________ __________. In addition to the above, the respiratory system (13) __________, (14) __________, and (15) __________ the air we breathe. Respiratory organs include the (16) __________, (17) __________, (18) __________, (19) __________, (20) __________, and the (21) __________. The respiratory system ends in millions of tiny, thin-walled sacs called (22) __________. (23) __________ of gases takes place in these sacs. Finally, (24)__________ __________ lines most of the air distribution tubes of the respiratory system. This membrane is covered by pseudostratified columnar epithelium rich in mucus-producing (25)__________ cells.

If you have had difficulty with this section, review pages 325-328.

NOSE, PHARYNX, LARYNX

Circle the one that does not *belong.*

26. Nares	Septum	Oropharynx	Conchae
27. Conchae	Frontal	Maxillary	Sphenoidal
28. Oropharynx	Throat	5 inches	Epiglottis
29. Pharyngeal	Adenoids	Uvula	Nasopharynx
30. Middle ear	Tubes	Nasopharynx	Larynx
31. Voice box	Thyroid cartilage	Pharyngeal	Vocal cords
32. Palatine	Eustachian tube	Tonsils	Oropharynx
33. Pharynx	Epiglottis	Adam's apple	Voice box

Choose the correct term from the options given and write the letter in the answer blank.

(A) Nose (B) Pharynx (C) Larynx

_____ 34. Warms and humidifies air

_____ 35. Air and food pass through here

_____ 36. Sinuses

_____ 37. Conchae

_____ 38. Septum

_____ 39. Tonsils

_____ 40. Middle ear infections

_____ 41. Epiglottis

If you have had difficulty with this section, review pages 328-331.

TRACHEA, BRONCHI, BRONCHIOLES, ALVEOLI, LUNGS, AND PLEURA

Fill in the blanks.

42. The windpipe is more properly referred to as the _______________.

43. _______________ keeps the framework of the trachea almost noncollapsible.

44. _______________ is a major cause of death in the U.S. and includes choking on food and other substances caught in the trachea.

45. The first branch or division of the trachea leading to the lungs is the _____________ _______________.

46. Each alveolar duct ends in several _____________ ___________.

47. The narrow part of each lung, up under the collarbone, is its _______________.

48. The _______________ covers the outer surface of the lungs and lines the inner surface of the rib cage.

49. Inflammation of the lining of the thoracic cavity is _______________.

50. The presence of air in the intrapleural space on one side of the chest is a(n) _______________.

If you have had difficulty with this section, review pages 331-336.

RESPIRATION

True or False

If the statement is true, write "T" in the answer blank. If the statement is false, correct the statement by circling the incorrect term and writing the correct term in the answer blank.

_______________ 51. Diffusion is the process that moves air into and out of the lungs.

_______________ 52. For inspiration to take place, the diaphragm and other respiratory muscles relax.

_______________ 53. Diffusion is a passive process that results in movement up a concentration gradient.

_______________ 54. The exchange of gases that occurs between blood in systemic capillaries and the body cells is external respiration.

_______________ 55. Many pulmonary volumes can be measured as a person breathes into a spirometer.

_______________ 56. Ordinarily we take about 2 pints of air into our lungs.

_______________ 57. The amount of air normally breathed in and out with each breath is called tidal volume.

_______________ 58. The largest amount of air that one can breathe out in one expiration is called residual volume.

_______________ 59. The inspiratory reserve volume is the amount of air that can be forcibly inhaled after a normal inspiration.

If you have had difficulty with this section, review pages 336-343.

Multiple Choice

Select the best answer.

60. The term that means the same thing as breathing is:
    A. Gas exchange
    B. Respiration
    C. Inspiration
    D. Expiration
    E. Pulmonary ventilation

61. Carbaminohemoglobin is formed when _______________ binds to hemoglobin.
    A. Oxygen
    B. Amino acids
    C. Carbon dioxide
    D. Nitrogen
    E. None of the above

62. Most of the oxygen transported by the blood is:
    A. Dissolved in white blood cells
    B. Bound to white blood cells
    C. Bound to hemoglobin
    D. Bound to carbaminohemoglobin
    E. None of the above

63. Which of the following would *not* assist inspiration?
    A. Elevation of the ribs
    B. Elevation of the diaphragm
    C. Contraction of the diaphragm
    D. Chest cavity becomes longer from top to bottom

64. A young adult male would have a vital capacity of about ___________ ml.
    A. 500
    B. 1200
    C. 3300
    D. 4800
    E. 6200

65. The amount of air that can be forcibly exhaled after expiring the tidal volume is known as the:
    A. Total lung capacity
    B. Vital capacity
    C. Inspiratory reserve volume
    D. Expiratory reserve volume
    E. None of the above

66. Which one of the following is correct?
    A. VC = TV – IRV + ERV
    B. VC = TV + IRV – ERV
    C. VC = TV + IRV x ERV
    D. VC = TV + IRV + ERV
    E. None of the above

If you have had difficulty with this section, review pages 336-343.

REGULATION OF RESPIRATION
RECEPTORS INFLUENCING RESPIRATION
TYPES OF BREATHING

Match the term on the left with the proper selection on the right.

_____	67. Respiratory control centers	A. Difficult breathing
_____	68. Chemoreceptors	B. Located in carotid bodies
_____	69. Pulmonary stretch receptors	C. Slow and shallow respirations
_____	70. Dyspnea	D. Normal respiratory rate
_____	71. Respiratory arrest	E. Located in the medulla
_____	72. Eupnea	F. Failure to resume breathing following a period of apnea
_____	73. Hypoventilation	G. Located throughout pulmonary airways and in the alveoli

If you have had difficulty with this section, review pages 342-345.

UNSCRAMBLE THE WORDS

Take the circled letters, unscramble them, and fill in the statement.

74. **SPUELIRY**

75. **CRNBOSITHI**

76. **SESXPTIAI**

77. **DDNEAOIS**

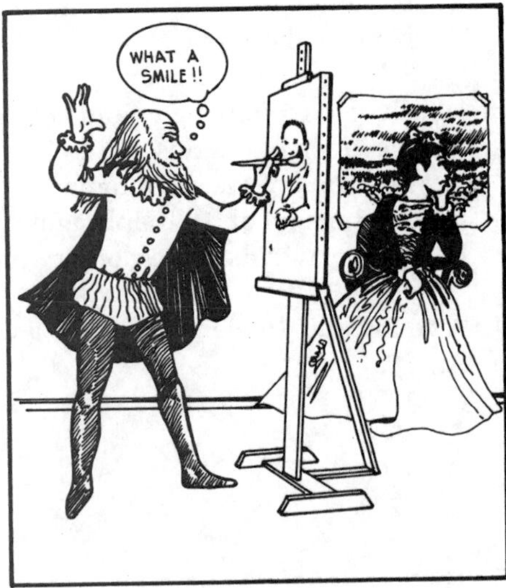

What Mona Lisa was to DaVinci.

78.

APPLYING WHAT YOU KNOW

79. Mr. Gorski is a heavy smoker. Recently he has noticed that when he gets up in the morning, he has a bothersome cough that brings up a large accumulation of mucus. This cough persists for several minutes and then leaves until the next morning. What is an explanation for this problem?

80. Michaela is 5 years old and is a mouth breather. She has had repeated episodes of tonsillitis and the pediatrician has suggested removal of her tonsils and adenoids. He has further suggested that the surgery would probably cure her mouth-breathing problem. Why is this a possibility?

81. WORD FIND

Can you find 14 terms from this chapter in the box of letters? Words may be spelled top to bottom, bottom to top, right to left, left to right, or diagonally.

```
N K S A Q B I L V A D T I X D
O X O O B F I F G I M N R G Y
I G N X W D E E F L B A U T S
T B K Y N H E F O I U T I R P
A T M H E O U T R C C C P V N
L L A E P S I R I Z A A N F E
I P T M I H G T I P R F P C A
T U B O G Q E V A Q O R V N W
N L N G L R J C C R T U P D C
E M U L O V L A U D I S E R E
V O V O T A N G J E D P Z U U
O N K B T C N U U E B O S J S
P A L I I K E U C N O Z K N A
Y R V N S D I O N E D A M F I
H Y O M L O A Z D T Y M N L K
```

Adenoids	Epiglottis	Residual volume
Carotid body	Hypoventilation	Surfactant
Cilia	Inspiration	URI
Diffusion	Oxyhemoglobin	Vital capacity
Dyspnea	Pulmonary	

DID YOU KNOW?

If the alveoli in our lungs were flattened out they would cover a half of a tennis court.

Sinusitis affects 37 million Americans causing difficulty in breathing and chronic headaches.

A person's nose and ears continue to grow throughout his or her life.

Approximately a half a liter of water per day is lost through breathing.

RESPIRATORY SYSTEM

Fill in the crossword puzzle.

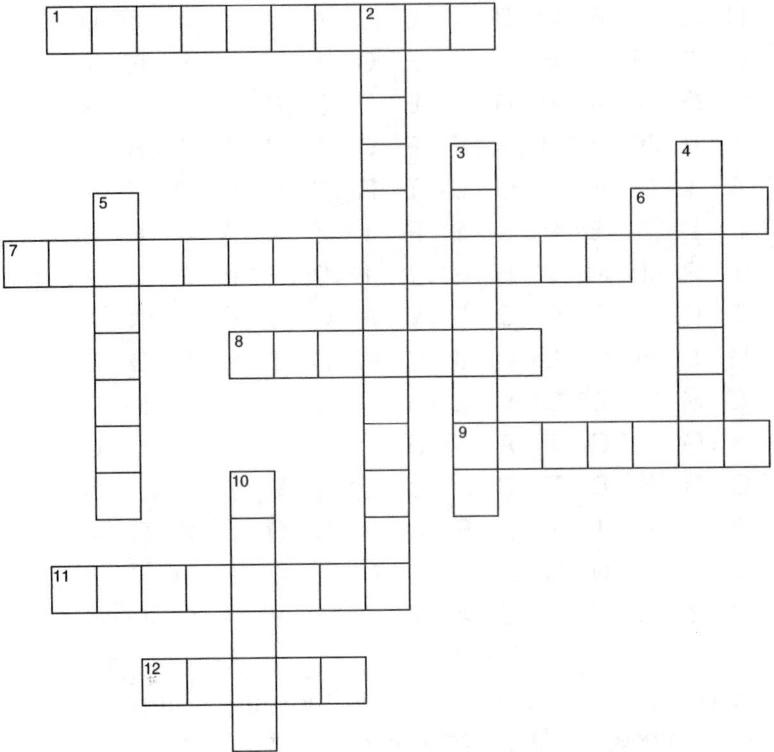

Across

1. Device used to measure the amount of air exchanged in breathing
6. Expiratory reserve volume (abbreviation)
7. Sphenoidal (two words)
8. Terminal air sacs
9. Shelf-like structures that protrude into the nasal cavity
11. Inflammation of pleura
12. Respirations stop

Down

2. Surgical procedure to remove tonsils
3. Doctor who developed lifesaving technique
4. Windpipe
5. Trachea branches into right and left structures
10. Voice box

CHECK YOUR KNOWLEDGE

Multiple Choice

Select the best answer.

1. The exchange of gases between the air and blood is made possible by the process of:
   A. Diffusion
   B. Osmosis
   C. Filtration
   D. Pinocytosis

2. Which of the following is *not* a paranasal sinus?
   A. Frontal
   B. Temporal
   C. Maxillary
   D. Sphenoidal

3. The respiratory system serves the body as a(n):
   A. Air distributor
   B. Gas exchanger
   C. Important homeostatic mechanism
   D. All of the above

4. Select the correct pathway that air takes on the way to the lungs.
   A. Primary bronchi, secondary bronchi, alveolar sacs, alveolar ducts
   B. Primary bronchi, secondary bronchi, alveolar sacs, alveoli
   C. Primary bronchi, bronchioles, secondary bronchi, alveolar ducts
   D. Bronchioles, primary bronchi, secondary bronchi, alveoli

5. During expiration:
   A. The thoracic cavity decreases in size
   B. The lungs expand
   C. The diaphragm flattens out and contracts
   D. All of the above

6. The pleura:
   A. Covers the outer surface of the lungs and lines the inner surface of the rib cage
   B. Is an extensive, thin, moist, slippery membrane
   C. Is made up of two membranes known as the *parietal pleura* and *visceral pleura*
   D. All of the above

7. The exchange of gases that occurs between blood in tissue capillaries and the body cells is called:
   A. Internal respiration
   B. External respiration
   C. Vital capacity
   D. Inspiratory reserve volume

8. Residual volume is the:
   A. Amount of air that can be forcibly inspired over and above a normal inspiration
   B. Amount of air that can be forcibly exhaled after expiring the tidal volume
   C. Air that remains in the lungs after the most forceful expiration
   D. Largest amount of air that we can breathe out in one expiration

9. *Eupnea* is a term used to describe:
   A. Labored breathing
   B. A temporary stop in breathing
   C. Rapid respirations
   D. A normal respiratory rate

10. The respiratory control centers are located in the:
   A. Cerebrum
   B. Medulla and pons of the brain
   C. Cerebellum
   D. Thalamus

Matching

Select the most correct answer from column B for each statement in column A. (Only one answer is correct.)

Column A	Column B
_____ 11. URI	A. Nostrils
_____ 12. Lower respiratory tract	B. Used to measure air exchange
_____ 13. External nares	C. Carotid and aortic bodies
_____ 14. Voice box	D. C-rings of cartilage
_____ 15. Trachea	E. Head cold
_____ 16. Spirometer	F. Slow, shallow respirations
_____ 17. Chemoreceptors	G. Larynx
_____ 18. Apnea	H. Respiratory arrest
_____ 19. Hypoventilation	I. Chest cold
_____ 20. Apex	J. Lung

SAGITTAL VIEW OF HEAD AND NECK

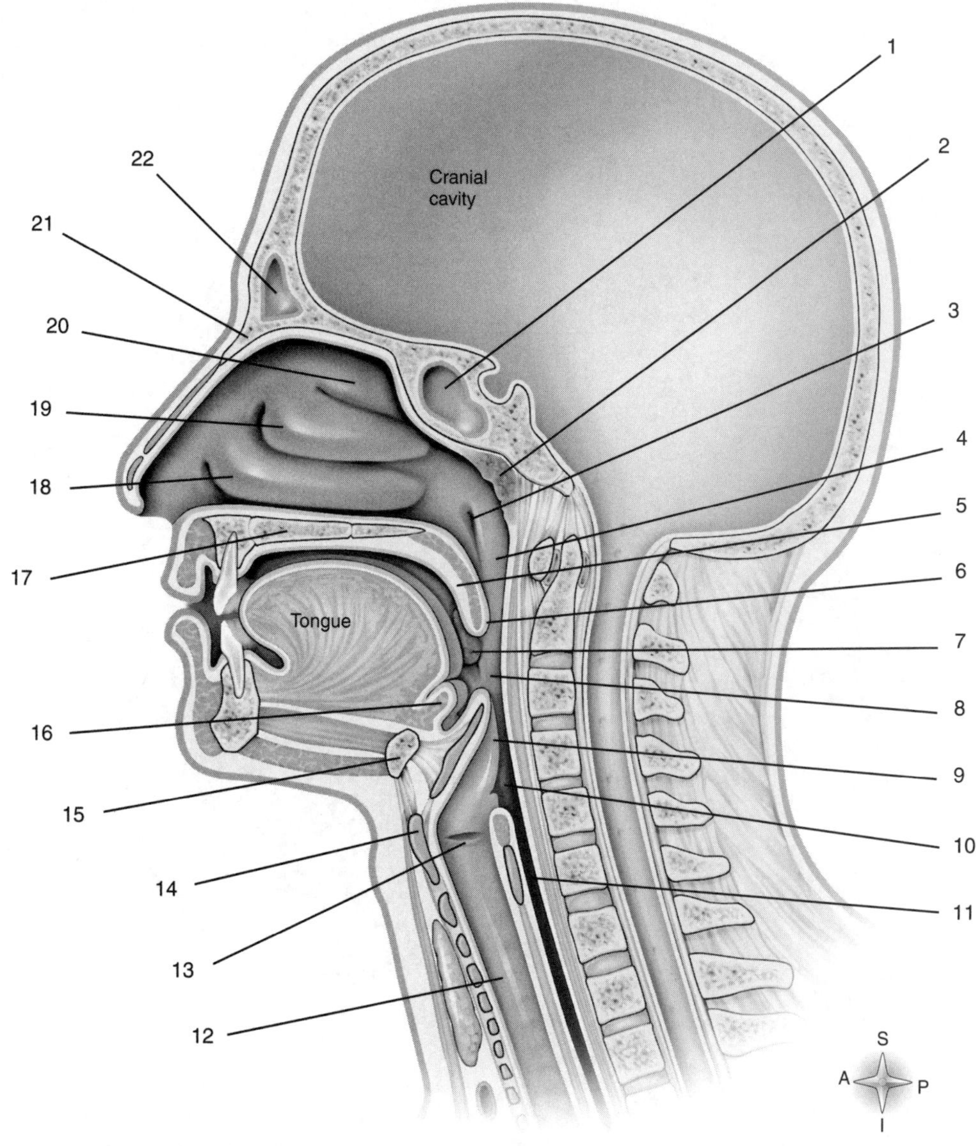

1. ______________________
2. ______________________
3. ______________________
4. ______________________
5. ______________________
6. ______________________
7. ______________________
8. ______________________
9. ______________________
10. ______________________
11. ______________________
12. ______________________
13. ______________________
14. ______________________
15. ______________________
16. ______________________
17. ______________________
18. ______________________
19. ______________________
20. ______________________
21. ______________________
22. ______________________

RESPIRATORY ORGANS

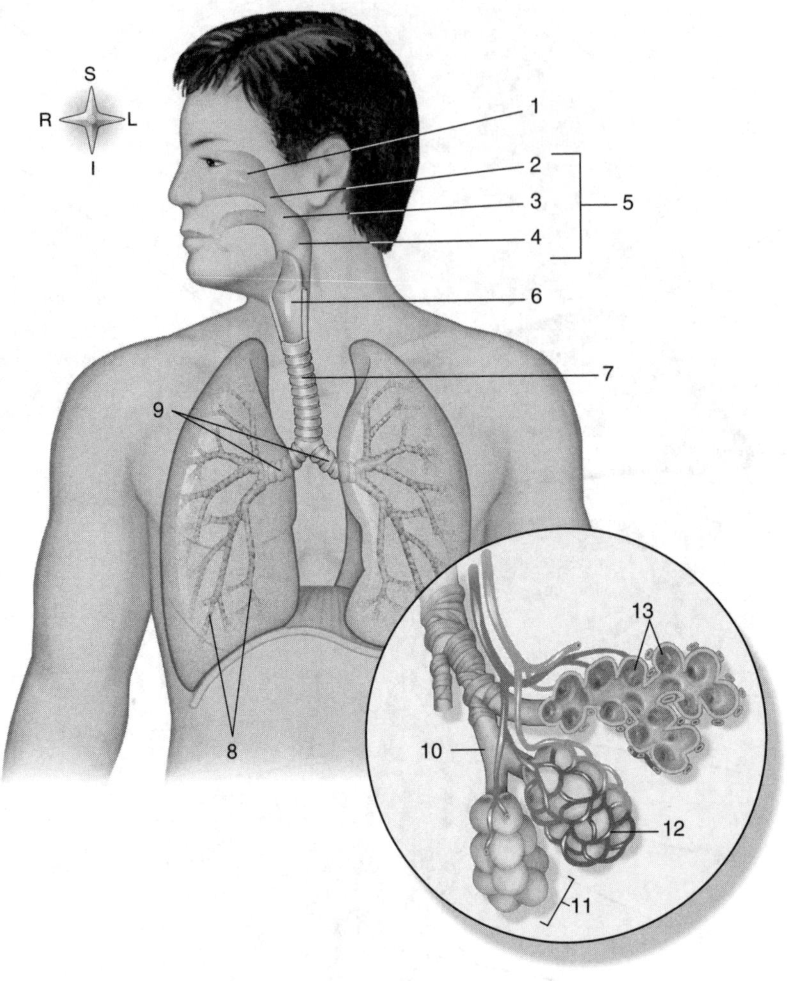

1. ______________________
2. ______________________
3. ______________________
4. ______________________
5. ______________________
6. ______________________
7. ______________________
8. ______________________
9. ______________________
10. ______________________
11. ______________________
12. ______________________
13. ______________________

PULMONARY VENTILATION VOLUMES

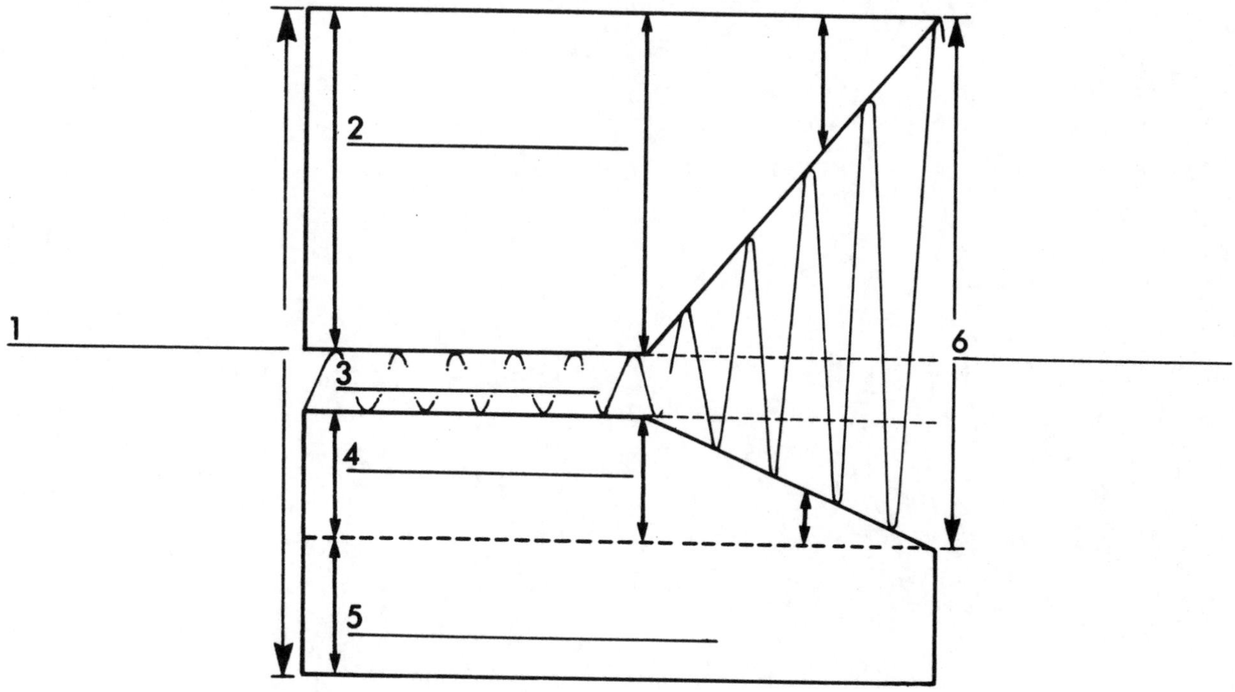

1. ______________________
2. ______________________
3. ______________________
4. ______________________
5. ______________________
6. ______________________

CHAPTER 15

The Digestive System

Think of the last meal you ate. Imagine the different shapes, sizes, tastes, and textures that you so recently enjoyed. Think of those items circulating in your bloodstream in those same original shapes and sizes. Impossible? Of course. And because of this impossibility you will begin to understand and marvel at the close relationship of the digestive system to the circulatory system. It is the digestive system that changes our food, both mechanically and chemically, into a form that is acceptable to the blood and the body.

This change begins the moment you take the very first bite. Digestion starts in the mouth, where food is chewed and mixed with saliva. The food then moves down the pharynx and esophagus by peristalsis and enters the stomach. In the stomach it is churned and mixed with gastric juices to become chyme. The chyme goes from the stomach to the duodenum where it is further broken down chemically by intestinal fluids, bile, and pancreatic juice. Those secretions prepare the food for absorption all along the course of the small intestine.

Products that are not absorbed pass on through the entire length of the small intestine (duodenum, jejunum, ileum). From there they enter into the cecum of the large intestine, then the ascending colon, transverse colon, descending colon, sigmoid colon, into the rectum and out the anus.

Products that are used in the cells undergo absorption. Absorption allows newly processed nutrients to pass through the walls of the digestive tract and into the bloodstream to be distributed to the cells.

Your review of this system will help you understand the mechanical and chemical processes necessary to convert food into energy sources and compounds necessary for survival.

TOPICS FOR REVIEW

Before progressing to Chapter 16, you should review the structure and function of all the organs of digestion. You should have an understanding of the process of digestion, both chemical and mechanical, and of the processes of absorption and metabolism.

WALL OF THE DIGESTIVE SYSTEM

Fill in the blanks.

1. The organs of the digestive system form an irregularly shaped tube called the *alimentary canal* or the _______________ _______________.
2. The churning of food in the stomach is an example of the _______________ digestive process of food.
3. _______________ breakdown occurs when digestive enzymes act on food as it passes through the digestive tract.
4. Waste material resulting from the digestive process is known as _______________.
5. The process of ingested food being broken down into simpler nutrients is known as _______________.
6. After the digestive processes have altered the physical and chemical composition of ingested food, the resulting nutrients are ready for the process of _______________.
7. The digestive tract extends from the _______________ to the _______________.
8. The inside or hollow space within the alimentary canal is called the _______________.
9. The inside layer of the digestive tract is the _______________.
10. The connective tissue layer that lies beneath the lining of the digestive tract is the _______________.
11. The muscularis contracts and moves food through the gastrointestinal tract by a process known as _______________.
12. The outermost covering of the digestive tube is the _______________.
13. The loops of the digestive tract are anchored to the posterior wall of the abdominal cavity by the _______________.

Choose the correct term from the choices given and write the letter in the answer blank.

(A) Main organ (B) Accessory organ

_____ 14. Mouth
_____ 15. Parotids
_____ 16. Liver
_____ 17. Stomach
_____ 18. Cecum
_____ 19. Esophagus
_____ 20. Rectum
_____ 21. Pharynx
_____ 22. Appendix
_____ 23. Teeth
_____ 24. Gallbladder
_____ 25. Pancreas

If you have had difficulty with this section, review pages 350-355.

MOUTH, TEETH, SALIVARY GLANDS

Select the best answer.

26. Which one of the following is *not* a part of the roof of the mouth?
    A. Uvula
    B. Palatine bones
    C. Maxillary bones
    D. Soft palate
    E. All of the above are part of the roof of the mouth

27. A thin membrane called the ________ attaches the tongue to the floor of the mouth.
    A. Filiform
    B. Fungiform
    C. Frenulum
    D. Root

28. The first baby tooth, on an average, appears at age:
    A. 2 months
    B. 1 year
    C. 3 months
    D. 1 month
    E. 6 months

29. The portion of the tooth that is covered with enamel is the:
    A. Pulp cavity
    B. Neck
    C. Root
    D. Crown
    E. None of the above

30. The wall of the pulp cavity is surrounded by:
    A. Enamel
    B. Dentin
    C. Cementum
    D. Connective tissue
    E. Blood and lymphatic vessels

31. A general term for mild, localized inflammation of the gums is:
    A. Periodontitis
    B. Dental caries
    C. Gingivitis
    D. Deciduitis

32. The leading cause of tooth loss among adults is:
    A. Dental caries
    B. Gingivitis
    C. Poor diet
    D. Periodontitis

33. The third molar appears between the ages of ______________.
    A. 10–14
    B. 5–8
    C. 11–16
    D. 17–24
    E. None of the above

34. Which one of the following will *not* significantly reduce caries?
    A. Good dental health practices
    B. Regular flossing
    C. Regular and thorough brushing
    D. Eating a carrot or stick of celery instead of brushing

35. The ducts of the ________________ glands open into the floor of the mouth.
    A. Sublingual
    B. Submandibular
    C. Parotid
    D. Carotid

36. The volume of saliva secreted per day is about:
    A. One-half pint
    B. One pint
    C. One liter
    D. One gallon

37. Mumps are an infection of the:
    A. Parotid gland
    B. Sublingual gland
    C. Submandibular gland
    D. Tonsils

38. Incisors are used during mastication to:
    A. Cut
    B. Pierce
    C. Tear
    D. Grind

39. Another name for the third molar is:
    A. Central incisor
    B. Wisdom tooth
    C. Canine
    D. Lateral incisor

40. After food has been chewed, it is formed into a small rounded mass called a:
    A. Moat
    B. Chyme
    C. Bolus
    D. Protease

If you have had difficulty with this section, review pages 355-358.

PHARYNX, ESOPHAGUS, STOMACH

Fill in the blanks.

The (41) ________________ is a tubelike structure that functions as part of both respiratory and digestive systems. It connects the mouth with the (42) ________________. The esophagus serves as a passageway for movement of food from the pharynx to the (43) ________________. Food enters the stomach by passing through the muscular (44) ________________ ________________ at the end of the esophagus. Contraction of the stomach mixes the food thoroughly with the gastric juices and breaks it down into a semisolid mixture called (45) ____________________.

The three divisions of the stomach are the (46) ________________, (47) ________________, and (48) ________________.

Food is held in the stomach by the (49) ________________ ________________ muscle long enough for partial digestion to occur. After food has been in the stomach for approximately 3 hours, the chyme will enter the (50) ________________ ____________________.

Match the term with the correct definition.

A. Esophagus
B. Chyme
C. Peristalsis
D. Rugae
E. Triple therapy
F. Greater curvature
G. Hiatal hernia
H. Antacid
I. Acid indigestion
J. Lesser curvature

_____ 51. Stomach folds

_____ 52. Upper right border of stomach

_____ 53. Condition that may result in backward movement or reflux of stomach contents into the lower portion of the esophagus

_____ 54. 10-inch passageway

_____ 55. Drug used to treat GERD

_____ 56. Semisolid mixture of stomach contents

_____ 57. Muscle contractions of the digestive system

_____ 58. Used to heal ulcers and prevent recurrences

_____ 59. Heartburn

_____ 60. Lower left border of stomach

If you have had difficulty with this section, review pages 358-360.

SMALL INTESTINE, LIVER AND GALLBLADDER, PANCREAS

Select the best answer.

61. Which one is *not* part of the small intestine?
    A. Jejunum
    B. Ileum
    C. Cecum
    D. Duodenum

62. Which one of the following structures does *not* increase the surface area of the intestine for absorption?
    A. Plicae
    B. Rugae
    C. Microvilli
    D. Villi

63. The union of the cystic duct and hepatic duct form the:
    A. Common bile duct
    B. Major duodenal papilla
    C. Minor duodenal papilla
    D. Pancreatic duct

64. Obstruction of the ________________ will lead to jaundice.
    A. Hepatic duct
    B. Pancreatic duct
    C. Cystic duct
    D. None of the above

65. Each villus in the intestine contains a lymphatic vessel or ________________ that serves to absorb lipid or fat materials from the chyme.
    A. Plica
    B. Lacteal
    C. Villa
    D. Microvilli

66. The middle third of the duodenum contains the:
    A. Islets
    B. Fundus
    C. Body
    D. Rugae
    E. Major duodenal papilla

67. Most gastric and duodenal ulcers result from infection with the bacterium:
    A. Biaxin
    B. Metronidazole
    C. Prilosec
    D. *Helicobacter pylori*

68. The liver is an:
    A. Enzyme
    B. Endocrine organ
    C. Endocrine gland
    D. Exocrine gland

69. Fats in chyme stimulate the secretion of the hormone:
    A. Lipase
    B. Cholecystokinin
    C. Protease
    D. Amylase

70. The largest gland in the body is the:
    A. Pituitary
    B. Thyroid
    C. Liver
    D. Thymus

If you have had difficulty with this section, review pages 360-364.

LARGE INTESTINE, APPENDIX, PERITONEUM

If the statement is true, write "T" in the answer blank. If the statement is false, correct the statement by circling the incorrect term and writing the correct term in the answer blank.

________ 71. Bacteria in the large intestine are responsible for the synthesis of vitamin E needed for normal blood clotting.

________ 72. Villi in the large intestine absorb salts and water.

________ 73. If waste products pass rapidly through the large intestine, constipation results.

________ 74. The ileocecal valve opens into the sigmoid colon.

________ 75. The splenic flexure is the bend between the ascending colon and the transverse colon.

________ 76. The splenic colon is the S-shaped segment that terminates in the rectum.

________ 77. The appendix serves no important digestive function in humans.

________ 78. For patients with suspected appendicitis, a physician will often evaluate the appendix by a digital rectal examination.

________ 79. The visceral layer of the peritoneum lines the abdominal cavity.

________ 80. The greater omentum is shaped like a fan and serves to anchor the small intestine to the posterior abdominal wall.

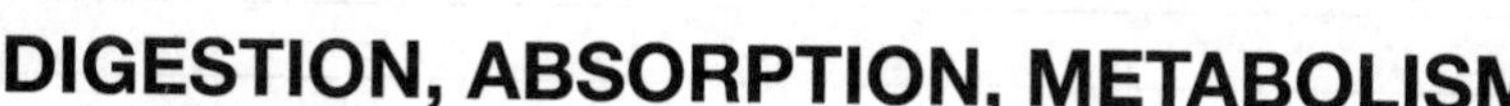
If you have had difficulty with this section, review pages 364-368.

DIGESTION, ABSORPTION, METABOLISM

Select the best answer.

81. Which one of the following substances does *not* contain any enzymes?
    A. Saliva
    B. Bile
    C. Gastric juice
    D. Pancreatic juice
    E. Intestinal juice

82. Which one of the following is a simple sugar?
    A. Maltose
    B. Sucrose
    C. Lactose
    D. Glucose
    E. Starch

83. Cane sugar is the same as:
    A. Maltose
    B. Lactose
    C. Sucrose
    D. Glucose
    E. None of the above

84. Most of the digestion of carbohydrates takes place in the:
   A. Mouth
   B. Stomach
   C. Small intestine
   D. Large intestine

85. Fats are broken down into:
   A. Amino acids
   B. Simple sugars
   C. Fatty acids
   D. Disaccharides

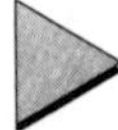
If you have had difficulty with this section, review pages 368-372 and page 353.

CHEMICAL DIGESTION

86. *Fill in the blank areas on the chart below.*

DIGESTIVE JUICES AND ENZYMES	SUBSTANCE DIGESTED (OR HYDROLYZED)	RESULTING PRODUCT
Saliva		
1. Amylase	1.	1. Maltose (disaccharide)
Gastric Juice		
2. Protease (pepsin) plus hydrochloric acid	2. Proteins	2.
Pancreatic Juice		
3. Proteases (e.g., trypsin)	3. Proteins (intact or partially digested)	3.
4. Lipases	4.	4. Fatty acids, monoglycerides, and glycerol
5. Amylase	5.	5. Maltose
Intestinal Enzymes		
6. Peptidases	6.	6. Amino acids
7.	7. Sucrose	7. Glucose and fructose
8. Lactase	8.	8. Glucose and galactose (simple sugars)
9. Maltase	9. Maltose	9.

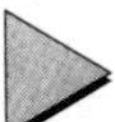
If you have had difficulty with this section, review page 371.

UNSCRAMBLE THE WORDS

Take the circled letters, unscramble them, and fill in the statement.

87. **SLBOU**

88. **EYCHM**

89. **LLAAPPI**

90. **PMERTEUION**

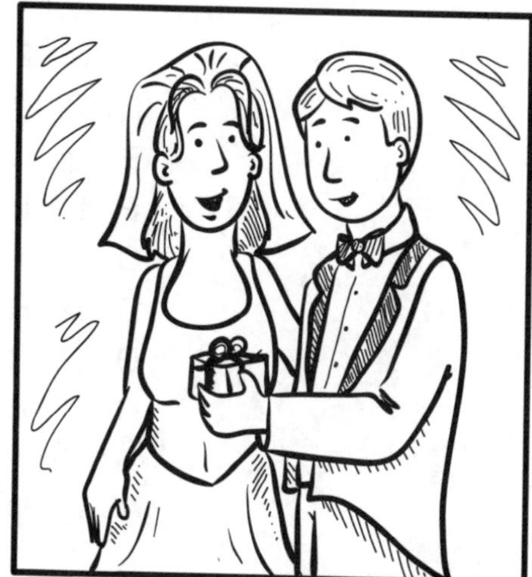

What the groom gave his bride after the wedding.

91.

APPLYING WHAT YOU KNOW

92. Dan was a successful businessman, but he worked too hard and was always under great stress. His doctor cautioned him that if he did not alter his style of living he would be subject to hyperacidity. What could be the resulting condition of hyperacidity?

93. Baby Shearer has been regurgitating his bottle-feeding at every meal. The milk is curdled, but does not appear to be digested. He has become dehydrated, and so his mother is taking him to the pediatrician. What is a possible diagnosis from your textbook reading?

94. Scott has gained a great deal of weight suddenly. He has also noticed that he is sluggish and always tired. What test might his physician order for him and for what reason?

95. WORD FIND

Can you find the 22 terms from the chapter in the box of letters? Words may be spelled top to bottom, bottom to top, right to left, left to right, or diagonally.

```
X M E T A B O L I S M X X W
R S D P E R I S T A L S I S
E V A M N O I T S E G I D R
E D E E U O Q T W Q O H N Q
Q Z H S R N I N T F E C E S
D H R E C C I T K C J A P E
Q W R N A T N V P Y R M P C
O C A T N R B A P R H O A I
U Y I E O W T A P A O T W D
B O D R L N P B F Q J S V N
N T S Y F I S L U M E E B U
W G J A L U V U N R N W O A
Q S N L X D U O D E N U M J
H C A V I T Y M U C O S A D
Y E A A P H V W S V C Q J C
```

Absorption	Emulsify	Mucosa
Appendix	Feces	Pancreas
Cavity	Fundus	Papillae
Crown	Heartburn	Peristalsis
Dentin	Jaundice	Stomach
Diarrhea	Mastication	Uvula
Digestion	Mesentery	
Duodenum	Metabolism	

DID YOU KNOW?

The liver performs over 500 functions and produces over 1000 enzymes to handle the chemical conversions necessary for survival.

The human stomach lining replaces itself every 3 days.

Even if the stomach, the spleen, 75% of the liver, 80% of the intestines, one kidney, one lung, and virtually every organ from the pelvic and groin area are removed, the human body can still survive!

Every day, approximately 11.5 liters of digested food, liquids, and digestive juices flow through an individual's digestive system, but only 100 mL of that is lost in feces.

DIGESTIVE SYSTEM

Fill in the crossword puzzle.

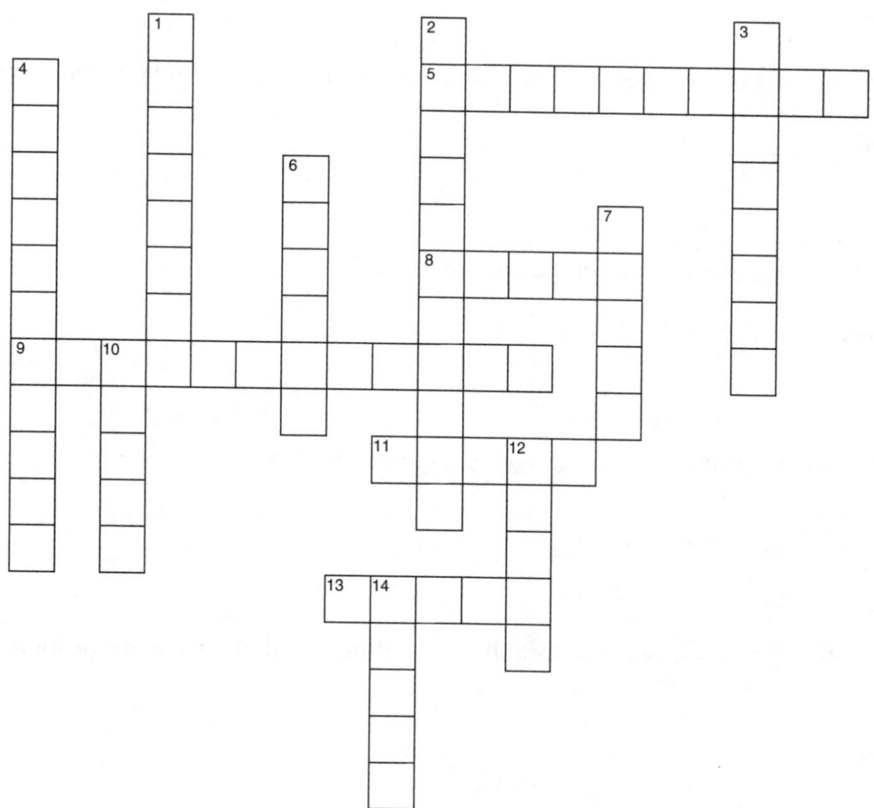

Across

5. Digested food moves from intestine to blood
8. Semisolid mixture
9. Inflammation of the appendix
11. Rounded mass of food
13. Stomach folds

Down

1. Yellowish skin discoloration
2. Process of chewing
3. Fluid stools
4. Movement of food through digestive tract
6. Vomitus
7. Waste product of digestion
10. Intestinal folds
12. Open wound in digestive area acted on by acid juices
14. Prevents food from entering nasal cavities

CHECK YOUR KNOWLEDGE

Multiple Choice

Select the best answer.

1. The principal structure of the digestive system is an irregular tube, open at both ends, that is called the:
   A. Alimentary canal
   B. Oral cavity
   C. Colon
   D. Esophagus

2. Which of the following is *not* a layer of the digestive tract?
   A. Mucosa
   B. Muscularis
   C. Lumen
   D. Serosa

3. Which of the following is *not* a main organ of the digestive system?
   A. Liver
   B. Stomach
   C. Cecum
   D. Colon

4. Which of the following classification of teeth have a cutting function during mastication?
   A. Canines
   B. Incisors
   C. Premolars
   D. Molars

5. Which of the following is an accurate description of the salivary glands?
   A. There are four pairs of salivary glands.
   B. Salivary amylase begins the chemical digestion of carbohydrates.
   C. They are located within the digestive tube.
   D. The submandibular glands are the ones involved when people have the mumps.

6. The act of swallowing moves a mass of food called a _______ from the mouth to the stomach.
   A. Dentin
   B. Bolus
   C. Chyme
   D. Frenulum

7. Stomach muscle contractions result in:
   A. Rugae
   B. Peristalsis
   C. Plicae
   D. None of the above

8. The stomach sphincter that keeps food from reentering the esophagus when the stomach contracts is known as the:
   A. Hiatal
   B. Pyloric
   C. Cardiac
   D. Fundus

9. Most of the chemical digestion occurs in the:
   A. Stomach
   B. Liver
   C. Duodenum
   D. Jejunum

10. The pancreas:
    A. Is both an endocrine and an exocrine gland
    B. Contains enzymes that digest proteins and fats only
    C. Contains an acid substance that elevates the pH of the gastric juice
    D. None of the above

COMPLETION

Complete the following statements.

11. Undigested and unabsorbed food materials enter the large intestine after passing through a sphincterlike structure called the ____________________ ____________________.

12. The subdivisions of the large intestine in the order in which food material or feces pass through them are: cecum, ascending colon, transverse colon, descending colon, ____________________ ____________________, rectum, and anal canal.

13. The vermiform appendix is directly attached to the ____________________.

14. The ____________________ is an extension between the parietal and visceral layers of the peritoneum and is shaped like a giant, pleated fan.

15. Chewing, swallowing, peristalsis, and defecation are the main processes of ________________ ________________.

16. The end products of carbohydrate digestion are ____________________.

17. The end products of protein digestion are____________________.

18. The end products of fat digestion are ____________________ and ____________________.

19. The process by which molecules of amino acids, glucose, fatty acids, and glycerol go from the inside of the intestines into the circulating fluids of the body is known as ____________________.

20. Three intestinal enzymes____________________, ____________________, and ____________________digest disaccharides by changing them into monosaccharides.

DIGESTIVE ORGANS

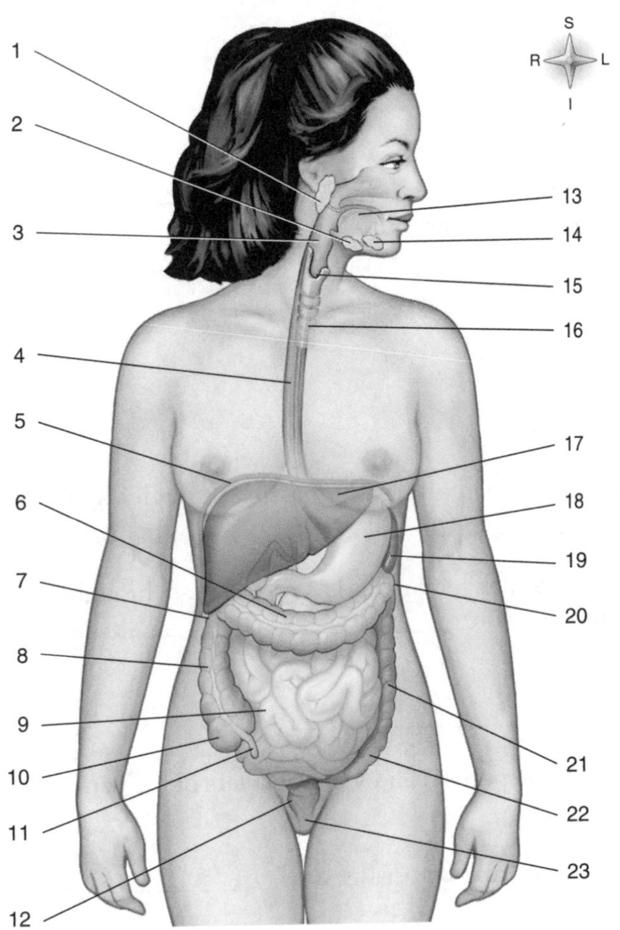

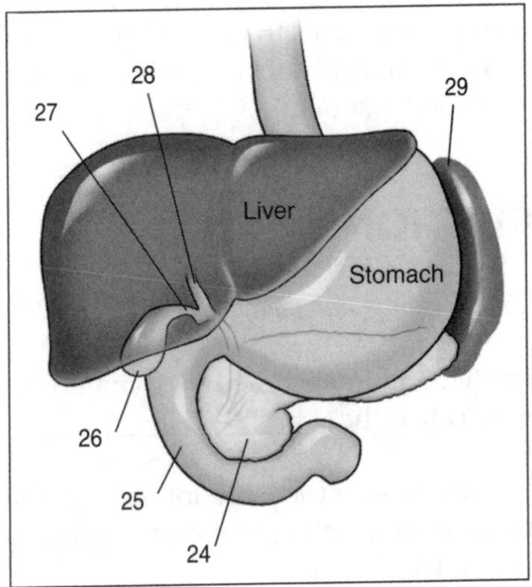

1. ____________________
2. ____________________
3. ____________________
4. ____________________
5. ____________________
6. ____________________
7. ____________________
8. ____________________
9. ____________________
10. ____________________
11. ____________________
12. ____________________
13. ____________________
14. ____________________
15. ____________________
16. ____________________
17. ____________________
18. ____________________
19. ____________________
20. ____________________
21. ____________________
22. ____________________
23. ____________________
24. ____________________
25. ____________________
26. ____________________
27. ____________________
28. ____________________
29. ____________________

TOOTH

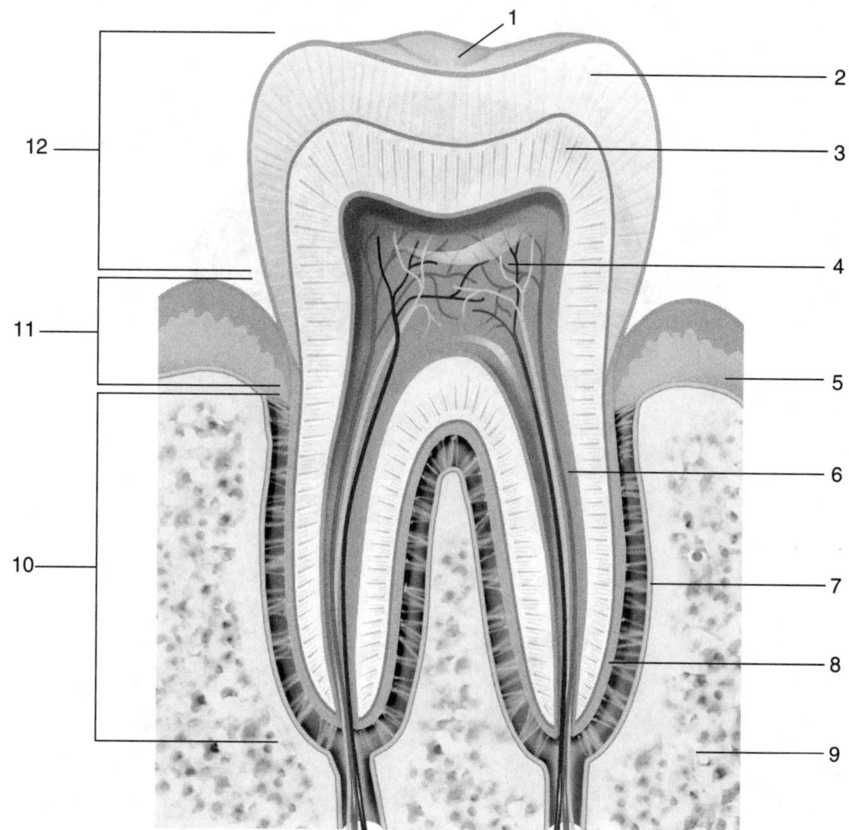

1. ______________________
2. ______________________
3. ______________________
4. ______________________
5. ______________________
6. ______________________
7. ______________________
8. ______________________
9. ______________________
10. ______________________
11. ______________________
12. ______________________

THE SALIVARY GLANDS

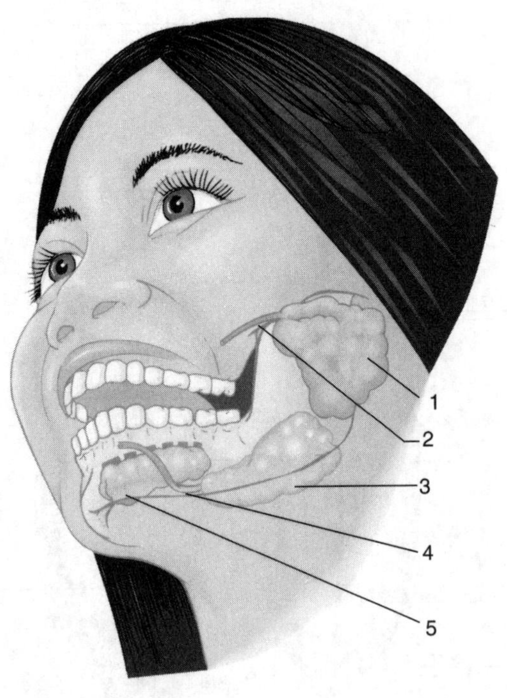

1. ______________________
2. ______________________
3. ______________________
4. ______________________
5. ______________________

STOMACH

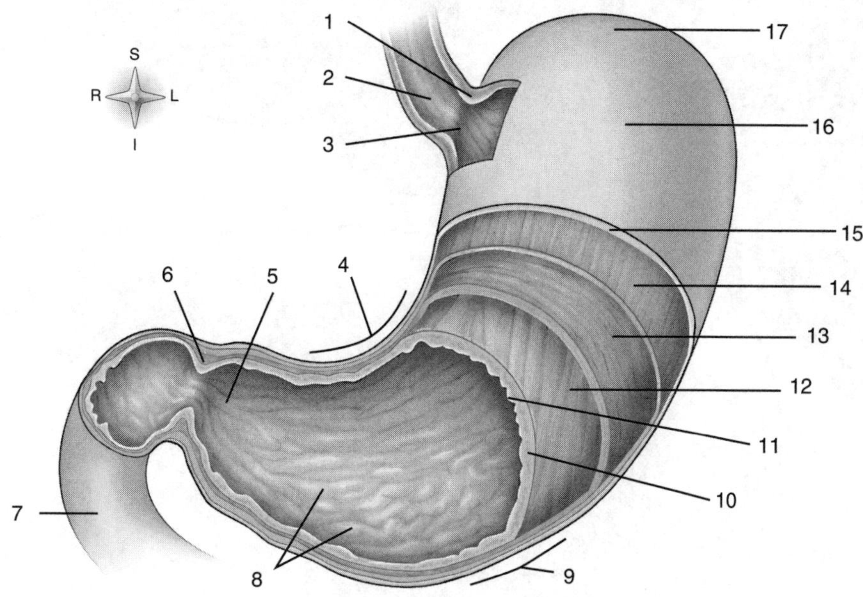

1. ______________________
2. ______________________
3. ______________________
4. ______________________
5. ______________________
6. ______________________
7. ______________________
8. ______________________
9. ______________________
10. ______________________
11. ______________________
12. ______________________
13. ______________________
14. ______________________
15. ______________________
16. ______________________
17. ______________________

GALLBLADDER AND BILE DUCTS

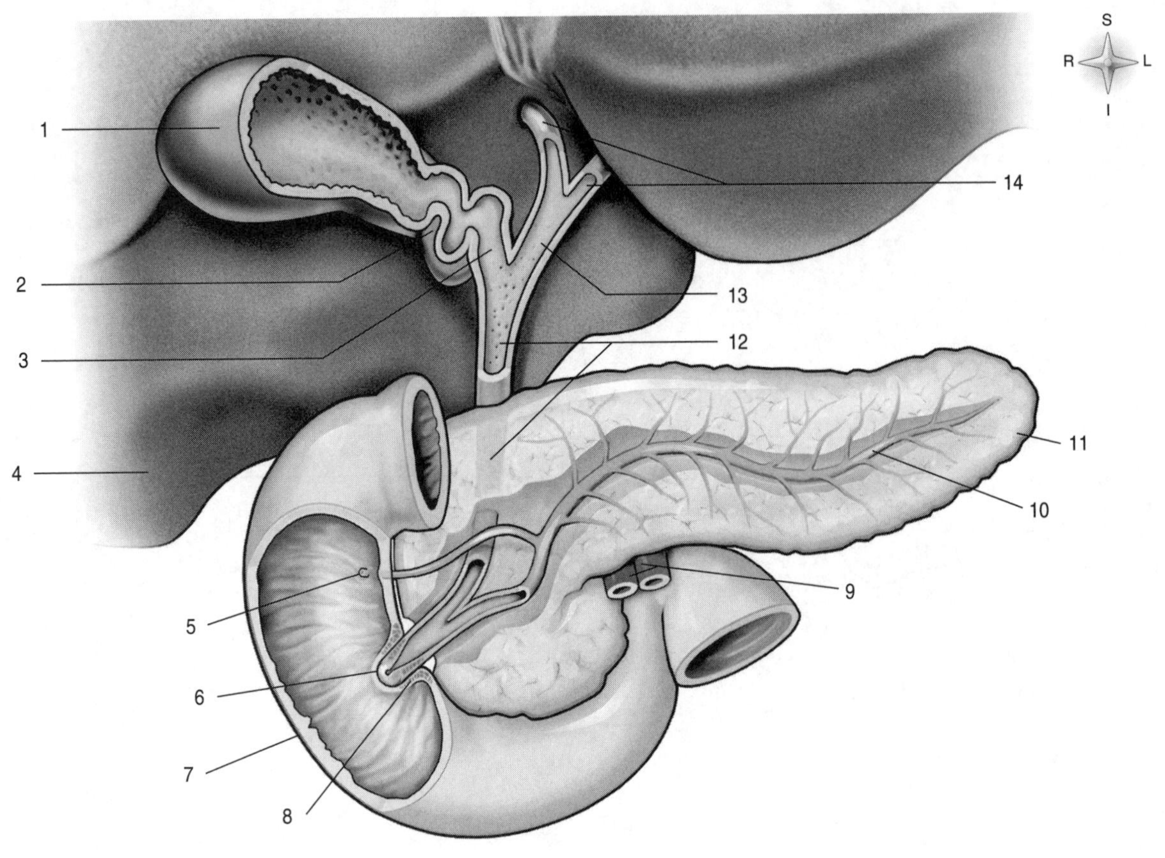

1. ______________________
2. ______________________
3. ______________________
4. ______________________
5. ______________________
6. ______________________
7. ______________________
8. ______________________
9. ______________________
10. ______________________
11. ______________________
12. ______________________
13. ______________________
14. ______________________

THE SMALL INTESTINE

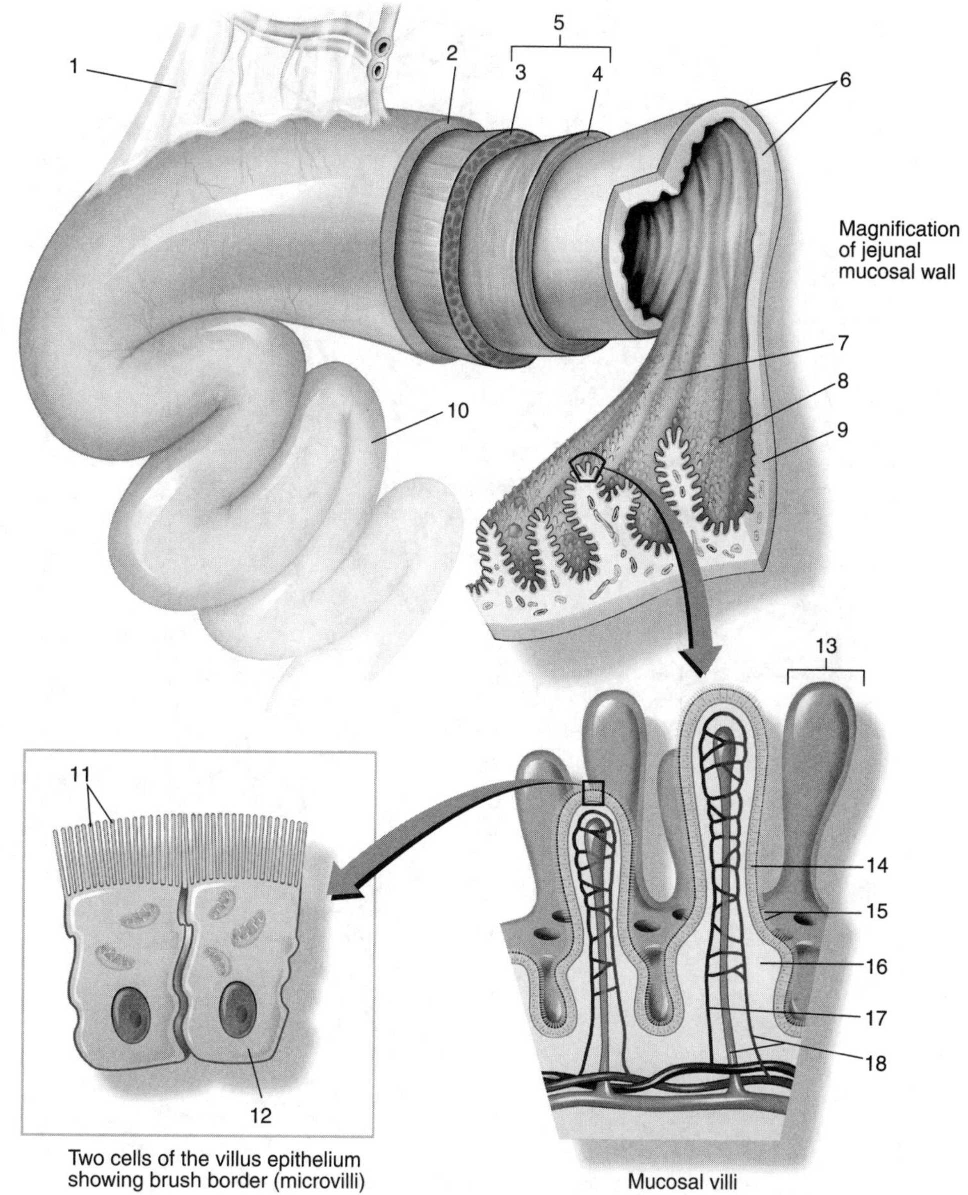

Two cells of the villus epithelium showing brush border (microvilli)

Mucosal villi

1. ______
2. ______
3. ______
4. ______
5. ______
6. ______
7. ______
8. ______
9. ______
10. ______
11. ______
12. ______
13. ______
14. ______
15. ______
16. ______
17. ______
18. ______

THE LARGE INTESTINE

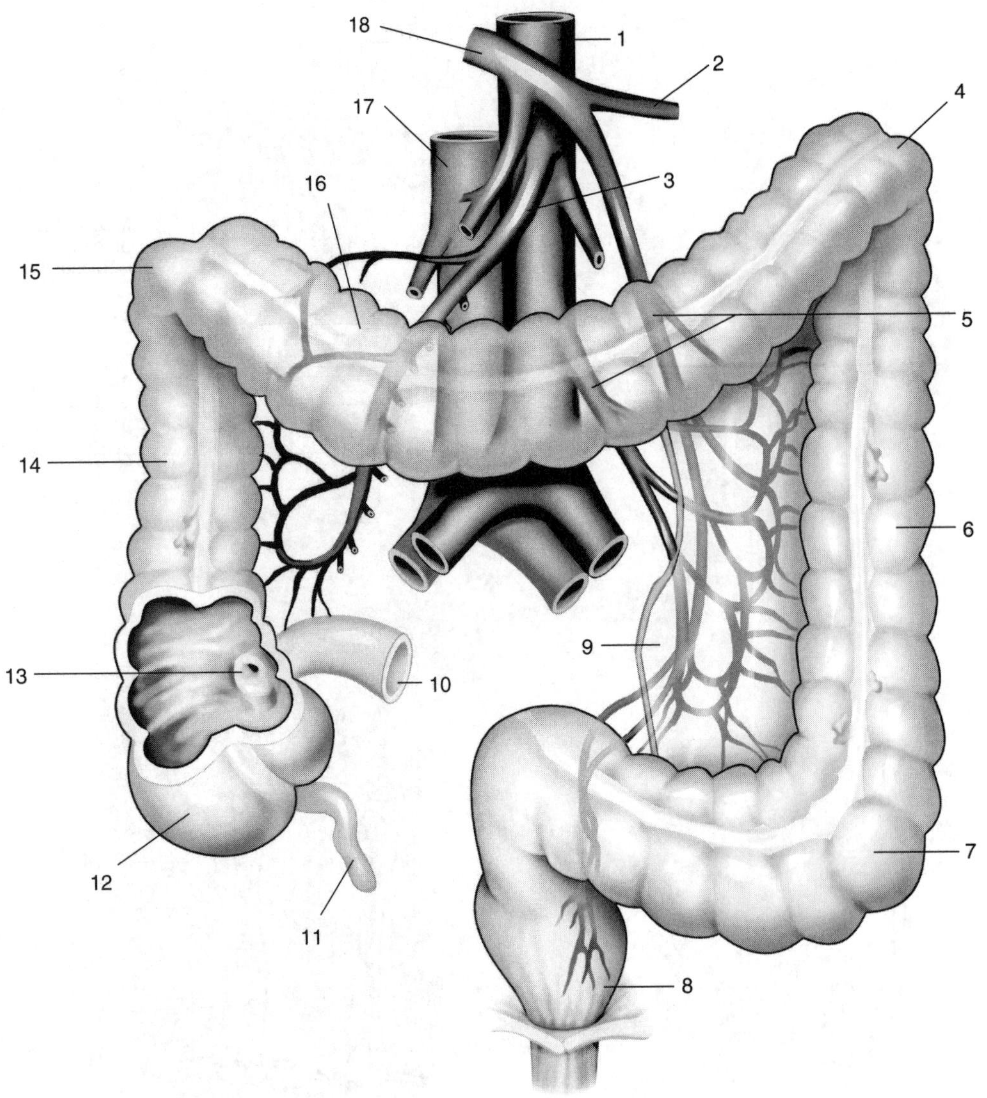

1. ______________________
2. ______________________
3. ______________________
4. ______________________
5. ______________________
6. ______________________
7. ______________________
8. ______________________
9. ______________________
10. ______________________
11. ______________________
12. ______________________
13. ______________________
14. ______________________
15. ______________________
16. ______________________
17. ______________________
18. ______________________

CHAPTER 16

Nutrition and Metabolism

Most of us love to eat, but do the foods we enjoy provide us with the basic food types necessary for good nutrition? The body, a finely tuned machine, requires fuel to function properly. A healthy balance of carbohydrates, fats, proteins, vitamins, and minerals is necessary to allow the body to perform at the highest level. These nutrients must be digested, absorbed, and circulated to cells constantly to accommodate the numerous activities that occur throughout the body. The use the body makes of foods once these processes are completed is called *metabolism.*

The liver plays a major role in the metabolism of food. It helps maintain a normal blood glucose level, removes toxins from the blood, processes blood immediately after it leaves the gastrointestinal tract, and initiates the first steps of protein and fat metabolism.

This chapter also discusses basal metabolic rate (BMR). The BMR is the rate at which food is catabolized under basal conditions. This test and the measurement of the amount of protein-bound iodine (PBI) are indirect measures of thyroid gland functioning. The total metabolic rate (TMR) is the amount of energy, expressed in calories, used by the body each day.

Finally, maintaining a constant body temperature is a function of the hypothalamus and a challenge for the metabolic mechanisms of the body. Review of this chapter is necessary to provide you with an understanding of the "fuel" or nutrition necessary to maintain your complex homeostatic machine—the body.

TOPICS FOR REVIEW

Before progressing to Chapter 17, you should be able to define and contrast catabolism and anabolism. Your review should include the metabolic roles of carbohydrates, fats, proteins, vitamins, and minerals. Your study should conclude with an understanding of the basal metabolic rate and physiological mechanisms that regulate body temperature.

THE ROLE OF THE LIVER

Fill in the blanks.

The liver plays an important role in the mechanical digestion of lipids because it secretes (1) ________________. It also produces two of the plasma proteins that play an essential role in blood clotting: (2) ______________ and (3) ______________. Additionally, liver cells store several substances, notably vitamins A and D and (4) ______________. Finally, the liver is assisted by a unique structural feature of the blood vessels that supply it. This arrangement, known as the (5) ________ ________ ________, allows toxins to be removed from the bloodstream before nutrients are distributed throughout the body.

If you have had difficulty with this section, review pages 378-380.

NUTRIENT METABOLISM

Match the term on the left with the proper selection on the right.

(A) Carbohydrates (B) Fats (C) Proteins (D) Vitamins (E) Minerals

_____ 6. Used if cells have inadequate amounts of glucose to catabolize
_____ 7. Preferred energy food
_____ 8. Amino acids
_____ 9. Fat soluble
_____ 10. Required for nerve conduction
_____ 11. Glycolysis
_____ 12. Inorganic elements found naturally in the earth
_____ 13. Pyruvic acid

Circle the one that does not *belong.*

14. Glycolysis	Citric acid cycle	ATP	Bile
15. Adipose	Amino acids	Triglycerides	Glycerol
16. A	D	M	K
17. Iron	Proteins	Amino acids	Essential
18. Hydrocortisone	Insulin	Growth hormone	Epinephrine
19. Sodium	Calcium	Zinc	Folic acid
20. Thiamine	Niacin	Ascorbic acid	Riboflavin

If you have had difficulty with this section, review pages 380-384.

METABOLIC RATES, BODY TEMPERATURE

Select the best answer.

21. The rate at which food is catabolized under basal conditions is the:
    A. TMR
    B. PBI
    C. BMR
    D. ATP

22. The total amount of energy used by the body per day is the:
    A. TMR
    B. PBI
    C. BMR
    D. ATP

23. Over ____________ of the energy released from food molecules during catabolism is converted to heat rather than being transferred to ATP.
    A. 20%
    B. 40%
    C. 60%
    D. 80%

24. Maintaining thermoregulation is a function of the:
    A. Thalamus
    B. Hypothalamus
    C. Thyroid
    D. Parathyroids

25. Transfer of heat energy to the skin and then to the external environment is known as:
    A. Radiation
    B. Conduction
    C. Convection
    D. Evaporation

26. A flow of heat waves away from the blood is known as:
    A. Radiation
    B. Conduction
    C. Convection
    D. Evaporation

27. A transfer of heat energy to air that is continually flowing away from the skin is known as:
    A. Radiation
    B. Conduction
    C. Convection
    D. Evaporation

28. Heat absorbed by the process of water vaporization is called:
    A. Radiation
    B. Conduction
    C. Convection
    D. Evaporation

29. A(n) ________________ is the amount of energy needed to raise the temperature of 1 gram of water 1° C.
    A. Calorie
    B. Kilocalorie
    C. ATP
    D. BMR

If you have had difficulty with this section, review pages 384-388.

UNSCRAMBLE THE WORDS

Take the circled letters, unscramble them, and fill in the statement.

30. **L R I E V**

31. **T A O B A L I C M S**

32. **O M N I A**

33. **Y P U R C V I**

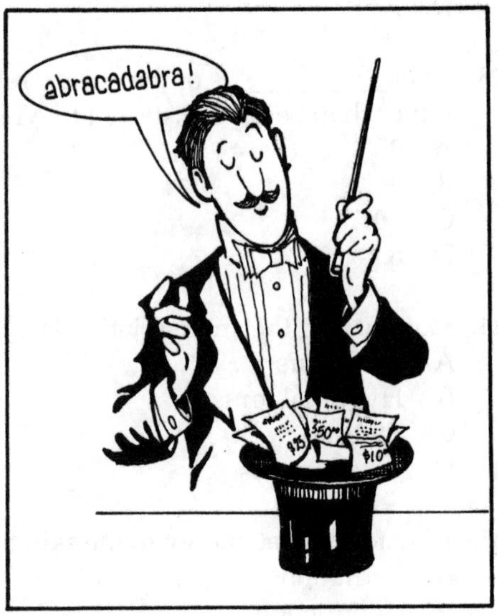

How the magician paid his bills.

34.

APPLYING WHAT YOU KNOW

35. Dr. Culp was concerned about Deborrah. Her daily food intake provided fewer calories than her TMR. If this trend continues, what will be the result? If it continues over a long period of time, what eating disorder might Deborrah develop?

36. Mrs. Bishop was experiencing fatigue and a blood test revealed that she was slightly anemic. What mineral will her doctor most likely prescribe? What dietary sources might you suggest that she emphasize in her daily intake?

37. Mrs. Hosmer was training daily for an upcoming marathon. Three days before the 26-mile event, she suddenly quit her daily routine of jogging and switched to a diet high in carbohydrates. Why did Mrs. Hosmer suddenly switch her routine of training?

38. WORD FIND

Can you find 18 terms from this chapter in the box of letters? Words may be spelled top to bottom, bottom to top, right to left, left to right, or diagonally.

```
C C C B W E F F L J V G G S
A T N L W E U O Z I E L I B
R K K P Z F R I T P O Y K L
B Q M I N E R A L S J C C P
O S S N C X M I D B D O W P
H S I Y O I T X H I N L S N
Y E L N N I K W W D S Y N S
D G O S O W T I U E H S C N
R M B Y T I W C Z N N I A A
A R A Q W A T B E I G S J M
T E T F N I F A E V E W T Y
E V A P O R A T I O N D T E
S I C N E S O P I D A O F E
H L Y K I R E B V P A H C J
I W E E P A D F T E A R G G
```

ATP	Conduction	Liver
Adipose	Convection	Minerals
BMR	Evaporation	Proteins
Bile	Fats	Radiation
Carbohydrates	Glycerol	TMR
Catabolism	Glycolysis	Vitamins

DID YOU KNOW?

Twenty-five years ago, 3%–5% of Americans were deficient in vitamin C. Today, about 15% don't get the amount they need for optimum health.

The human body has enough fat to produce 7 bars of soap.

Forty to fifty percent of body heat can be lost through the head (no hat) as a result of its extensive circulatory network.

NUTRITION/METABOLISM

Fill in the crossword puzzle.

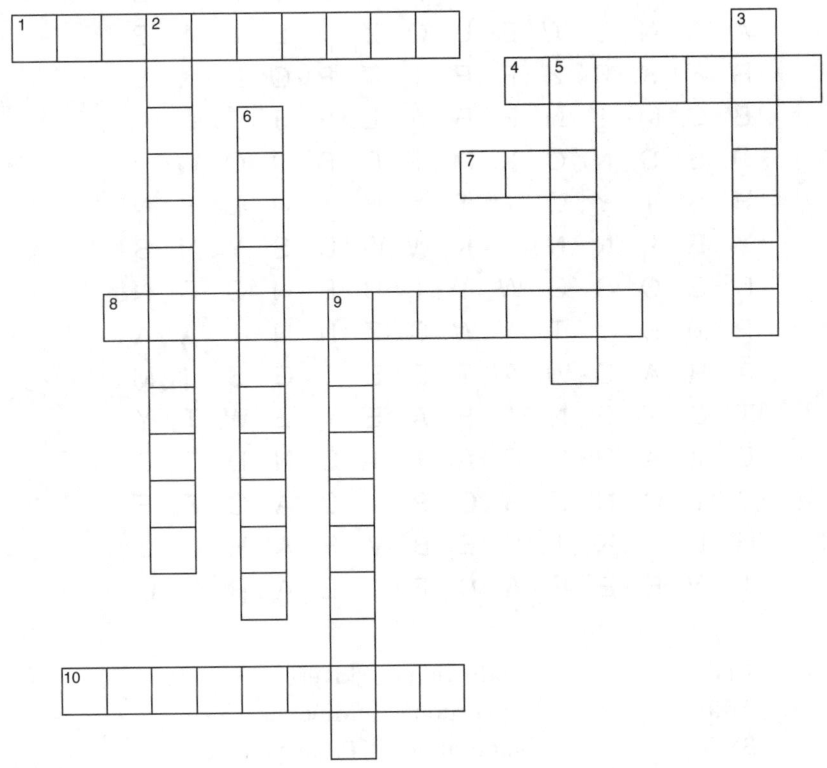

Across

1. Breaks food molecules down releasing stored energy
4. Amount of energy needed to raise the temperature of one gram of water 1° Celsius
7. Rate of metabolism when a person is lying down, but awake (abbreviation)
8. A series of reactions that join glucose molecules together to form glycogen
10. Builds food molecules into complex substances

Down

2. Occurs when food molecules enter cells and undergo many chemical changes there
3. Organic molecule needed in small quantities for normal metabolism throughout the body
5. Oxygen-using
6. A unit of measure for heat, also known as a large calorie
9. Takes place in the cytoplasm of a cell and changes glucose to pyruvic acid

CHECK YOUR KNOWLEDGE

Multiple Choice

Select the best answer.

1. *Metabolism* is a term that refers to the:
   A. Nutrients that we eat
   B. Use of foods
   C. Building blocks
   D. None of the above

2. Glycolysis changes glucose into:
   A. Pyruvic acid
   B. Carbon dioxide
   C. ATP
   D. None of the above

3. An anaerobic process:
   A. Is an oxygen-using process
   B. Is an oxygen-storing process
   C. Uses no oxygen
   D. Both A and B

4. The amount of nutrients in the blood:
   A. Changes significantly when we exercise
   B. Changes significantly when we go without food for many hours
   C. Does not change very much and remains relatively constant
   D. Both A and B

5. Which of the following hormones lowers blood glucose levels?
   A. Growth hormone
   B. Insulin
   C. Hydrocortisone
   D. Epinephrine

6. Fats not needed for catabolism are anabolized to form:
   A. Nonessential amino acids
   B. Triglycerides
   C. Glycogen
   D. ATP

7. Essential amino acids:
   A. Must be in the diet
   B. Can be made by the body
   C. Make up the majority of the 20 amino acids
   D. All of the above

8. A good source of iron in the diet is:
   A. Meat
   B. Dairy products
   C. Seafood
   D. Fruits

9. The flow of heat waves away from the blood is known as:
   A. Conduction
   B. Radiation
   C. Convection
   D. Evaporation

10. The liver:
    A. Plays an important role in the mechanical digestion of lipids because it secretes bile
    B. Detoxifies various poisonous substances such as bacterial products and certain drugs
    C. Synthesizes several kinds of protein compounds
    D. All of the above

Completion

Complete the following statements.

11. The preferred energy food of the body is ______________________.

12. An anaerobic process is ____________________.

13. An aerobic process is the ______________ ______________ ______________.

14. A deficiency of ________________ may result in a goiter.

15. The rate at which food is catabolized under basal conditions is known as the ______________ ______________ ______________.

16. The total amount of energy used by the body per day is the ______________ ______________ ______________.

17. Maintaining homeostasis of temperature is the function of the ________________.

18. All the chemical reactions that release energy from food molecules make up the process of ______________.

19. The many chemical reactions that build food molecules into more complex chemical compounds constitute the process of ____________________.

20. Four fat-soluble vitamins that can be stored in the liver for later use are: ____________, ____________, ______________, and ______________.

CHAPTER 17

The Urinary System

Living produces wastes. Wherever people live or work or play, wastes accumulate. To keep these areas healthy, there must be a method—such as a sanitation department—of disposing of these wastes.

Wastes accumulate in your body also. The conversion of food and gases into substances and energy necessary for survival results in waste products. A large percentage of these wastes is removed by the urinary system.

Two vital organs, the kidneys, cleanse the blood of the many waste products that are continually produced as a result of the metabolism of food in the body cells. They eliminate these wastes in the form of urine.

Urine formation is the result of three processes: filtration, reabsorption, and secretion. These processes occur in successive portions of the microscopic units of the kidneys known as *nephrons*. The amount of urine produced by the nephrons is controlled primarily by the hormones ADH and aldosterone.

After urine is produced it is drained from the renal pelvis by the ureters to flow into the bladder. The bladder then stores the urine until it is voided through the urethra.

If waste products are allowed to accumulate in the body they soon become poisonous, a condition called *uremia*. Knowledge of the urinary system is necessary to understand how the body rids itself of waste and avoids toxicity.

TOPICS FOR REVIEW

Before progressing to Chapter 18 you should have an understanding of the structure and function of the organs of the urinary system. Your review should include knowledge of the nephron and its role in urine production. Your study should conclude with a review of the three main processes involved in urine production and the mechanisms that control urine volume.

KIDNEYS

Multiple Choice

Select the best answer.

1. The outermost portion of the kidney is known as the:
   A. Medulla
   B. Papilla
   C. Pelvis
   D. Pyramid
   E. Cortex

2. The saclike structure that surrounds the glomerulus is the:
   A. Renal pelvis
   B. Calyx
   C. Bowman's capsule
   D. Cortex
   E. None of the above

3. The renal corpuscle is made up of the:
   A. Bowman's capsule and proximal convoluted tubule
   B. Glomerulus and proximal convoluted tubule
   C. Bowman's capsule and the distal convoluted tubule
   D. Glomerulus and the distal convoluted tubule
   E. Bowman's capsule and the glomerulus

4. Which of the following functions is *not* performed by the kidneys?
   A. Maintenance of homeostasis
   B. Removal of wastes from the blood
   C. Production of ADH
   D. Removal of electrolytes from the blood

5. ____________ percent of the glomerular filtrate is reabsorbed.
   A. Twenty
   B. Forty
   C. Seventy-five
   D. Eighty-five
   E. Ninety-nine

6. The glomerular filtration rate is ________________ ml per minute.
   A. 1.25
   B. 12.5
   C. 125.0
   D. 1250.0
   E. None of the above

7. Glucose is reabsorbed in the:
   A. Loop of Henle
   B. Proximal convoluted tubule
   C. Distal convoluted tubule
   D. Glomerulus
   E. None of the above

8. Reabsorption does *not* occur in the:
   A. Loop of Henle
   B. Proximal convoluted tubule
   C. Distal convoluted tubule
   D. Collecting tubules
   E. Calyx

9. The greater the amount of salt intake, the:
   A. Less salt excreted in the urine
   B. More salt is reabsorbed
   C. More salt excreted in the urine
   D. None of the above

10. Which one of the following substances is secreted by diffusion?
    A. Sodium ions
    B. Certain drugs
    C. Ammonia
    D. Hydrogen ions
    E. Potassium ions

11. Which of the following statements about ADH is *not* true?
    A. It is stored by the pituitary gland.
    B. It makes the collecting tubules less permeable to water.
    C. It makes the distal convoluted tubules more permeable.
    D. It is produced by the hypothalamus.

12. Which of the following statements about aldosterone is *not* true?
    A. It is secreted by the adrenal cortex.
    B. It is a water-retaining hormone.
    C. It is a salt-retaining hormone.
    D. All of the above are correct.

If you have had difficulty with this section, review pages 392-403.

Matching

Choose the correct term and write the letter in the space next to the appropriate definition below.

A. Medulla
B. Cortex
C. Pyramids
D. Papilla
E. Pelvis
F. Calyx
G. Nephrons
H. Uremia
I. Proteinuria
J. Bowman's capsule
K. Glomerulus
L. Loop of Henle
M. CAPD
N. Glycosuria

G 13. Functioning unit of urinary system
I 14. Abnormally large amounts of plasma proteins in the urine
H 15. Uremic poisoning
B 16. Outer part of kidney
K 17. Together with Bowman's capsule forms renal corpuscle
F 18. Division of the renal pelvis
J 19. Cup-shaped top of a nephron
D 20. Innermost end of a pyramid
L 21. Extension of proximal tubule
C 22. Triangular-shaped divisions of the medulla of the kidney
M 23. Used in the treatment of renal failure
A 24. Inner portion of kidney

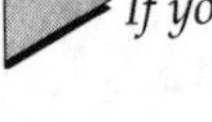
If you have had difficulty with this section, review pages 392-403.

URETERS, URINARY BLADDER, URETHRA

Indicate which organ is identified by the following descriptions by writing the appropriate letter in the answer blank.

(A) Ureters (B) Bladder (C) Urethra

B 25. Rugae
C 26. Lowermost part of urinary tract
A 27. Lining membrane richly supplied with sensory nerve endings
B 28. Lies behind pubic symphysis
C 29. Dual function in male
C 30. 1½ inches long in female
A 31. Drains renal pelvis
C 32. Surrounded by prostate in male
B 33. Elastic fibers and involuntary muscle fibers
A 34. 10–12 inches long
B 35. Trigone

Fill in the blanks.

36. ______________ ______________ is the description of the pain caused by the passage of a kidney stone.

37. The urinary tract is lined with ______________ ______________.

38. Another name for kidney stones is ______________ ______________.

39. A technique that uses ______________ to pulverize stones, thus avoiding surgery, is being used to treat kidney stones.

40. Older people generally have a lower overall lean body mass, and therefore, a(n) ______________ production of waste products that must be excreted from the body.

41. The ______________ ______________ is the basinlike upper end of the ureter located inside the kidney.

42. In the male, the urethra serves as a passageway for both urine and ______________.

43. The external opening of the urethra is the ______________ ______________.

If you have had difficulty with this section, review pages 403-407.

MICTURITION

Fill in the blanks.

The terms (44) ______________, (45) ______________ and (46) ______________ all refer to the passage of urine from the body or the emptying of the bladder. The sphincters guard the bladder. The (47) ______________ ______________ sphincter is located at the bladder (48) ______________ and is involuntary. The external urethral sphincter is formed of (49) ______________ muscle and is under (50) ______________ control.

As the bladder fills, nervous impulses are transmitted to the spinal cord and a(n) (51) ______________ ______________ is initiated. Urine then enters the (52) ______________ to be eliminated.

Urinary (53) ______________ is a condition in which no urine is voided. Urinary (54) ______________ is when the kidneys do not produce any urine, but the bladder retains its ability to empty itself. The term (55) ______________ ______________ refers to the urge for frequent urination with or without incontinence.

If you have had difficulty with this section, review pages 405-407.

UNSCRAMBLE THE WORDS

Take the circled letters, unscramble them, and fill in the statement.

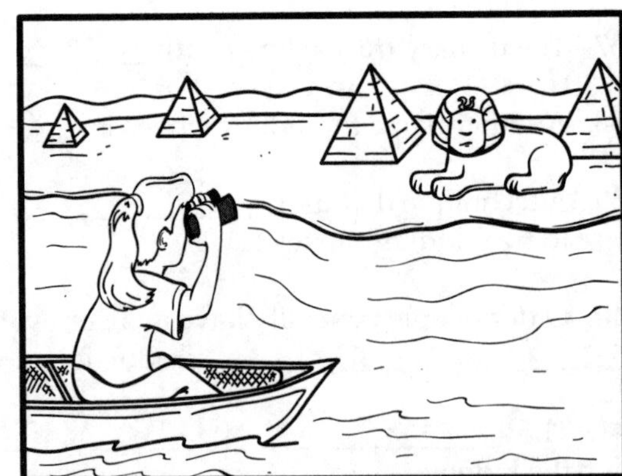

56. **AYXLC**

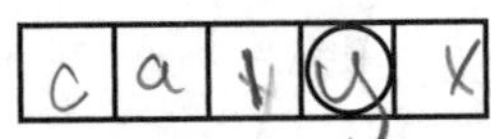

57. **GVNOIDI**

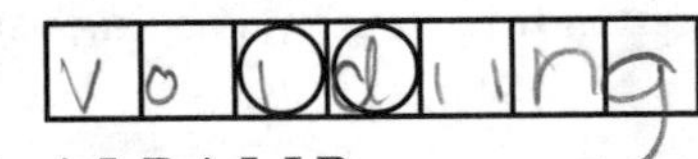

58. **ALPALIP**

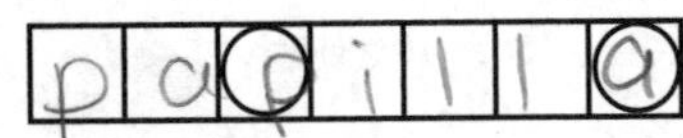

59. **SGULLOUMRE**

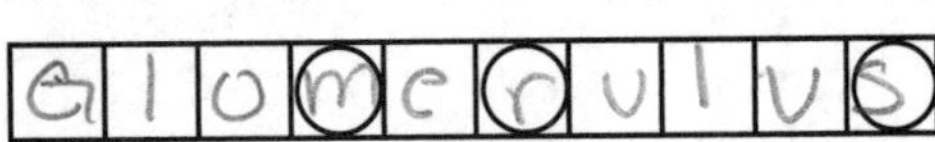

What Betty saw while cruising down the Nile.

60.

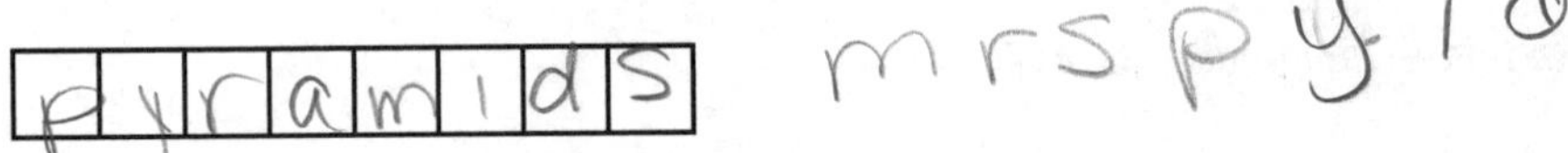

mrspyid

APPLYING WHAT YOU KNOW

61. John suffered from low levels of ADH. What primary urinary symptom would he notice?

polyuria

62. Bud was in a diving accident and his spinal cord was severed. He was paralyzed from the waist down and as a result was incontinent. His physician was concerned about the continuous residual urine build-up. What was the reason for concern?

often a cause of repeated cystitis

63. Caryl had a prolonged surgical procedure and experienced problems with urinary retention postoperatively. A urinary catheter was inserted into her bladder for the elimination of urine. Several days later Caryl developed cystitis. What might be a possible cause?

poor insertion techniques

64. WORD FIND

Can you find 18 terms from the chapter in the box of letters? Words may be spelled top to bottom, bottom to top, right to left, left to right, or diagonally.

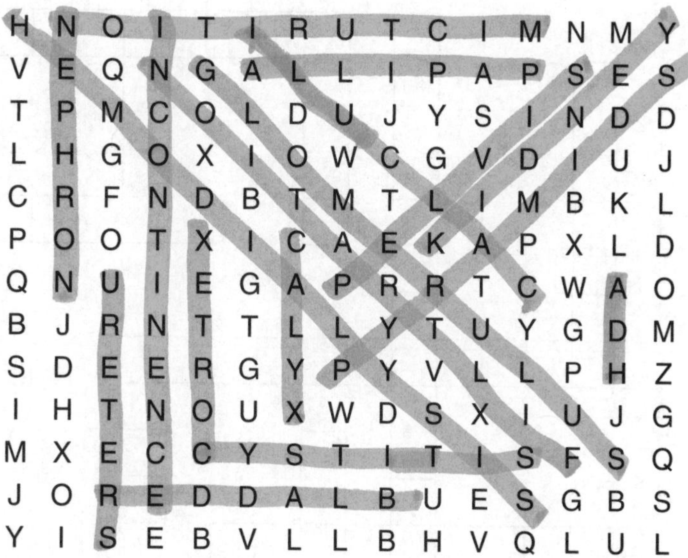

ADH	Filtration	Micturition
Bladder	Glomerulus	Nephron
Calculi	Hemodialysis	Papilla
Calyx	Incontinence	Pelvis
Cortex	Kidney	Pyramids
Cystitis	Medulla	Ureters

DID YOU KNOW?

If the tubules in a kidney were stretched out and untangled, there would be 70 miles of them.

While examining urine, German chemist Hennig Brand discovered phosphorus.

People adrift at sea or lost in the desert for long periods often resort to drinking their urine when no rainwater is available. This, however, will not prevent you from dying of dehydration, especially if it causes vomiting.

URINARY SYSTEM

Fill in the crossword puzzle.

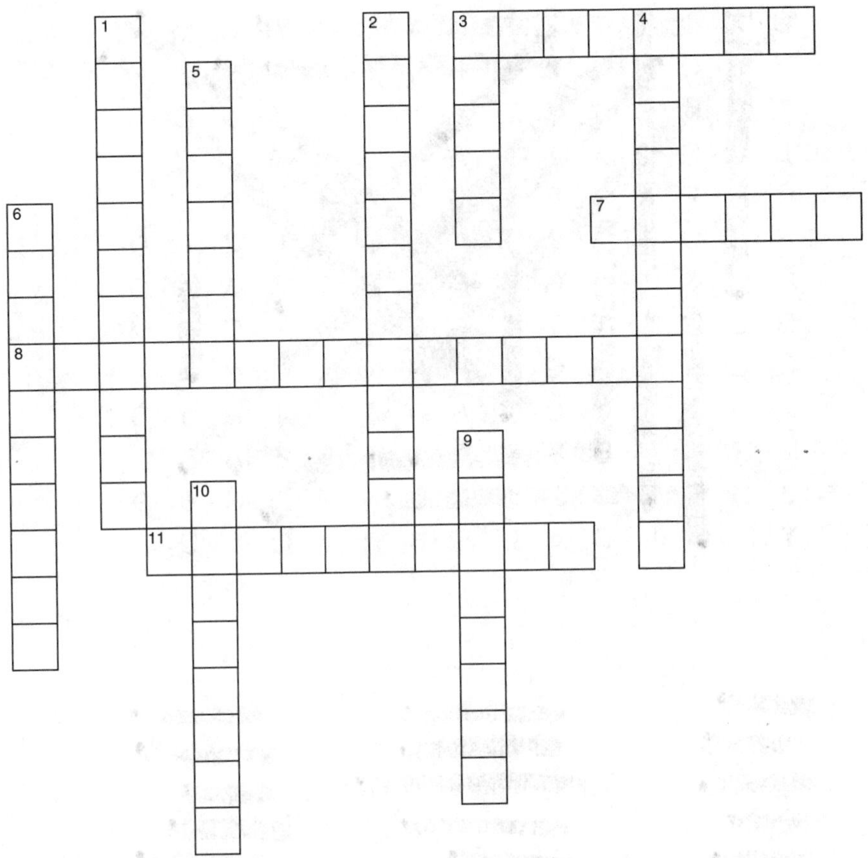

Across

3. Bladder infection
7. Absence of urine
8. Passage of a tube into the bladder to withdraw urine
11. Network of blood capillaries tucked into Bowman's capsule

Down

1. Urination
2. Ultrasound generator used to break up kidney stones
3. Division of the renal pelvis
4. Voiding involuntarily
5. Area on posterior bladder wall free of rugae
6. Glucose in the urine
9. Large amount of urine
10. Scanty urine

CHECK YOUR KNOWLEDGE

Multiple Choice

Select the best answer.

1. Which of the following is *not* true of the kidneys?
   A. The right kidney is lower than the left.
   B. They are retroperitoneal.
   C. The rate of blood flow through the kidneys is among the highest in the body.
   D. All of the above are true.

2. Bowman's capsule and the glomerulus make up the:
   A. Renal tubule
   B. Renal corpuscle
   C. Loop of Henle
   D. Collecting tubule

3. The kidneys serve the body by:
   A. Maintaining homeostasis
   B. Excreting toxins and waste products containing nitrogen
   C. Regulating the proper balance between body water content and salt
   D. All of the above

4. Urine formation begins with:
   A. Glomerular filtration
   B. The proximal convoluted tubule
   C. The distal convoluted tubule
   D. The loop of Henle

5. A well-known sign of diabetes mellitus is:
   A. Proteinuria
   B. Oliguria
   C. Glycosuria
   D. Anuria

6. A lithotriptor is used for:
   A. Diabetes mellitus
   B. Incontinence
   C. Renal calculi
   D. Oliguria

7. Aldosterone:
   A. Assists in controlling the kidney tubules' excretion of salt
   B. Stimulates the tubules to reabsorb sodium salts at a faster rate
   C. Decreases tubular water reabsorption
   D. Is a salt- and water-losing hormone

8. Control of urine volume is maintained primarily by the:
   A. Bowman's capsule
   B. Loop of Henle
   C. ADH from the posterior pituitary gland
   D. Kidney tubule

9. Which is *not* a part of the kidney?
   A. Cortex
   B. Trigone
   C. Medulla
   D. Pyramids

10. Which of the following is *not* a primary process in urine formation?
   A. Active transport
   B. Filtration
   C. Reabsorption
   D. Secretion

Matching

Select the most correct answer from column B for each statement in column A. (Only one answer is correct.)

Column A	Column B
E 11. Uremia	A. Urinary bladder infection
C 12. Nephrons	B. Triangular divisions of medulla of kidney
F 13. Renal tubule	C. Microscopic units of kidney
D 14. Juxtaglomerular apparatus	D. Blood pressure regulation
J 15. Secretion	E. Uremic poisoning
H 16. CAPD	F. Loop of Henle
A 17. Cystitis	G. Relaxation of internal sphincter
G 18. Emptying reflex	H. Renal failure
I 19. Calyces	I. Divisions of renal pelvis
B 20. Pyramids	J. Hydrogen and potassium ions

URINARY SYSTEM

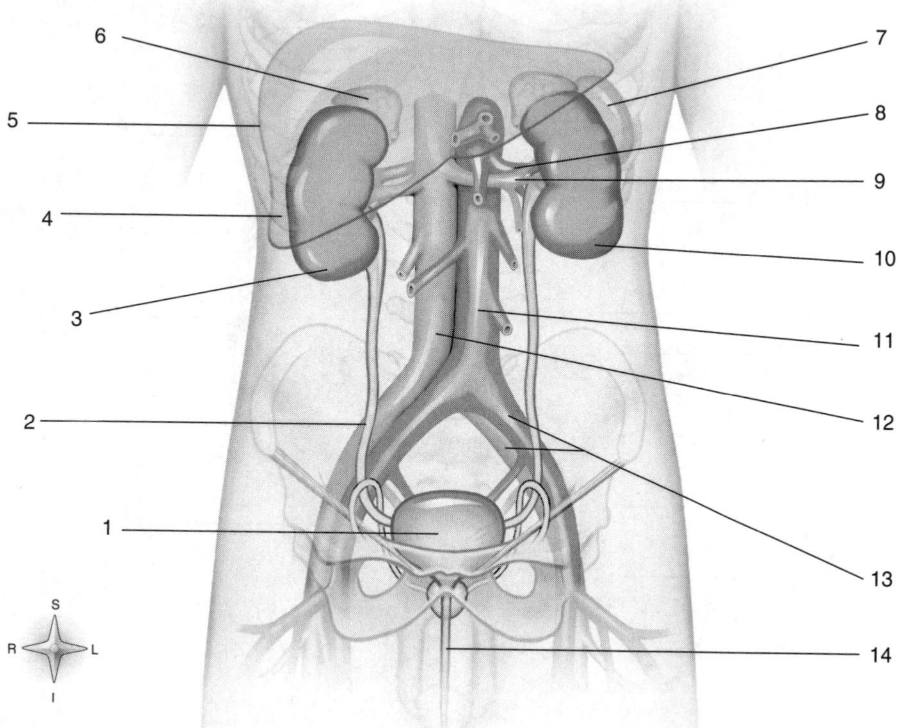

1. bladder
2. ureter
3. kidney (R)
4. 12 rib
5. liver
6. adronal gland
7. Spleen
8. Renal artery
9. Renal vein
10. kidney (L)
11. arota
12. Inferior vena cava
13. common illiac vein/artery
14. urethra.

KIDNEY

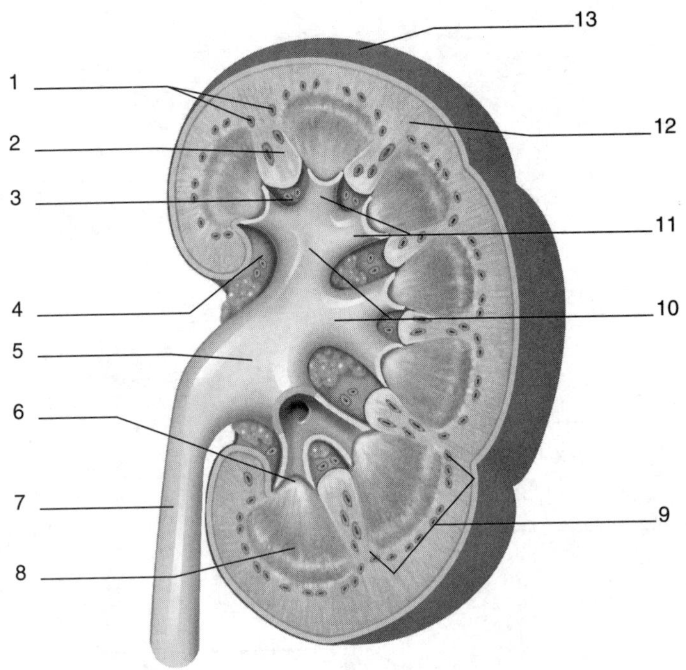

1. arteries
2. renal colum
3. renal sinuses
4. Hilum
5. renal pelvis
6. renal pyramid
7. urtere
8. medulla
9. medulla pyramid
10. mayor calyces
11. minor calyces
12. curtex
13. capsule

NEPHRON

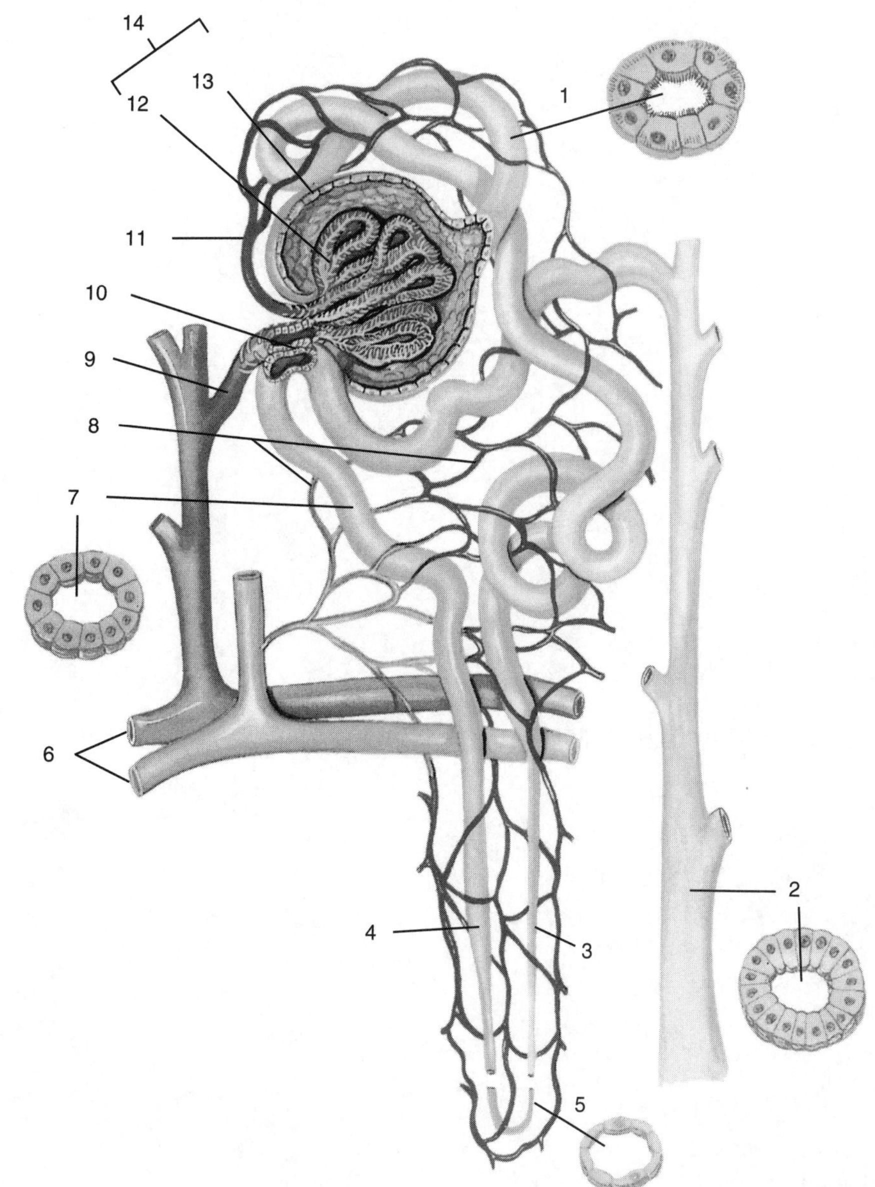

1. convolated tubule
2. collecting duct
3. a luup of henle
4. d luup of henle
5. arterics & veins
6. distal tubule
7. peritubular capillanes
8. peritubular capillanes
9. afferent atriole
10.
11. efferent arteria
12. glomerulus
13. bowmans capsule
14. renal corpuse

CHAPTER 18

Fluid and Electrolyte Balance

In the very first chapter of the text, you learned that survival depends on the body's ability to maintain or restore homeostasis. Specifically, *homeostasis* means that the body fluids remain constant within very narrow limits. These fluids are classified as either intracellular fluid (ICF) or extracellular fluid (ECF). As the names imply, intracellular fluid lies within the cells and extracellular fluid is located outside the cells. A balance between these two fluids is maintained by certain body mechanisms: (a) the adjustment of fluid output to fluid intake under normal circumstances; (b) the concentration of electrolytes in the extracellular fluid; (c) the capillary blood pressure; and (d) the concentration of proteins in the blood.

Comprehension of how these mechanisms maintain and restore fluid balance is necessary for an understanding of the complexities of homeostasis and its relationship to the survival of the individual.

TOPICS FOR REVIEW

Before progressing to Chapter 19, you should review the types of body fluids and their subdivisions. Your study should include the mechanisms that maintain fluid balance and the nature and importance of electrolytes in body fluids. You should be able to give examples of common fluid imbalances and have an understanding of the role of fluid and electrolyte balance in the maintenance of homeostasis.

BODY FLUIDS

Circle the correct answer.

1. The largest volume of body fluid by far lies (inside or outside) cells.

2. Interstitial fluid is (intracellular or extracellular).

3. Plasma is (intracellular or extracellular).

4. Obese people have a (lower or higher) water content per pound of body weight than thin people.

5. Infants have (more or less) water in comparison to body weight than adults of either sex.

6. There is a rapid (increase or decline) in the proportion of body water to body weight during the first 10 years of life.

7. The female body contains slightly (more or less) water per pound of weight.

8. In general, as age increases, the amount of water per pound of body weight (increases or decreases).

9. Excluding adipose tissue, approximately (55% or 85%) of body weight is water.

10. The term (fluid balance or fluid compartments) means the volumes of ICF, IF, plasma, and the total volume of water in the body all remain relatively constant.

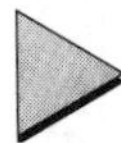
If you have had difficulty with this section, review pages 413-415.

MECHANISMS THAT MAINTAIN FLUID BALANCE

Multiple Choice

Select the best answer.

11. Which one of the following is a positively charged ion?
    A. Sodium
    B. Chloride
    C. Phosphate
    D. Bicarbonate

12. Which one of the following is a negatively charged ion?
    A. Sodium
    B. Potassium
    C. Calcium
    D. Chloride

13. The most abundant electrolytes in the blood plasma are:
    A. NaCl
    B. KMg
    C. HCO_3
    D. HPO_4
    E. $CaPO_4$

14. If the blood sodium concentration increases, then blood volume will:
    A. Increase
    B. Decrease
    C. Remain the same
    D. None of the above

15. The smallest amount of water comes from:
    A. Water in foods that are eaten
    B. Ingested liquids
    C. Water formed from catabolism
    D. None of the above

16. The greatest amount of water lost from the body is from the:
    A. Lungs
    B. Skin, by diffusion
    C. Skin, by sweat
    D. Feces
    E. Kidneys

17. Which one of the following is *not* a major factor that influences extracellular and intracellular fluid volumes?
    A. The concentration of electrolytes in the extracellular fluid
    B. The capillary blood pressure
    C. The concentration of proteins in blood
    D. All of the above are major factors

18. The type of fluid output that changes the most is:
    A. Water loss in the feces
    B. Water loss across the skin
    C. Water loss via the lungs
    D. Water loss in the urine
    E. None of the above

19. The chief regulators of sodium within the body is (are) the:
    A. Lungs
    B. Sweat glands
    C. Kidneys
    D. Large intestine
    E. None of the above

20. Which of the following is *not* correct?
    A. Fluid output must equal fluid intake.
    B. ADH controls salt reabsorption in the kidney.
    C. Water follows sodium.
    D. Renal tubule regulation of salt and water is the most important factor in determining urine volume.

21. Diuretics work on all of the following *except*:
    A. Proximal tubule
    B. Loop of Henle
    C. Distal tubule
    D. Collecting ducts
    E. Diuretics work on all of the above

22. Of all the sodium-containing secretions, the one with the largest volume is:
    A. Saliva
    B. Gastric secretions
    C. Bile
    D. Pancreatic juice
    E. Intestinal secretions

23. The higher the capillary blood pressure, the ____________ the amount of interstitial fluid.
    A. Smaller
    B. Larger
    C. There is no relationship between capillary blood pressure and volume of interstitial fluid

24. An increase in capillary blood pressure will lead to ____________ in blood volume.
    A. An increase
    B. A decrease
    C. No change
    D. None of the above

25. Which one of the fluid compartments varies the most in volume?
    A. Intracellular
    B. Interstitial
    C. Extracellular
    D. Plasma

26. Which one of the following will *not* cause edema?
    A. Retention of electrolytes in the extracellular fluid
    B. Increase in capillary blood pressure
    C. Burns
    D. Decrease in plasma proteins
    E. All of the above may cause edema

True or False

If the statement is true, write "T" in the answer blank. If the statement is false, correct the statement by circling the incorrect term and writing the correct term in the answer blank.

__________ 27. The three sources of fluid intake are the liquids we drink, the foods we eat, and the water formed by the anabolism of foods.

__________ 28. The body maintains fluid balance mainly by changing the volume of urine excreted to match changes in the volume of fluid intake.

__________ 29. Some output of fluid will occur as long as life continues.

__________ 30. Glucose is an example of an electrolyte.

__________ 31. Where sodium goes, water soon follows.

__________ 32. Excess aldosterone leads to hypovolemia.

__________ 33. Diuretics have their effect on glomerular function.

__________ 34. Typical daily intake and output totals should be approximately 1200 ml.

__________ 35. Bile is a sodium-containing internal secretion.

__________ 36. The average daily diet contains about 500 mEq of sodium.

If you have had difficulty with this section, review pages 415-421.

FLUID IMBALANCES

Fill in the blanks.

(37)__________ is the fluid imbalance seen most often. In this condition, interstitial fluid volume (38) __________ first, but eventually, if treatment has not been given, intracellular fluid and plasma volumes (39) __________. (40) __________ can also occur, but is much less common.

Giving (41) __________ __________ too rapidly or in too large amounts can put too heavy a burden on the (42) __________.

If you have had difficulty with this section, review pages 421-422.

UNSCRAMBLE THE WORDS

Take the circled letters, unscramble them, and fill in the statement.

43. **MDEEA**

44. **DFILU**

45. **NIO**

46. **SOUITNVAREN**

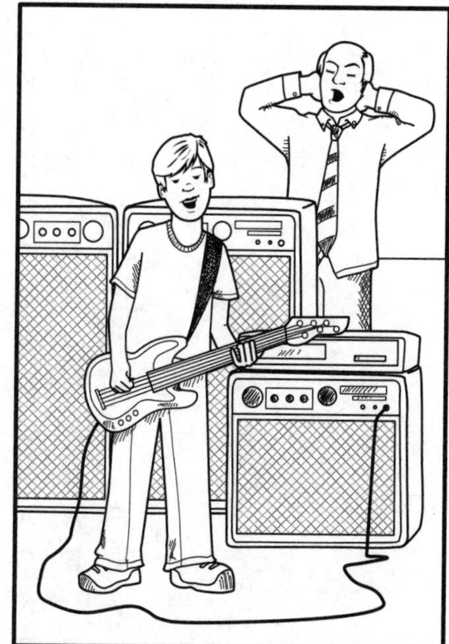

What Gary's dad disliked most about his music.

47.

APPLYING WHAT YOU KNOW

48. Mrs. Titus was asked to keep an accurate record of her fluid intake and output. She was concerned because the two did not balance. What is a possible explanation for this?

49. Nurse Briker was caring for a patient who was receiving diuretics. What special nursing implications should be followed for patients on this therapy?

50. WORD FIND

Can you find the 12 terms from this chapter in the box of letters? Words may be spelled top to bottom, bottom to top, right to left, left to right, or diagonally.

```
S T V H O M E O S T A S I S H
I E D E M A S Q A L P U E G L
M M L U F L U I D O Y O I S L
W S B E A E C O L D P N I E R
L I T A C V S H Q O C E H B C
L L X J L T E A W Y B V Q Q O
I O O P E A R U C T C A A R I
N B H R X S N O I I P R T C N
S A O X M G J C L N J T B A H
I N X X D V U D E Y K N Y O C
E A A J Q D I U R E T I C S X
I F C J A M P V E N B E Y F W
V F K T Q X R M D D S I V O T
E T T Z N T R P X I M L J F I
S W Y A P V Q N S K T K W B P
```

Aldosterone	Edema	Imbalance
Anabolism	Electrolyte	Intravenous
Catabolism	Fluid	Ions
Diuretics	Homeostasis	Kidney

DID YOU KNOW?

The best fluid replacement drink is 1/4 teaspoon of table salt to 1 quart of water.

If all of the water were drained from the body of an average 160-pound man, the body would weigh 64 pounds.

The average person can live up to 11 days without water, assuming a mean environmental temperature of 60° F.

FLUID/ELECTROLYTES

Fill in the crossword puzzle.

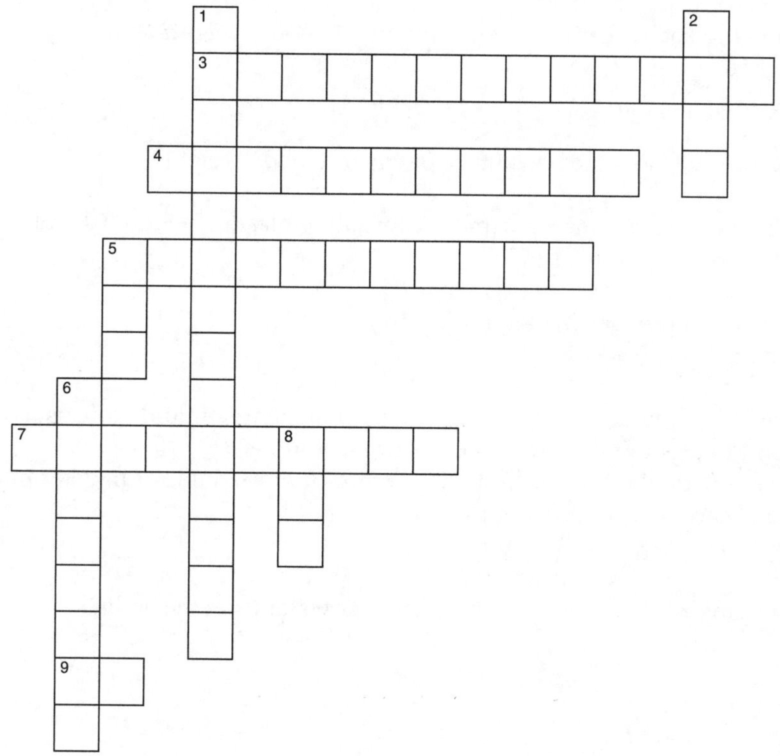

Across

3. Result of rapidly given intravenous fluids
4. Result of large loss of body fluids
5. Compound that dissociates in solution into ions
7. To break up
9. A subdivision of extracellular fluid (abbreviation)

Down

1. Organic substance that doesn't dissociate in solution
2. Dissociated particles of an electrolyte that carry an electrical charge
5. Fluid outside cells (abbreviation)
6. "Causing urine"
8. Fluid inside cells (abbreviation)

CHECK YOUR KNOWLEDGE

Multiple Choice

Select the best answer.

1. Which of the following have the most water compared to body weight?
   A. Infants
   B. Females
   C. Males
   D. All of the above have the same percentage of water to body weight

2. Which of the following acts as a mechanism for controlling plasma, IF, and ICF volumes?
   A. The concentration of electrolytes in ECF
   B. The capillary blood pressure
   C. The concentration of proteins in blood
   D. All of the above

3. Which of the following statements is true regarding maintenance of fluid homeostasis?
   A. The type of fluid output that changes most is urine volume.
   B. Renal tubule regulation of salt and water is the most important factor in determining urine volume.
   C. The presence of sodium causes water to move.
   D. All of the above are true.

4. Which of the following is *not* a normal portal of exit for water from the body?
   A. Diffusion
   B. Lungs
   C. Water formed by catabolism
   D. Intestines

5. The fluid imbalance that is seen most often is:
   A. Dehydration
   B. Increased plasma volumes
   C. Overhydration
   D. Sunstroke

6. Congestive heart failure is the most common cause of:
   A. Overhydration
   B. Edema
   C. Dehydration
   D. Decreased capillary hydrostatic pressure

7. The kidney acts as the chief regulator of:
   A. Aldosterone
   B. Ingested liquids
   C. Perspiration
   D. Sodium in body fluids

8. Excess aldosterone leads to:
   A. Hypervolemia
   B. Hypovolemia
   C. Hypertension
   D. Hypotension

9. Which of the following is the most abundant body fluid in a young adult male?
   A. Intracellular fluid
   B. Interstitial fluid
   C. Plasma
   D. Blood

10. The average ingested liquid intake per day is:
    A. 500 ml
    B. 750 ml
    C. 1000 ml
    D. 1500 ml

Matching

Select the most correct answer from column B for each statement in column A. (Only one answer is correct.)

Column A	Column B
_____ 11. Extracellular	A. Glucose
_____ 12. Intracellular	B. Inside cells
_____ 13. Nonelectrolyte	C. Homeostasis
_____ 14. Electrolyte	D. Stimulates production of urine
_____ 15. Diuretic	E. Plasma
_____ 16. Fluid balance	F. Fluid imbalance
_____ 17. Edema	G. Dehydration
_____ 18. Prolonged diarrhea	H. Overhydration
_____ 19. Rapid IV fluids	I. "Water-pushing" force
_____ 20. Capillary blood pressure	J. Table salt
_____ 21. Kwashiorkor	K. Positively charged ions
_____ 22. ANH	L. Hormone
_____ 23. Anions	M. Negatively charged ions
_____ 24. Pitting edema	N. Subcutaneous swelling in ankles and feet
_____ 25. Cations	O. Decrease in concentration of plasma proteins

CHAPTER 19

Acid-Base Balance

It has been established in previous chapters that an equilibrium between intracellular and extracellular fluid volume must exist for homeostasis to be maintained. Equally important to homeostasis is the chemical acid-base balance of the body fluids. The degree of acidity or alkalinity of a body fluid is expressed in pH value. The neutral point, where a fluid would be neither acid nor alkaline, is pH 7. Increasing acidity is expressed as less than 7, and increasing alkalinity is expressed as greater than 7. Examples of body fluids that are acidic are gastric juice (1.6) and urine (6.0). Blood, on the other hand, is considered alkaline with a pH of 7.45.

Buffers are substances that prevent a sharp change in the pH of a fluid when an acid or base is added to it. They are one of several mechanisms that are constantly monitoring the pH of fluids in the body. If, for any reason, these mechanisms do not function properly, a pH imbalance occurs. These two kinds of imbalances are known as *alkalosis* and *acidosis*.

Maintaining the acid-base balance of body fluids is a matter of vital importance. If this balance varies even slightly, necessary chemical and cellular reactions cannot occur. Your review of this chapter is necessary to understand the delicate acid-base balance necessary to survival.

TOPICS FOR REVIEW

Before progressing to Chapter 20 you should have an understanding of the pH of body fluids and the mechanisms that control the pH of these fluids in the body. Your study should conclude with a review of the metabolic and respiratory types of pH imbalances.

pH OF BODY

Choose the correct term from the options given and write the letter in the answer blank.

(A) Acid (B) Base

_____ 1. Lower concentration of hydrogen ions than hydroxide ions

_____ 2. Higher concentration of hydrogen ions than hydroxide ions

_____ 3. Gastric juice

_____ 4. Saliva

_____ 5. Arterial blood

_____ 6. Venous blood

_____ 7. Baking soda

_____ 8. Beer

_____ 9. Ammonia

_____ 10. Pancreatic fluid

If you have had difficulty with this section, review pages 426-429.

MECHANISMS THAT CONTROL pH OF BODY FLUIDS pH IMBALANCES

Multiple Choice

Select the best answer.

11. When carbon dioxide enters the blood, it reacts with the enzyme carbonic anhydrase to form:
    A. Sodium bicarbonate
    B. Water and carbon dioxide
    C. Ammonium chloride
    D. Bicarbonate ion
    E. Carbonic acid

12. The lungs remove _______________ liters of carbonic acid each day.
    A. 10
    B. 15
    C. 20
    D. 25
    E. 30

13. When a buffer reacts with a strong acid it changes the strong acid to a:
    A. Weak acid
    B. Strong base
    C. Weak base
    D. Water
    E. None of the above

14. Which one of the following is *not* a change in the blood that results from the buffering of fixed acids in tissue capillaries?
    A. The amount of carbonic acid increases slightly.
    B. The amount of bicarbonate in blood decreases.
    C. The hydrogen ion concentration of blood increases slightly.
    D. The blood pH decreases slightly.
    E. All of the above are changes that result from the buffering of fixed acids in tissue capillaries.

15. The most abundant acid in the body is:
    A. HCl
    B. Lactic acid
    C. Carbonic acid
    D. Acetic acid
    E. Sulfuric acid

16. The normal ratio of sodium bicarbonate to carbonic acid in arterial blood is:
    A. 5:1
    B. 10:1
    C. 15:1
    D. 20:1
    E. None of the above

17. Which of the following would *not* be a consequence of holding your breath?
    A. The amount of carbonic acid in the blood increases.
    B. The blood pH decreases.
    C. The body develops an alkalosis.
    D. No carbon dioxide leaves the body.

18. Which of the following is *not* true of the kidneys?
    A. They can eliminate larger amounts of acid than the lungs.
    B. More bases than acids are usually excreted by the kidneys.
    C. If the kidneys fail, homeostasis of acid-base balance fails.
    D. They are the most effective regulators of blood pH.

19. The pH of the urine may be as low as:
    A. 1.6
    B. 2.5
    C. 3.2
    D. 4.8
    E. 7.4

20. In the distal tubule cells, the product of the reaction aided by carbonic anhydrase is:
    A. Water
    B. Carbon dioxide
    C. Water and carbon dioxide
    D. Hydrogen ions
    E. Carbonic acid

21. In the distal tubule, ________________ leaves the tubule cells and enters the blood capillaries.
    A. Carbon dioxide
    B. Water
    C. HCO_3
    D. NaH_2PO_4
    E. $NaHCO_3$

True or False

If the statement is true, write "T" in the answer blank. If the statement is false, correct the statement by circling the incorrect term and writing the correct term in the answer blank.

_______________ 22. The body has three mechanisms for regulating the pH of its fluids. They are the heart mechanism, the respiratory mechanism, and the urinary mechanism.

_______________ 23. Buffers consist of two kinds of substances and are, therefore, often called duobuffers.

_______________ 24. Ordinary baking soda is one of the main buffers of the normally occurring "fixed" acids in the blood.

_______________ 25. The accumulation of ketone bodies in the blood results from excessive metabolism of fats most often seen in uncontrolled type 1 diabetes.

_______________ 26. Anything that causes an excessive increase in respirations will in time produce acidosis.

_______________ 27. The lungs are the body's most effective regulator of blood pH.

_______________ 28. More acids than bases are usually excreted by the kidneys because more acids than bases usually enter the blood.

_______________ 29. Blood levels of sodium bicarbonate can be regulated by the lungs.

_______________ 30. Blood levels of carbonic acid can be regulated by the kidneys.

If you have had difficulty with this section, review pages 429-434.

pH IMBALANCES
METABOLIC AND RESPIRATORY DISTURBANCES
VOMITING

Write the letter of the correct term on the blank next to the appropriate definition.

A. Metabolic acidosis
B. Metabolic alkalosis
C. Respiratory acidosis
D. Respiratory alkalosis
E. Vomiting
F. Normal saline
G. Ketoacidosis
H. Hyperventilation
I. Hypersalivation
J. Anxiety

_____ 31. Emesis
_____ 32. Uncontrolled type 1 diabetes
_____ 33. Chloride-containing solution
_____ 34. Bicarbonate deficit
_____ 35. Present during emesis
_____ 36. Bicarbonate excess
_____ 37. Rapid breathing
_____ 38. Carbonic acid excess
_____ 39. Carbonic acid deficit
_____ 40. Hyperventilation syndrome

If you have had difficulty with this section, review pages 434-437.

ACID/BASE BALANCE

Fill in the crossword puzzle.

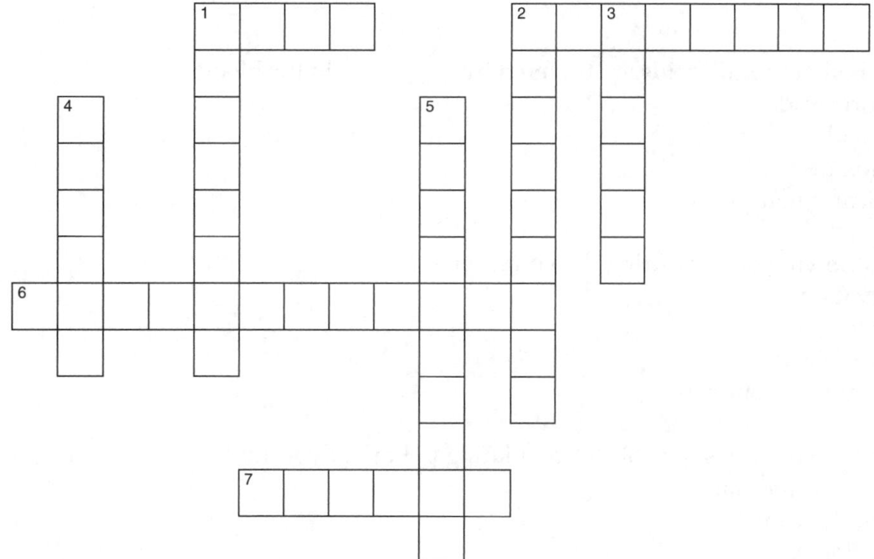

Across

1. Substance with a pH lower than 7.0
2. Acid-base imbalance
6. Results from the excessive metabolism of fats in uncontrolled diabetics (2 words)
7. Vomitus

Down

1. Substance with a pH higher than 7.0
2. Serious complication of vomiting
3. Emetic
4. Prevents a sharp change in the pH of fluids
5. Released as a waste product from working muscles (2 words)

CHECK YOUR KNOWLEDGE

Multiple Choice

Select the best answer.

1. A pH lower than 7.0 indicates:
   A. An acid solution
   B. An alkaline solution
   C. A lower concentration of hydrogen than hydroxide ions
   D. Both A and C

2. The overall pH range is expressed numerically on what is called a(n):
   A. pH calculator
   B. Acid-base numerator
   C. Logarithmic scale of 1–14
   D. Hydrogen-hydroxide value indicator

3. Chemical substances that prevent a sharp change in the pH of a fluid when an acid or base is added to it are called:
   A. Buffers
   B. Ketone bodies
   C. Enzymes
   D. Fixed acids

4. Lactic acid and other "fixed" acids are buffered by ________ in the blood.
   A. Hydrochloric acid
   B. Carbonic acid
   C. Carbon dioxide
   D. Sodium bicarbonate

5. Which of the following occurs during the vomit reflex?
   A. Hypersalivation
   B. Glottis opens
   C. Diaphragm relaxes
   D. Cardiac sphincter contracts

6. Which of the following is responsible for regulating pH of body fluids?
   A. Respiratory mechanism
   B. Urinary mechanism
   C. Buffer mechanism
   D. All of the above

7. Which of the following statements regarding metabolic disturbances is correct?
   A. Metabolic acidosis is a bicarbonate deficit.
   B. Metabolic alkalosis is a bicarbonate excess.
   C. Metabolic alkalosis is a complication of severe vomiting.
   D. All of the above are correct.

8. Which of the following statements regarding respiratory disturbances is correct?
   A. Depression of the respiratory center by drugs or disease can cause respiratory acidosis.
   B. Hyperventilation can result in respiratory alkalosis.
   C. Excess carbon dioxide in the arterial blood contributes to respiratory acidosis.
   D. All of the above are correct.

9. The key to acid-base balance is the:
   A. CO_2 ratio
   B. Buffer mechanism
   C. Ratio of respirations to blood pH levels
   D. Ratio of $NaHCO_3$ to H_2CO_3

10. A rare, but serious, complication of the medication Glucophage for type 2 diabetes is:
    A. Lactic acidosis
    B. Respiratory alkalosis
    C. Metabolic alkalosis
    D. None of the above

Matching

Select the most correct answer from column B for each statement in column A. (Only one answer is correct.)

Column A	Column B
_____ 11. Blood	A. Excessive fat metabolism
_____ 12. Gastric juice	B. Red blood cell enzyme
_____ 13. Aerobic respiration	C. Acid
_____ 14. "Fixed" acid	D. pH imbalance
_____ 15. Buffer	E. Lactic acid
_____ 16. Ketone bodies	F. Baking soda
_____ 17. Carbonic anhydrase	G. Alkaline
_____ 18. Acidosis	H. Respiratory acidosis
_____ 19. Hyperventilation	I. Cellular respiration
_____ 20. Emphysema	J. Respiratory alkalosis

CHAPTER 20

Reproductive Systems

The reproductive system consists of those organs that participate in perpetuating the species. It is a unique body system in that its organs differ between the two sexes and yet they work toward the same goal: creating a new life. Of interest also is the fact that this system is the only one not necessary to the survival of the individual, and yet survival of the species depends on its proper functioning. The male reproductive system is divided into the external genitals, the testes, the duct system, and accessory glands. The testes, or gonads, are considered essential organs because they produce the sex cells, sperm, that join with the female sex cells, ova, to form a new human being. They also secrete the male sex hormone, testosterone, which is responsible for the physical transformation of a boy to a man.

Sperm are formed in the testes by the seminiferous tubules. From there they enter a long narrow duct, the epididymis. They continue onward through the vas deferens into the ejaculatory duct, down the urethra, and out of the body. Throughout this journey, various glands secrete substances that add motility to the sperm and create a chemical environment conducive to reproduction.

The female reproductive system is truly extraordinary and diverse. It produces ova, receives the penis and sperm during intercourse, serves as the site of conception, houses and feeds the embryo during prenatal development, and nourishes the infant after birth.

Because of its diversity, the physiology of the female is generally considered to be more complex than that of the male. Much of the activity of this system revolves around the menstrual cycle and the monthly preparation that the female undergoes for a possible pregnancy.

The organs of the female system are divided into essential organs and accessory organs of reproduction. The essential organs of the female are the ovaries. Just as with the male, the essential organs of the female are referred to as the *gonads*. The gonads of both sexes produce the sex cells. In the male, the gonads produce the sperm and in the female they produce the ova. The gonads are also responsible for producing the hormones in each sex necessary for the appearance of the secondary sex characteristics.

The menstrual cycle of the female typically covers a period of 28 days. Each cycle consists of three phases: the menstrual period, the postmenstrual phase, and the premenstrual phase. Changes in the blood levels of the hormones that are responsible for the menstrual cycle also cause physical and emotional changes in the female. Knowledge of these phenomena and this system, in both the male and the female, are necessary to complete your understanding of the reproductive system.

TOPICS FOR REVIEW

Before progressing to Chapter 21 you should familiarize yourself with the structure and function of the organs of the male and female reproductive systems. Your review should include emphasis on the gross and microscopic structure of the testes and the production of sperm and testosterone. Your study should continue by tracing and understanding the pathway of a sperm cell from formation to expulsion from the body.

You should then familiarize yourself with the structure and function of the organs of the female reproductive system. Your review should include emphasis on the development of a mature ovum from ovarian follicles, and should additionally concentrate on the phases and occurrences in a typical 28-day menstrual cycle.

MALE REPRODUCTIVE SYSTEM STRUCTURAL PLAN

Match the term on the left with the proper selection on the right.

Group A

_____ 1. Testes — A. Fertilized ovum

_____ 2. Spermatozoa — B. Accessory organ

_____ 3. Ova — C. Male sex cell

_____ 4. Penis — D. Gonads

_____ 5. Zygote — E. Gamete

Group B

_____ 6. Testes — A. Cowper's gland

_____ 7. Bulbourethral — B. Scrotum

_____ 8. Asexual — C. Essential organ

_____ 9. External genitalia — D. Single parent

_____ 10. Prostate — E. Accessory organ

If you have had difficulty with this section, review pages 440-442.

TESTES

Multiple Choice

Select the best answer.

11. The testes are surrounded by a tough membrane called the:
    A. Ductus deferens
    B. Tunica albuginea
    C. Septum
    D. Seminiferous membrane

12. The ______________ lie near the septa that separate the lobules.
    A. Ductus deferens
    B. Sperm
    C. Interstitial cells
    D. Nerves

13. Sperm are found in the walls of the:
    A. Seminiferous tubule
    B. Interstitial cells
    C. Septum
    D. Blood vessels

14. An undescended testicle is called a(n):
    A. Orchidalgia
    B. Orchidorrhaphy
    C. Orchichorea
    D. Cryptorchidism

15. The structure(s) that produce(s) testosterone is (are) the:
    A. Seminiferous tubules
    B. Prostate gland
    C. Bulbourethral gland
    D. Pituitary gland
    E. Interstitial cells

16. The part of the sperm that contains genetic information that will be inherited is the:
    A. Tail
    B. Neck
    C. Middle piece
    D. Head
    E. Acrosome

17. Which one of the following is *not* a function of testosterone?
    A. It causes a deepening of the voice.
    B. It promotes the development of the male accessory glands.
    C. It has a stimulatory effect on protein catabolism.
    D. It causes greater muscular development and strength.

18. Sperm production is called:
    A. Spermatogonia
    B. Spermatids
    C. Spermatogenesis
    D. Spermatocyte

19. The section of the sperm that contains enzymes that enable it to break down the covering of the ovum and permit entry should contact occur is the:
    A. Acrosome
    B. Midpiece
    C. Tail
    D. Stem

20. Descent of the testes usually occurs about:
    A. Two months after birth
    B. Two months before birth
    C. Two months after conception
    D. Two years after birth
    E. None of the above

Completion

Fill in the blanks.

The (21) ____________________ are the gonads of the male. From puberty on, the seminiferous tubules are continuously forming (22) ____________________. Any of these cells may join with the female sex cell, the (23) ____________________, to become a new human being.

Another function of the testes is to secrete the male hormone (24) ____________________ which transforms a boy to a man. This hormone is secreted by the (25) ________________ ________________ of the testes. A good way to remember testosterone's functions is to think of it as "the (26) ____________________ hormone" and "the (27) ____________________ hormone."

If you have had difficulty with this section, review pages 442-447.

REPRODUCTIVE DUCTS
ACCESSORY OR SUPPORTIVE SEX GLANDS
EXTERNAL GENITALIA

Choose the correct term and write the letter in the space next to the appropriate definition below.

A. Epididymis
B. Vas deferens
C. Ejaculatory duct
D. Prepuce
E. Seminal vesicles
F. Prostate gland
G. Cowper's gland
H. Prostatectomy
I. Semen
J. Scrotum

_____ 28. Continuation of ducts that start in epididymis

_____ 29. Procedure performed for benign prostatic hypertrophy

_____ 30. Also known as *bulbourethral*

_____ 31. Coiled tube that lies along the top and behind the testes

_____ 32. Doughnut-shaped gland beneath bladder

_____ 33. Continuation of ductus deferens

_____ 34. Mixture of sperm and secretions of accessory sex glands

_____ 35. Contributes 60% of the seminal fluid volume

_____ 36. Removed during circumcision

_____ 37. External genitalia

If you have had difficulty with this section, review pages 447-450.

FEMALE REPRODUCTIVE SYSTEM STRUCTURAL PLAN

Match the term on the left with the proper selection on the right.

_____ 38. Ovaries — A. External genitals
_____ 39. Vagina — B. Accessory sex gland
_____ 40. Bartholin — C. Accessory duct
_____ 41. Vulva — D. Gonads
_____ 42. Ova — E. Sex cells

Select the correct term from the options given and write the letter in the answer blank.

(A) External structure (B) Internal structure

_____ 43. Mons pubis
_____ 44. Vagina
_____ 45. Labia majora
_____ 46. Uterine tubes
_____ 47. Vestibule
_____ 48. Clitoris
_____ 49. Labia minora
_____ 50. Ovaries

If you have had difficulty with this section, review pages 450-451 and pages 454 and 455.

OVARIES

Fill in the blanks.

The ovaries are the (51) _______________ of the female. They have two main functions. The first is the production of the female sex cell. This process is called (52) _______________. The specialized type of cell division that occurs during sexual cell reproduction is known as (53) _______________. The ovum is the body's largest cell and has (54) ___________ ___________ the number of chromosomes found in other body cells. At the time of (55) _______________, the sex cells from both parents fuse and (56) _______________ chromosomes are united.

The second major function of the ovaries is to secrete the sex hormones (57) _______________ and (58) _______________. Estrogen is the sex hormone that causes the development and maintenance of the female (59) ___________ ___________ ___________. Progesterone acts with estrogen to help initiate the (60) ___________ ___________ in girls entering (61) _______________.

If you have had difficulty with this section, review pages 451-452.

FEMALE REPRODUCTIVE DUCTS

Select the correct term from the options given and write the letter in the answer blank.

(A) Uterine tubes (B) Uterus (C) Vagina

_____ 62. Ectopic pregnancy

_____ 63. Lining known as *endometrium*

_____ 64. Terminal end of birth canal

_____ 65. Site of menstruation

_____ 66. Approximately 4 inches in length

_____ 67. Consists of body, fundus, and cervix

_____ 68. Site of fertilization

_____ 69. Also known as *oviduct*

_____ 70. Entranceway for sperm

_____ 71. Total hysterectomy

If you have had difficulty with this section, review pages 452-454 and page 458.

ACCESSORY OR SUPPORTIVE SEX GLANDS EXTERNAL GENITALS OF THE FEMALE

Match the term on the left with the proper selection on the right.

Group A

_____ 72. Bartholin's gland — A. Colored area around nipple

_____ 73. Breasts — B. Grapelike clusters of milk-secreting cells

_____ 74. Alveoli — C. Drain alveoli

_____ 75. Lactiferous ducts — D. Secretes lubricating fluid

_____ 76. Areola — E. Primarily fat tissue

Group B

_____ 77. Mons pubis — A. "Large lips"

_____ 78. Labia majora — B. Area between labia minora

_____ 79. Clitoris — C. Surgical procedure

_____ 80. Vestibule — D. Composed of erectile tissue

_____ 81. Episiotomy — E. Pad of fat over the symphysis pubis

If you have had difficulty with this section, review pages 454-455.

MENSTRUAL CYCLE

True or False

If the statement is true, insert "T" in the answer blank. If the statement is false, correct the statement by circling the incorrect term and writing the correct term in the answer blank.

__________ 82. "Climacteric" is the scientific name for the beginning of the menses.

__________ 83. As a general rule, several ovum mature each month during the 30–40 years that a woman has menstrual periods.

__________ 84. Ovulation occurs 28 days before the next menstrual period begins.

__________ 85. The first day of ovulation is considered the first day of the cycle.

__________ 86. A woman's fertile period lasts only a few days out of each month.

__________ 87. The control of the menstrual cycle lies in the posterior pituitary gland.

Matching

Write the letter of the correct hormone in the blank next to the appropriate description.

(A) FSH (B) LH

_____ 88. Ovulating hormone

_____ 89. Secreted during first days of menstrual cycle

_____ 90. Secreted after estrogen level of blood increases

_____ 91. Causes final maturation of follicle and ovum

_____ 92. Birth control pills suppress this hormone

If you have had difficulty with this section, review pages 455-458.

UNSCRAMBLE THE WORDS

Take the circled letters, unscramble them, and fill in the statement.

93. **ULAVV**

94. **TSTSEE**

95. **MNSSEE**

96. **AIEIFMBR**

97. **CUERPPE**

Where Kathleen displayed the flowers from her husband.

98.

APPLYING WHAT YOU KNOW

99. Mr. Belinki is going into the hospital for the surgical removal of his testes. As a result of this surgery, will Mr. Belinki be impotent?

100. When baby Ross was born, the pediatrician discovered that his left testicle had not descended into the scrotum. If this situation is not corrected soon, might baby Ross be sterile or impotent?

101. Ms. Satin contracted gonorrhea. By the time she made an appointment to see her doctor, it had spread to her abdominal organs. How is this possible when gonorrhea is a disease of the reproductive system?

102. Mrs. Harlan was having a bilateral oophorectomy. Is this a sterilization procedure? Will she experience menopause?

103. Delceta had a total hysterectomy. Will she experience menopause?

104. WORD FIND

Can you find 18 terms from this chapter in the box of letters? Words may be spelled top to bottom, bottom to top, right to left, left to right, or diagonally.

M	K	O	V	I	D	U	C	T	S	E	D	H	G
S	E	I	R	A	V	O	I	F	U	T	G	L	L
I	N	H	Z	H	M	P	M	K	O	H	I	C	W
D	D	V	A	S	D	E	F	E	R	E	N	S	H
I	O	A	C	C	I	P	J	V	E	H	Y	D	S
H	M	G	R	R	B	M	N	X	F	G	Y	I	O
C	E	I	O	O	E	Z	Y	T	I	C	S	T	E
R	T	N	S	T	P	S	D	D	N	O	V	A	D
O	R	A	O	U	W	E	B	A	I	J	S	M	Z
T	I	C	M	M	E	Y	N	E	M	D	L	R	V
P	U	A	E	U	D	G	M	I	E	H	I	E	H
Y	M	O	T	C	E	T	A	T	S	O	R	P	B
R	P	E	E	R	M	N	E	G	O	R	T	S	E
C	O	W	P	E	R	S	I	N	X	K	E	A	P

Acrosome	Meiosis	Scrotum
Cowpers	Ovaries	Seminiferous
Cryptorchidism	Oviducts	Sperm
Endometrium	Penis	Spermatids
Epididymis	Pregnancy	Vagina
Estrogen	Prostatectomy	Vas deferens

DID YOU KNOW?

The testes produce approximately 500 million sperm per day. Every 2–3 months they produce enough cells to populate the entire earth.

There are an estimated 925,000 daily occurrences of STD transmission and 550,000 daily pregnancies worldwide.

During menstruation, the sensitivity of a woman's middle finger is reduced.

The lifespan of a sperm on the average is 36 hours. The lifespan of an ovum on the average is 12-24 hours.

REPRODUCTIVE SYSTEMS

Fill in the crossword puzzle.

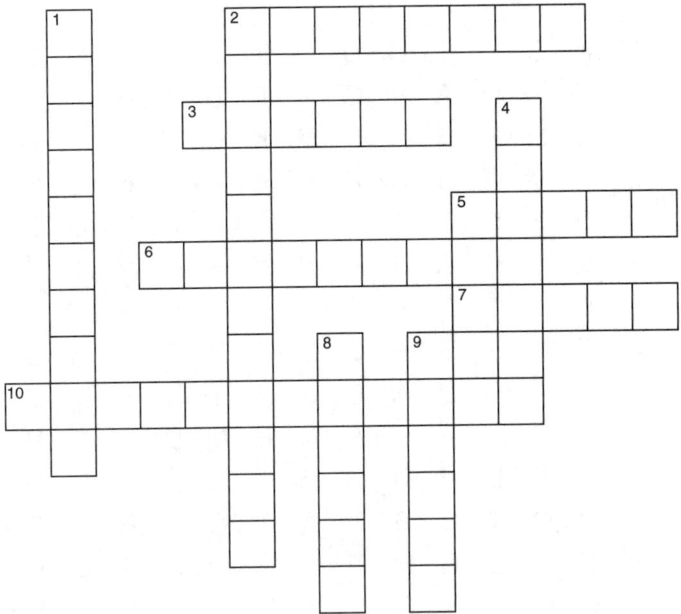

Across

2. Female erectile tissue
3. Colored area around nipple
5. Male reproductive fluid
6. Sex cells
7. External genitalia
10. Male sex hormone

Down

1. Failure to have a menstrual period
2. Surgical removal of foreskin
4. Foreskin
8. Menstrual period
9. Essential organs of reproduction

CHECK YOUR KNOWLEDGE

Multiple Choice

Select the best answer.

1. Which of the following is *not* an accessory organ of the male reproductive system?
   A. Gonads
   B. Prostate gland
   C. Scrotum
   D. Seminal vesicle

2. The acrosome:
   A. Contains the ATP to provide energy for the sperm
   B. Lies within the nucleus of the sperm
   C. Is responsible for sperm reproduction
   D. Contains enzymes that enable the sperm to enter the ovum

3. Which of the following contribute to the production of seminal fluid?
   A. Seminal vesicles
   B. Prostate gland
   C. Bulbourethral glands
   D. All of the above

4. Sperm mature and develop their ability to move or swim in the:
   A. Ductus deferens
   B. Ejaculatory duct
   C. Epididymis
   D. Cowper's glands

5. The bulbourethral glands:
   A. Are shaped like a doughnut
   B. Contribute 60% of the seminal fluid
   C. Secrete "pre-ejaculate"
   D. Pass through the inguinal canal as part of the spermatic cord

6. A mature ovum in its sac is sometimes called a(n):
   A. Graafian follicle
   B. Corpus luteum
   C. Oocyte
   D. Oogenesis

7. Progesterone:
   A. Initiates the first menstrual cycle
   B. Is produced by the corpus luteum
   C. Is responsible for the appearance of pubic hair and breast development
   D. All of the above

8. The external genitalia include all of the following *except:*
   A. Hymen
   B. Clitoris
   C. Lactiferous ducts
   D. Labia minora

9. Testosterone is produced by the:
   A. Interstitial cells
   B. Seminiferous tubules
   C. Process of meiosis
   D. Tunica albuginea

10. Which of the following analogous features of the reproductive systems is correct?
    A. Ovaries to testes
    B. Estrogen and progesterone to testosterone
    C. Clitoris and vulva to penis and scrotum
    D. All of the above

Matching

Select the most correct answer from column B for each statement in column A. (Only one answer is correct.)

Column A	Column B
_____ 11. Sex cells	A. Spermatogonia
_____ 12. Sperm stem cells	B. FSH
_____ 13. Testosterone	C. Gametes
_____ 14. Penis	D. Menarche
_____ 15. Scrotum	E. LH
_____ 16. Ovulating hormone	F. Male external genitalia
_____ 17. Sperm formation	G. Prepuce
_____ 18. Menses	H. Masculinizes
_____ 19. Breasts	I. Female external genitalia
_____ 20. Vestibule	J. Areola

MALE REPRODUCTIVE ORGANS

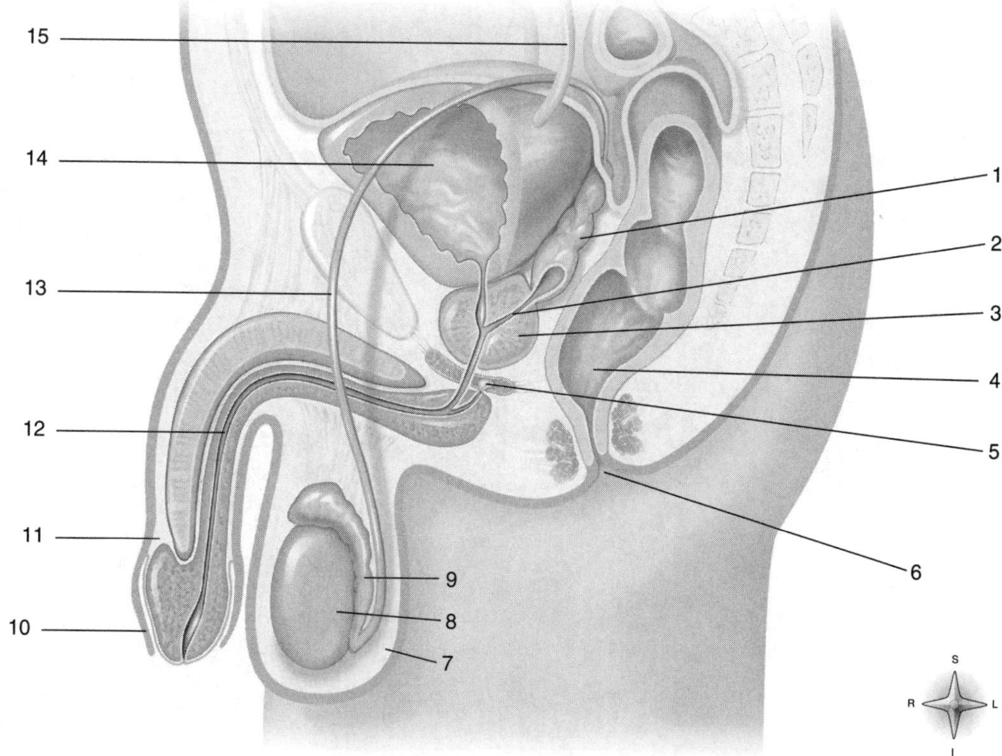

1. ______________________
2. ______________________
3. ______________________
4. ______________________
5. ______________________
6. ______________________
7. ______________________
8. ______________________
9. ______________________
10. ______________________
11. ______________________
12. ______________________
13. ______________________
14. ______________________
15. ______________________

TUBULES OF TESTIS AND EPIDIDYMIS

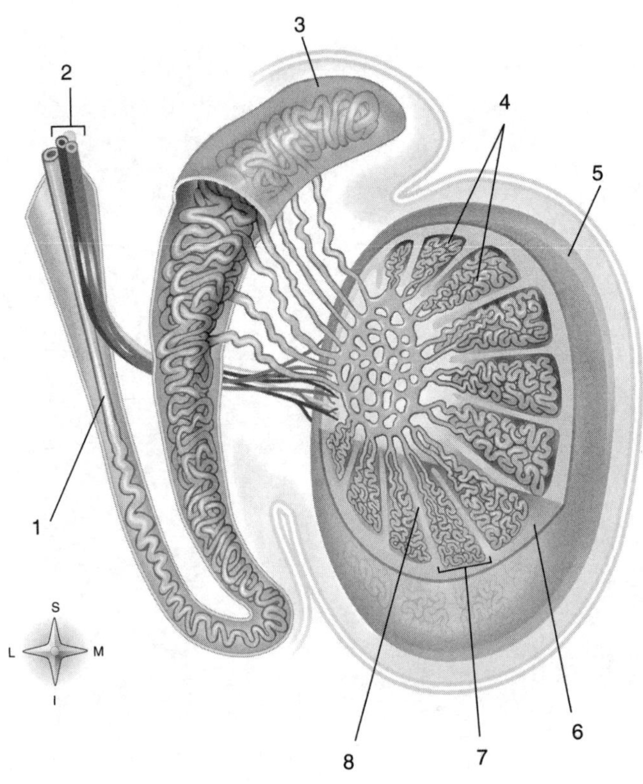

1. ______________________
2. ______________________
3. ______________________
4. ______________________
5. ______________________
6. ______________________
7. ______________________
8. ______________________

VULVA

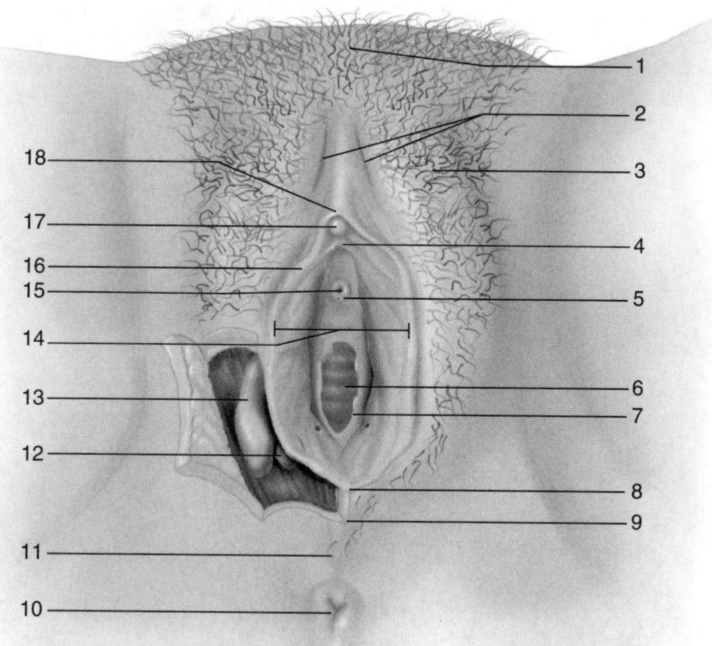

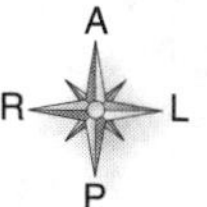

1. ______________________
2. ______________________
3. ______________________
4. ______________________
5. ______________________
6. ______________________
7. ______________________
8. ______________________
9. ______________________
10. ______________________
11. ______________________
12. ______________________
13. ______________________
14. ______________________
15. ______________________
16. ______________________
17. ______________________
18. ______________________

BREAST

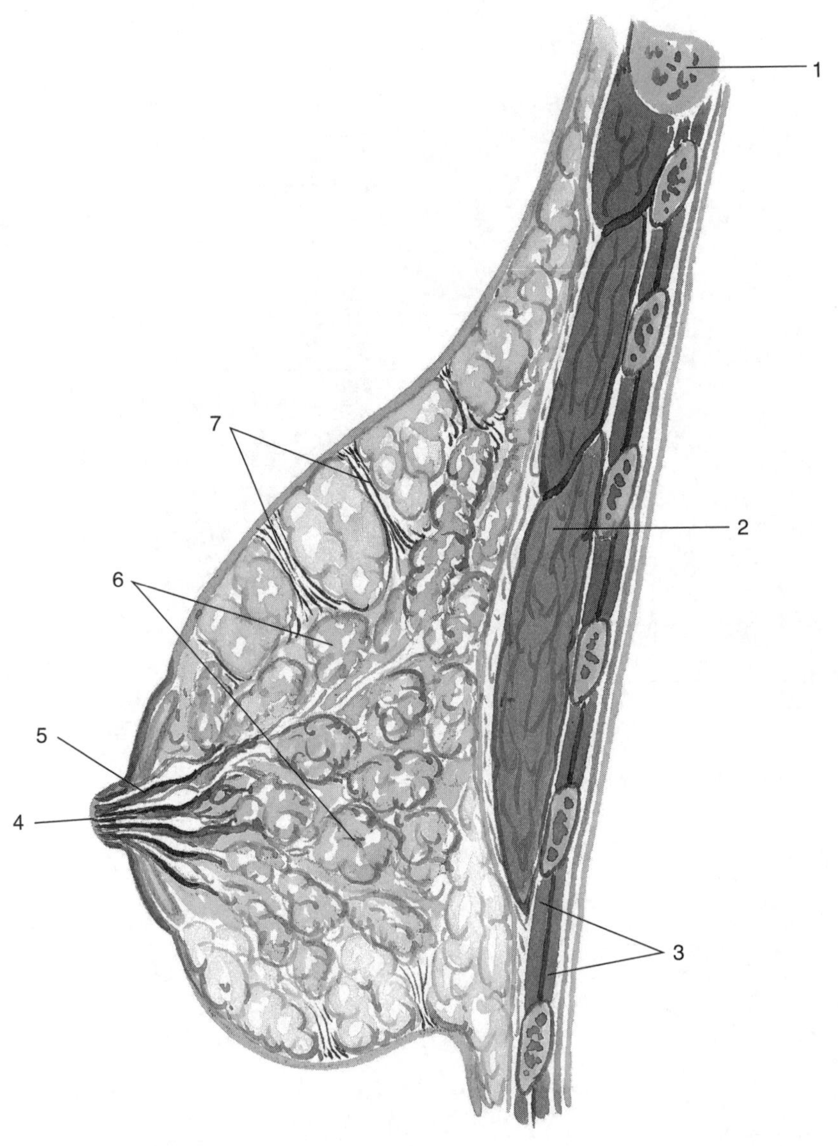

1. ______________________
2. ______________________
3. ______________________
4. ______________________
5. ______________________
6. ______________________
7. ______________________

FEMALE PELVIS

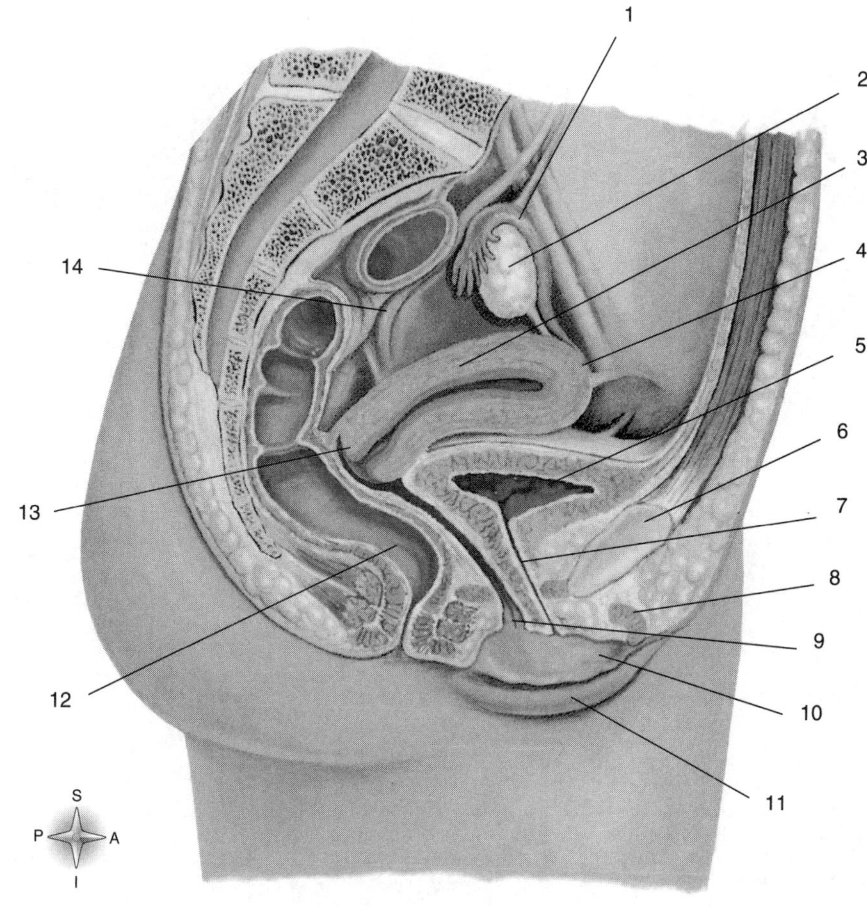

1. ____________________
2. ____________________
3. ____________________
4. ____________________
5. ____________________
6. ____________________
7. ____________________
8. ____________________
9. ____________________
10. ____________________
11. ____________________
12. ____________________
13. ____________________
14. ____________________

UTERUS AND ADJACENT STRUCTURES

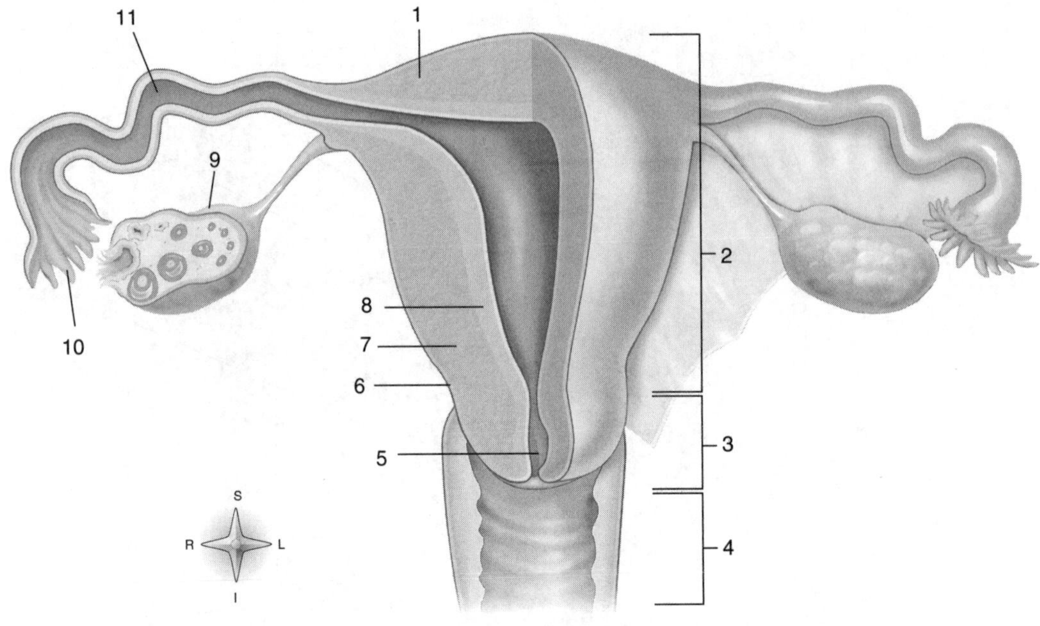

1. ______________________
2. ______________________
3. ______________________
4. ______________________
5. ______________________
6. ______________________
7. ______________________
8. ______________________
9. ______________________
10. ______________________
11. ______________________

CHAPTER 21

Growth and Development

Millions of fragile microscopic sperm swim against numerous obstacles to reach the ova and create a new life. At birth, the newborn will fill his lungs with air and cry lustily, signaling to the world that he is ready to begin the cycle of life. This cycle will be marked by ongoing changes, periodic physical growth, and continuous development.

This chapter reviews the more significant events that occur in the normal growth and development of an individual from conception to death. Realizing that each individual is unique, we nonetheless can discover, amid all the complexities of humanity, some constants that are understandable and predictable.

Knowledge of human growth and development is essential in understanding the commonalities that influence individuals as they pass through the cycle of life.

TOPICS FOR REVIEW

Your review of this chapter should include an understanding of the concept of development as a biological process. You should familiarize yourself with the major developmental changes from conception through older adulthood. Your study should conclude with a review of the effects of aging on the body systems.

PRENATAL PERIOD

Completion

Fill in the blanks.

The prenatal stage of development begins at the time of (1) __________________ and continues until (2) __________________. The science of the development of the offspring before birth is called (3) __________________.

Fertilization takes place in the outer third of the (4) __________________. The fertilized ovum or (5) __________________ begins to divide and in approximately 3 days forms a solid mass called a (6) __________________. By the time it enters the uterus, it is a hollow ball of cells called a (7) __________________.

As it continues to develop, it forms a structure with two cavities. The (8) ________________ ________________ will become a fluid-filled sac for the embryo. The (9) ________________________ will develop into an important fetal membrane in the (10) ________________________.

Matching

Choose the correct term and write the letter in the space next to the appropriate definition below.

A. Laparoscope
B. Gestation
C. Antenatal
D. Histogenesis
E. Quickening
F. Endoderm
G. In vitro
H. Parturition
I. Embryonic phase
J. Ultrasonogram

_____ 11. "Within a glass"

_____ 12. Inside germ layer

_____ 13. Before birth

_____ 14. Length of pregnancy

_____ 15. Fiberoptic viewing instrument

_____ 16. Process of birth

_____ 17. First fetal movement

_____ 18. Study of how the primary germ layers develop into many different kinds of tissues

_____ 19. Fertilization until the end of the eighth week of gestation

_____ 20. Monitors the progress of the developing fetus

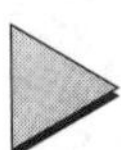 *If you have had difficulty with this section, review pages 467-476 and page 478.*

POSTNATAL PERIOD

Multiple Choice

Select the best answer.

21. During the postnatal period:
    A. The head becomes proportionately smaller
    B. Thoracic and abdominal contours change from round to elliptical
    C. The legs become proportionately longer
    D. The trunk becomes proportionately shorter
    E. All of the above

22. The period of infancy starts at birth and lasts about:
    A. 4 weeks
    B. 4 months
    C. 10 weeks
    D. 12 months
    E. 18 months

23. The lumbar curvature of the spine appears ____________ months after birth.
    A. 1–10
    B. 5–8
    C. 8–12
    D. 11–15
    E. 12–18

24. During the first 4 months, the birth weight will:
    A. Double
    B. Triple
    C. Quadruple
    D. None of the above

25. At the end of the first year, the weight of the baby will have:
    A. Doubled
    B. Tripled
    C. Quadrupled
    D. None of the above

26. The infant is capable of following a moving object with its eyes at:
    A. 2 days
    B. 2 weeks
    C. 2 months
    D. 4 months
    E. 10 months

27. The infant can lift its head and raise its chest at:
    A. 2 months
    B. 3 months
    C. 4 months
    D. 10 months

28. The infant can crawl at the age of:
    A. 2 months
    B. 3 months
    C. 4 months
    D. 10 months
    E. 12 months

29. The infant can stand alone at the age of:
    A. 2 months
    B. 3 months
    C. 4 months
    D. 10 months
    E. 12 months

30. The permanent teeth, with the exception of the third molar, have all erupted by age _______ years.
    A. 6
    B. 8
    C. 12
    D. 14
    E. None of the above

31. Puberty starts at age ____________ years in boys.
    A. 10–13
    B. 12–14
    C. 14–16
    D. None of the above

32. Most girls begin breast development at about age:
    A. 8
    B. 9
    C. 10
    D. 11
    E. 12

33. The growth spurt is generally complete by age __________ in males.
    A. 14
    B. 15
    C. 16
    D. 18

34. An average age at which girls begin to menstruate is __________ years.
    A. 10–12
    B. 11–12
    C. 12–13
    D. 13–14
    E. 14–15

35. The first sign of puberty in boys is:
    A. Facial hair
    B. Increased muscle mass
    C. Pubic hair
    D. Deepening of the voice
    E. Increased testicular enlargement

Matching

Write the letter of the correct word in the blank next to the appropriate definition.

A. Neonatology
B. Neonatal
C. Adolescence
D. Deciduous
E. Puberty
F. Postnatal
G. Infancy
H. Childhood
I. Senescence

_____ 36. Begins at birth and lasts until death
_____ 37. Concerned with the diagnosis and treatment of disorders of the newborn
_____ 38. Teenage years
_____ 39. From the end of infancy to puberty
_____ 40. Baby teeth
_____ 41. First 4 weeks of infancy
_____ 42. Secondary sexual characteristics occur
_____ 43. Begins at birth and lasts about 18 months
_____ 44. Older adulthood

If you have had difficulty with this section, review pages 476-481.

EFFECTS OF AGING

Fill in the blanks.

45. Old bones develop indistinct and shaggy margins with spurs, a process called ________________.

46. A degenerative joint disease common in the older adults is ________________.

47. The number of ____________________ units in the kidney decreases by almost 50% between the ages of 30 and 75.

48. In older adulthood, respiratory efficiency decreases, and a condition known as ________________ ________________ results.

49. Fatty deposits accumulate in blood vessels as we age, and the result is ____________________, which narrows the passageway for the flow of blood.

50. Hardening of the arteries or ____________________ occurs during the aging process.

51. Another term for high blood pressure is ____________________.

52. Hardening of the lens is ____________________.

53. If the lens becomes cloudy and impairs vision, it is called a(n) ____________________.

54. ____________________ causes an increase in the pressure within the eyeball and may result in blindness.

If you have had difficulty with this section, review pages 481-483.

UNSCRAMBLE THE WORDS

Take the circled letters, unscramble them, and fill in the statement.

55. **A N N F C Y I**

56. **N A A L T T S O P**

57. **O G S S N E G R A O N E I**

58. **G T E Y Z O**

59. **H D O O L H C I D**

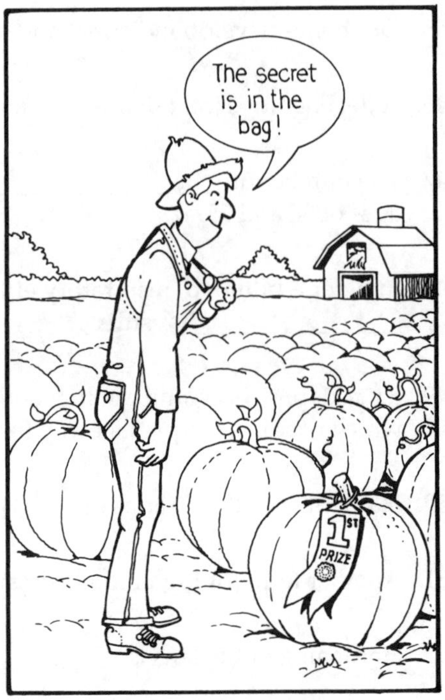

The secret to Farmer Brown's prize pumpkin crop.

60.

APPLYING WHAT YOU KNOW

61. Heather's mother told the pediatrician during her 1-year visit that Heather had tripled her birth weight, was crawling actively, and could stand alone. Is Heather's development normal, retarded, or advanced?

62. Sharon is 70 years old. She has always enjoyed food and has had a hearty appetite. Lately, however, she has complained that food "just doesn't taste as good anymore." What might be a possible explanation?

63. Mr. Hines, age 78, has noticed hearing problems, but only under certain circumstances. He has difficulty with certain tones, especially high or low tones, but has no problem with everyday conversation. What might be a possible explanation?

64. WORD FIND

Can you find 14 terms from the chapter in the box of letters? Words may be spelled top to bottom, bottom to top, right to left, left to right, or diagonally.

```
F T P N O I T A T S E G K F U
Z E P O C S O R A P A L H E A
E O R I L T O H H O C J V J T
C M V T N T I M L N L Z P U O
M A B I I F R M R E D O T C E
H Q C R D L A M E S O D E R M
N N M U Y U I N M F O W G O P
K N V T C O C Z C H H F R C N
H G Y R Y K L T A Y D U C V P
L A T A N T S O P T L U N Q G
Q N K P Y Y S W G A I K E M T
U G P Q N H O Y X Y H O Z B N
I Y T R E B U P L A C E N T A
```

Childhood	Infancy	Parturition
Ectoderm	Laparoscope	Placenta
Embryology	Mesoderm	Postnatal
Fertilization	Morula	Puberty
Gestation	Oviduct	

DID YOU KNOW?

Brain cells do not regenerate. One beer permanently destroys 10,000 cells.

A 3-week-old embryo is no larger than a sesame seed. A 1-month-old fetus' body is no heavier than an envelope and a sheet of paper. Its hand is no bigger than a teardrop.

During pregnancy, the uterus expands to 500 times its normal size.

From birth to adolescence, selected bones in the human body fuse together. The last bone to fuse is the collarbone, and this occurs between the ages of 18 and 25.

GROWTH/DEVELOPMENT

Fill in the crossword puzzle.

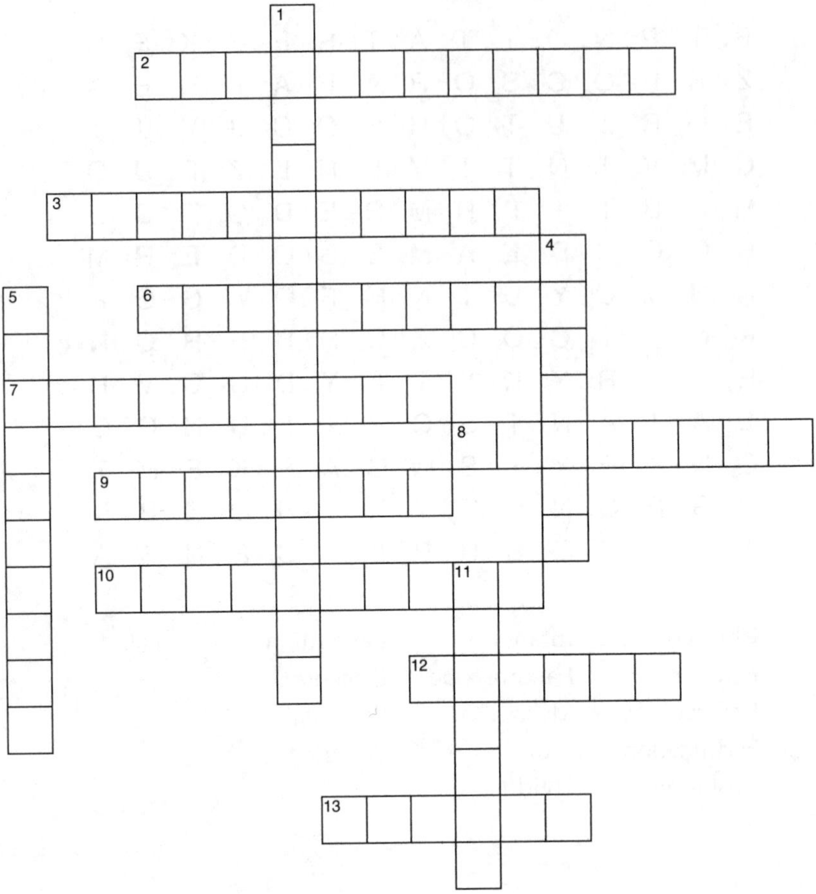

Across

2. Study of how germ layers develop into tissues
3. Process of birth
6. Name of zygote after implantation
7. Science of the development of the individual before birth
8. Eye disease marked by increased pressure in the eyeball
9. Cloudy lens
10. Old age
12. Name of zygote after 3 days
13. Fertilized ovum

Down

1. Fatty deposit buildup on walls of arteries
4. First 4 weeks of infancy
5. Hardening of the lens
11. Will develop into a fetal membrane in the placenta

CHECK YOUR KNOWLEDGE

Multiple Choice

Select the best answer.

1. The prenatal period begins:
   A. After implantation
   B. 4 weeks after gestation
   C. At conception
   D. 10 days after conception

2. By the time the developing embryo reaches the uterus, it is a:
   A. Morula
   B. Zygote
   C. Fetus
   D. Blastocyst

3. The chorion develops into the:
   A. Morula
   B. Zygote
   C. Fetus
   D. Placenta

4. Fertilization most often occurs in the:
   A. Outer one-third of the oviduct
   B. Inner one-third of the oviduct
   C. Uterus
   D. Vagina

5. The embryonic phase of development extends from fertilization until the end of week _______ of gestation.
   A. 2
   B. 4
   C. 6
   D. 8

6. The primary germ layers include the:
   A. Endoderm
   B. Ectoderm
   C. Mesoderm
   D. All of the above

7. The stage of labor that begins from the onset of uterine contractions until dilation of the cervix is complete is called:
   A. Parturition
   B. Transition
   C. Stage one
   D. Stage two

8. All organ systems are complete and in place by:
   A. 4 months of gestation
   B. 35 days of gestation
   C. 7 months of gestation
   D. 8 months of gestation

9. The initial stimulus to breathe when an infant is born results from the:
   A. Doctor shocking the baby by slapping the buttocks
   B. Cold new environment shocking the respiratory system
   C. Increasing amounts of carbon dioxide that accumulate in the blood after the umbilical cord is cut following delivery
   D. Baby's sudden change of position after delivery

10. Adulthood is characterized by:
    A. A period of rapid growth
    B. Maintenance of existing body tissues
    C. Senescence
    D. None of the above

Matching

Select the most correct answer from column B for each statement in column A. (Only one answer is correct.)

Column A	Column B
_____ 11. Embryology	A. Study of aging
_____ 12. Zygote	B. First 18 months of life
_____ 13. Gestation period	C. Trimesters
_____ 14. Older adult	D. Fetal movement
_____ 15. Teratogens	E. Prenatal science
_____ 16. Quickening	F. "Old eye"
_____ 17. Lipping	G. Fertilized ovum
_____ 18. Presbyopia	H. Factors that cause birth defects
_____ 19. Gerontology	I. Senescence
_____ 20. Infancy	J. Bone spurs

FERTILIZATION AND IMPLANTATION

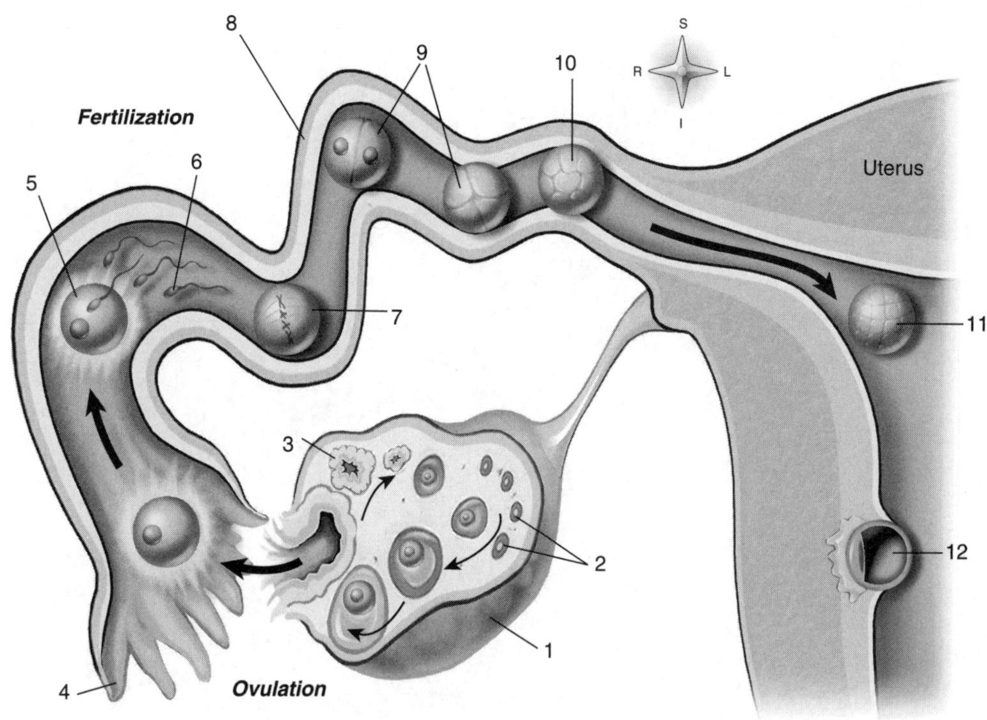

1. ______________________
2. ______________________
3. ______________________
4. ______________________
5. ______________________
6. ______________________
7. ______________________
8. ______________________
9. ______________________
10. ______________________
11. ______________________
12. ______________________

Answer Key

CHAPTER 1
AN INTRODUCTION TO THE STRUCTURE AND FUNCTION OF THE BODY

Fill in the Blanks

1. Scientific method, p. 1
2. Hypothesis, p. 1
3. Experimentation, p. 1
4. Test group p. 1
5. Control group, p. 1

True or False

6. T
7. F, a meter is 39.37 inches
8. T
9. T
10. F, a micron is another name for a micrometer

Matching

11. D, p. 3
12. E, p. 3
13. A, p. 3
14. C, p. 3
15. B, p. 3

Matching

16. C, p. 5
17. A, p. 5
18. E, p. 5
19. D, p. 5
20. B, p. 5

Crossword

21. Inferior
22. Transverse
23. Medial
24. Superior
25. Ventral
26. Lateral
27. Distal

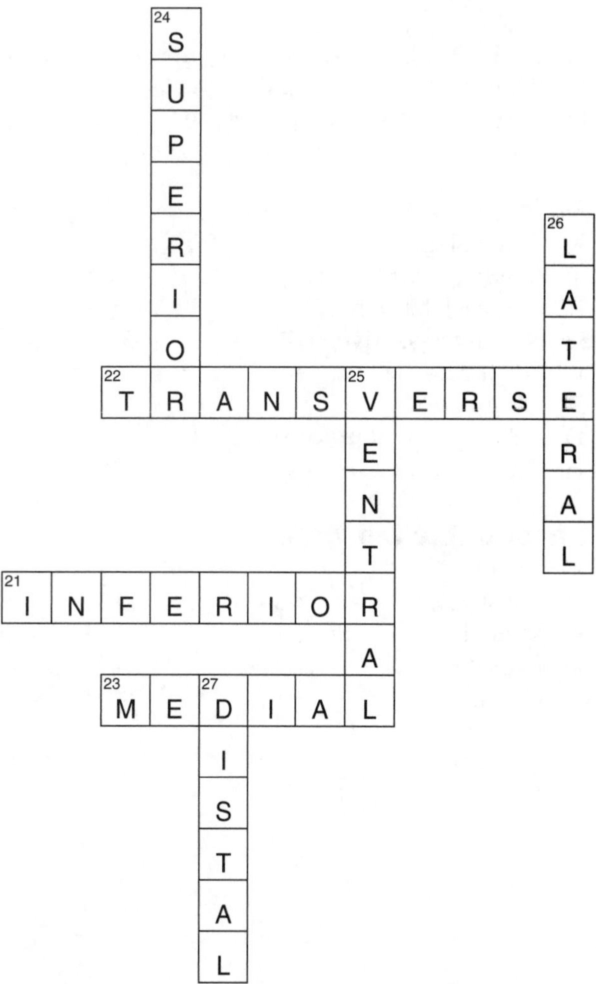

Did you notice that the answers were arranged as they appear on the human body?

Circle the correct answer

28. Inferior, p. 5
29. Anterior, p. 5
30. Lateral, p. 5
31. Proximal, p. 5
32. Superficial, p. 6
33. Equal, p. 7
34. Anterior and posterior, p. 7
35. Upper and lower, p. 7
36. Frontal, p. 7

Select the correct term

37. A, p. 7
38. B, p. 9
39. A, p. 7
40. A, p. 7
41. A, p. 7
42. B, p. 9
43. A, p. 7

Circle the one that does not belong

44. Extremities (all others are part of the axial portions)
45. Cephalic (all others are part of the arm)
46. Plantar (all others are part of the face)
47. Carpal (all others are part of the leg or foot)
48. Tarsal (all others are part of the skull)

Fill in the blanks

49. Survival, p. 12
50. Internal environment, p. 12
51. Feedback loop, p. 12
52. Negative, positive, p. 12
53. Stabilize, p. 13
54. Stimulatory, p. 13
55. Developmental processes, p. 14
56. Aging processes, p. 14

Unscramble the words

57. Axial
58. Physiology
59. Frontal
60. Dorsal
61. Organ

Applying what you know

62. #1 on diagram
63. #2 on diagram
64. #3 on diagram

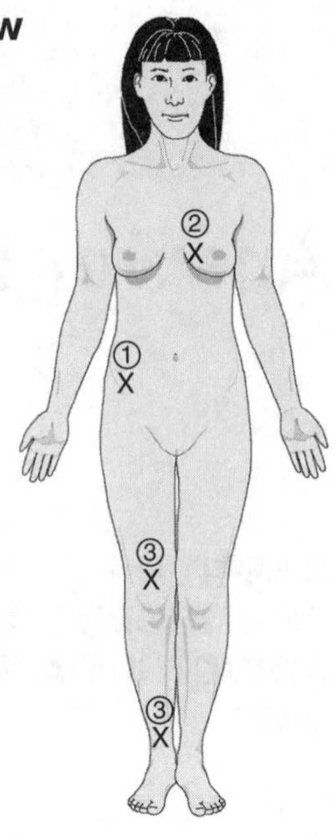

65. WORD FIND

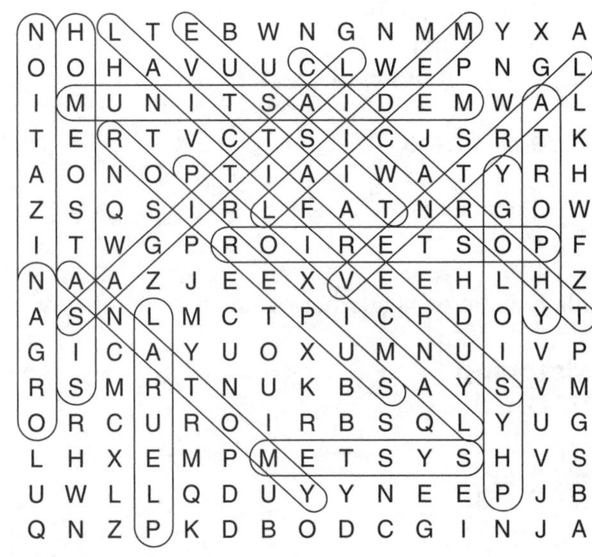

Check your knowledge

Multiple choice

1. A, p. 12
2. D, p. 8
3. B, p. 10
4. D, p. 7
5. A, p. 1
6. C, p. 7
7. C, p. 3
8. A, p. 7
9. C, p. 10
10. B, p. 8
11. D, p. 10
12. B, p. 10
13. C, p. 3

14. A, p. 7
15. D, p. 5
16. C, p. 5
17. D, p. 11
18. D, p. 7
19. A, p. 11
20. C, p. 5

Matching

21. F, p. 7
22. B, p. 11
23. J, p. 7
24. G, p. 1
25. H, p. 6
26. C, p. 7
27. D, p. 11
28. I, p. 5
29. A, p. 7
30. E, p. 3

Dorsal and ventral body cavities

1. cranial cavity
2. spinal cavity
3. thoracic cavity
4. pleural cavity
5. mediastinum
6. diaphragm
7. abdominal cavity
8. abdominopelvic
9. pelvic

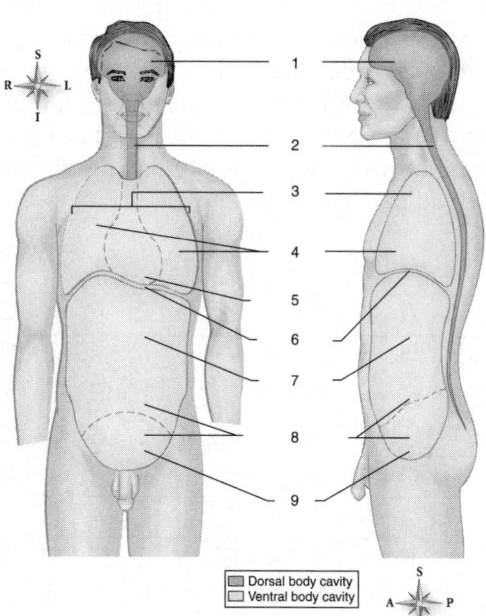

Directions and planes of the body

1. Superior
2. Proximal
3. Posterior (dorsal)
4. Anterior (ventral)
5. Inferior
6. Sagittal plane
7. Frontal plane
8. Lateral

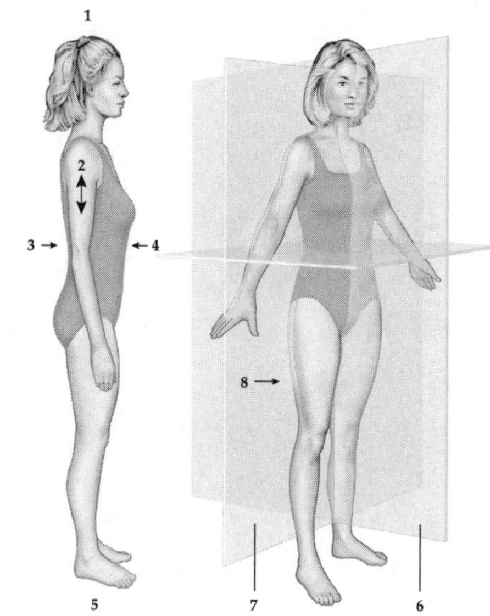

Regions of the abdomen

1. Right hypochondriac region
2. Epigastric region
3. Left hypochondriac region
4. Right lumbar region
5. Umbilical region
6. Left lumbar region
7. Right iliac (inguinal) region
8. Hypogastric region
9. Left iliac (inguinal) region

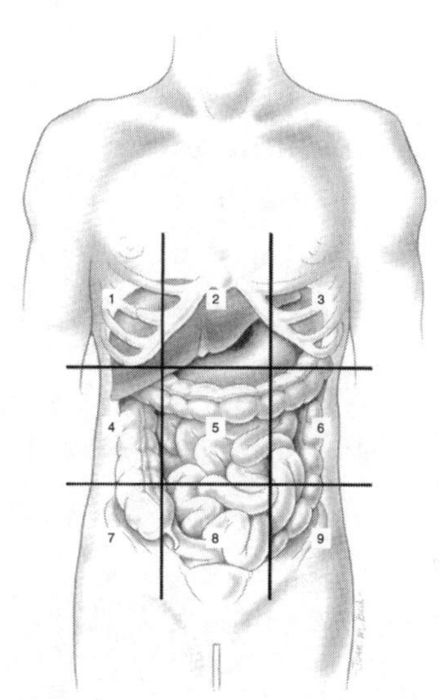

CHAPTER 2
CHEMISTRY OF LIFE

Multiple choice
1. C, p. 21
2. B, p. 19
3. C, p. 19
4. A, p. 19
5. D, p. 20
6. C, p. 20
7. A, p. 20

True or false
8. T, p. 19
9. molecules, p. 19
10. uncharged neutrons, p. 19
11. T, p. 19
12. T, p. 20

Multiple choice
13. C, p. 21
14. B, p. 22
15. A, p. 22
16. B, p. 22
17. A, p. 23
18. C, p. 22

Matching
19. H, p. 23
20. B, p. 23
21. E, p. 23
22. A, p. 23
23. G, p. 24
24. L, p. 24
25. J, p. 24
26. C, p. 24
27. D, p. 25
28. F, p. 25
29. K, p. 25
30. I, p. 25

Select the best answer
31. A, p. 26
32. B, p. 26
33. D, p. 29
34. B, p. 26
35. C, p. 26
36. A, p. 26
37. A, p. 26
38. B, p. 26
39. C, p. 28
40. D, p. 29

Crossword

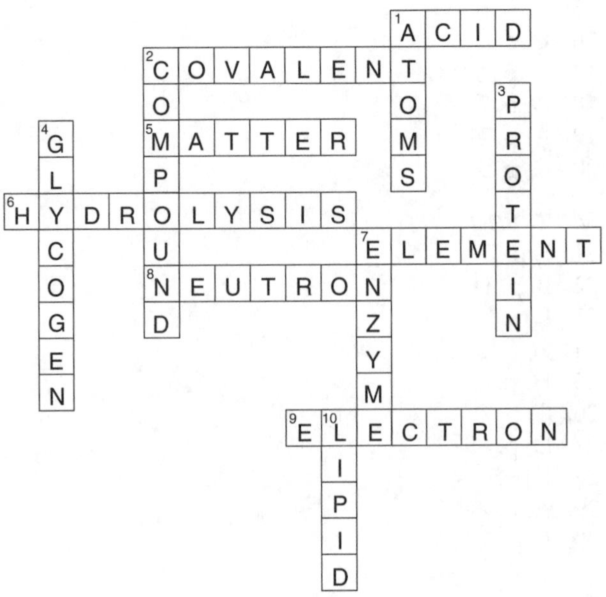

Unscramble the words
41. Matter
42. Elements
43. Molecules
44. Organic
45. Electrolyte
46. Energy

Applying what you know
47. Some fats can become solid at room temperature, such as the fat in butter and lard.
48. Radioactive isotopes will be used to measure Carol's thyroid activity. A diagnosis of hyperthyroidism or hypothyroidism will be based upon how rapidly or slowly the thyroid absorbs the radioactive iodine and emits radiation.

49. WORD FIND

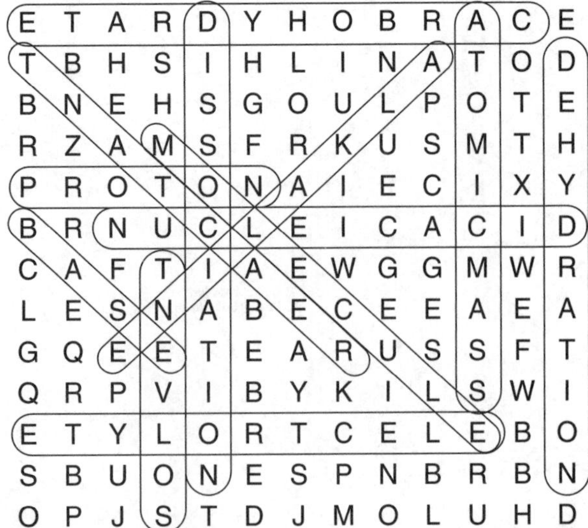

Check your knowledge
1. Biochemistry, p. 19
2. Neutrons, p. 19
3. Higher, p. 20
4. Elements; compounds, p. 20
5. Stable, p. 21
6. Ion, p. 21
7. Inorganic, p. 23
8. Dehydration synthesis, p. 24
9. Chemical equation, p. 24
10. CO_2, p. 25
11. Acids, p. 25
12. Buffers, p. 26
13. Carbohydrate, p. 26
14. Cholesterol, p. 28
15. Structural, p. 28

Multiple choice
16. A, p. 21
17. A, p. 21
18. B, p. 24
19. D, p. 26
20. C, p. 30

CHAPTER 3
CELLS AND TISSUES

Matching

Group A
1. C, p. 38
2. E, p. 38
3. A, p. 38
4. B, p. 43
5. D, p. 42

Group B
6. D, p. 40
7. E, p. 40
8. A, p. 41
9. B, p. 42
10. C, p. 41

Fill in the blanks
11. Organelles, p. 38
12. Tissue typing, p. 39
13. Cilia, p. 42
14. Cellular respiration, p. 42
15. Ribosomes, p. 40
16. Mitochondria, p. 41
17. Lysosomes, p. 42
18. Golgi apparatus, p. 41
19. Centrioles, p. 42
20. Chromatin granules, p. 43

Circle the correct choice
21. A, p. 44
22. D, p. 44
23. B, p. 44
24. D, p. 46
25. C, p. 46
26. A, p. 46
27. B, p. 46
28. C, p. 46
29. D, p. 47
30. A, p. 48
31. B, p. 49
32. A, p. 49

Circle the one that does not belong
33. Uracil (RNA contains the base uracil, not DNA)
34. Telophase (the others are complementary base pairings of DNA)
35. Anaphase (the others refer to genes and heredity)
36. Thymine (the others refer to RNA)
37. Interphase (the others refer to translation)
38. Prophase (the others refer to anaphase)
39. Prophase (the others refer to interphase)
40. Metaphase (the others refer to telophase)
41. Gene (the others refer to stages of cell division)

42. Fill the missing areas

TISSUE	LOCATION	FUNCTION
Epithelial		
1.	1A.	1A. Absorption by diffusion of respiratory gases between alveolar air and blood
	1B.	1B. Absorption by diffusion, filtration, and osmosis
2.	2A. Surface of lining of mouth and esophagus	2A.
	2B. Surface of skin	2B.
3.	3. Surface layer of lining of stomach, intestines, and parts of respiratory tract	3.
4. Stratified transitional	4.	4.
5.	5. Surface of lining of trachea	5.
6.	6.	6. Secretion; absorption
Connective		
1.	1. Between other tissues and organs	1.
2. Adipose	2.	2.
3.	3.	3. Flexible but strong connection
4.	4. Skeleton	4.
5.	5. Part of nasal septum, larynx, rings in trachea and bronchi, disks between vertebrae, external ear	5.
6.	6.	6. Transportation
7. Hemopoietic tissue	7.	7.
Muscle		
1.	1. Muscles that attach to bones, eyeball muscles, upper third of esophagus	1.
2. Cardiac	2.	
3.	3. Walls of digestive, respiratory, and genitourinary tracts; walls of blood and large lymphatic vessels; ducts of glands; intrinsic eye muscles; arrector muscles of hair	3.
Nervous		
1. Nerve cells	1. Brain and spinal cord, nerves	1.

Unscramble the words

43. Translation
44. Interphase
45. Gene
46. Osmosis
47. Diffusion
48. Tissues

Applying what you know

49.

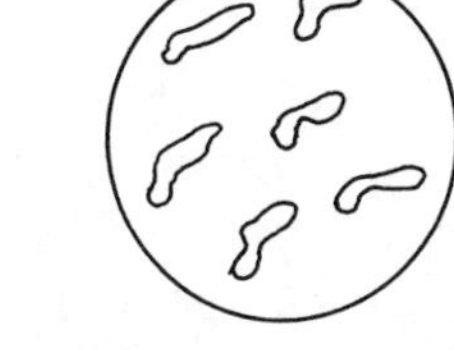

50. Diffusion
51. Absorption of oxygen into Ms. Bence's blood.
52. Merrily may have exceeded the 18–24% desirable body fat composition. Fitness depends more on the percentage and ratio of specific tissue types than the overall amount of tissue present.

53. WORD FIND

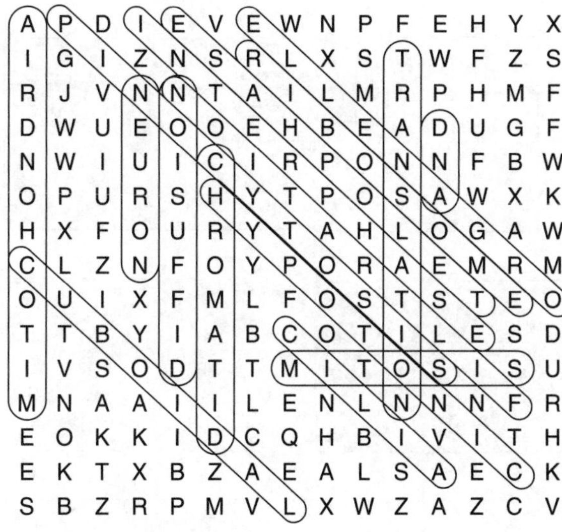

Crossword

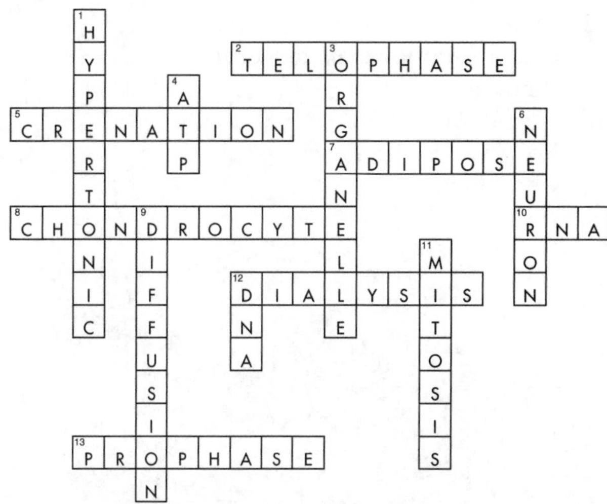

Check your knowledge

Multiple choice

1. A, p. 39
2. B, p. 40
3. B, p. 41
4. A, p. 42
5. C, p. 46
6. A, p. 49
7. D, p. 50
8. B, p. 52
9. C, p. 61
10. D, p. 55

Matching

11. F, p. 40
12. G, p. 42
13. J, p. 44
14. C, p. 44
15. A, p. 47
16. B, p. 49
17. I, p. 51
18. H, p. 54
19. D, p. 54
20. E, p. 59

Cell structure

1. Nucleolus
2. Nuclear envelope
3. Nucleus
4. Nuclear pores
5. Plasma membrane
6. Cytoplasm
7. Centrioles
8. Mitochondrion
9. Lysosome
10. Golgi apparatus

11. Free ribosome
12. Microvilli
13. Cilia
14. Smooth endoplasmic reticulum
15. Ribosome
16. Flagellum
17. Rough endoplasmic reticulum
18. Chromatin

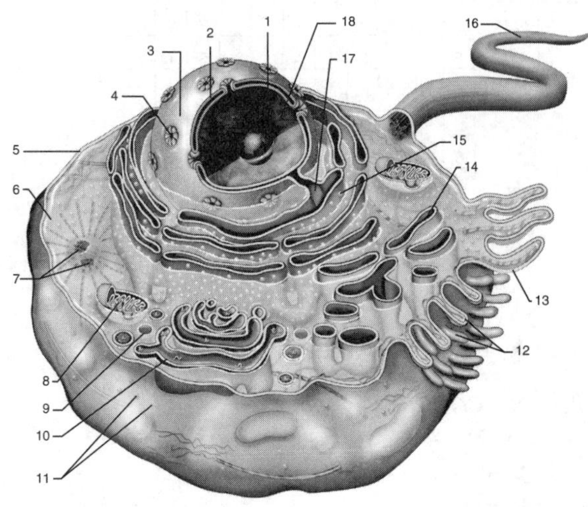

Mitosis
1. Interphase
2. Prophase
3. Metaphase
4. Anaphase
5. Telophase
6. Daughter cells (interphase)

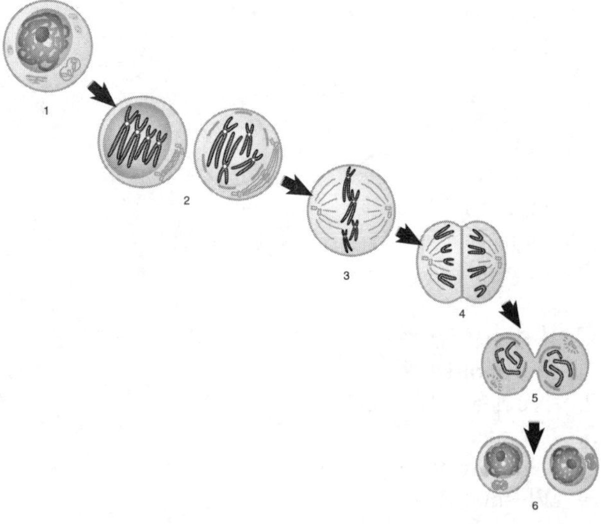

Tissues
1. Stratified squamous epithelium
2. Adipose tissue
3. Simple columnar epithelium
4. Dense fibrous connective tissue
5. Stratified transitional epithelium
6. Bone tissue
7. Cartilage
8. Cardiac muscle
9. Blood
10. Smooth muscle
11. Skeletal muscle
12. Nervous tissue

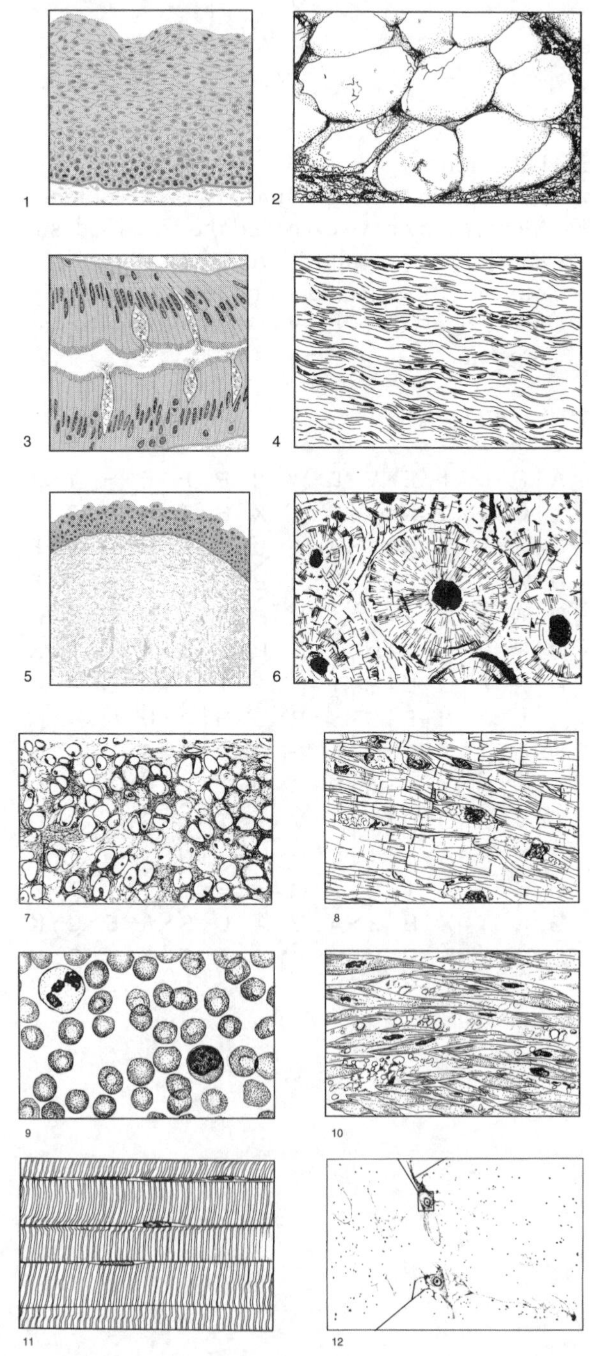

CHAPTER 4
ORGAN SYSTEMS OF THE BODY

Matching

Group A
1. A, p. 72
2. E, p. 72
3. D, p. 74
4. B, p. 74
5. C, p. 76

Group B
6. F, p. 76
7. E, p. 77
8. B, p. 78
9. A, p. 78
10. C, p. 77
11. D, p. 81

Circle the one that does not belong
12. Mouth (the others refer to the respiratory system)
13. Rectum (the others refer to the reproductive system)
14. Pancreas (the others refer to the circulatory system)
15. Pineal (the others refer to the urinary system)
16. Joints (the others refer to the muscular system)
17. Pituitary (the others refer to the nervous system)
18. Tendons (the others refer to the skeletal system)
19. Appendix (the others refer to the endocrine system)
20. Thymus (the others refer to the integumentary system)
21. Trachea (the others refer to the digestive system)
22. Liver (the others refer to the lymphatic system)

Fill in the missing areas

SYSTEM	ORGANS	FUNCTIONS
		23. Protection, regulation of body temperature, synthesis of chemicals and hormones, serves as a sense organ
	24. Bones, joints	
		25. Movement, maintains body posture, produces heat
26. Nervous		
	27. Pituitary, thymus, pineal, adrenal, hypothalamus, thyroid, pancreas, parathyroid, ovaries, testes	
		28. Transportation, immunity
	29. Lymph nodes, lymph vessels, thymus, spleen, tonsils	
30. Urinary		
	31. Mouth, pharynx, esophagus, stomach, small and large intestine, rectum, anal canal, teeth, salivary glands, tongue, liver, gallbladder, pancreas, appendix	
32. Respiratory		
	33. a. Gonads—testes and ovaries	
	b. Accessory organs, ducts, and glands (p. 73)	

Unscramble the words

34. Heart
35. Pineal
36. Nerve
37. Esophagus
38. Nervous

Applying what you know

39. Endocrinology (endocrine system); gynecology (reproductive system)
40. The skin protects the underlying tissue against invasion by harmful bacteria. With a large percentage of Brian's skin destroyed, he was vulnerable to bacteria, and so he was placed in the cleanest environment possible—isolation. Jenny is required to wear special attire so that the risk of her bringing bacteria to the patient is reduced.
41. WORD FIND

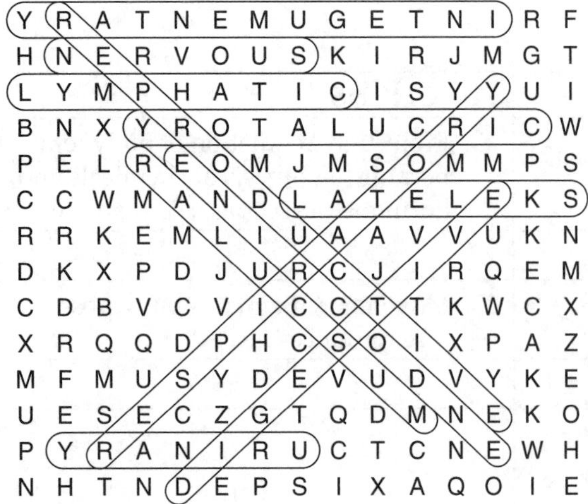

Crossword

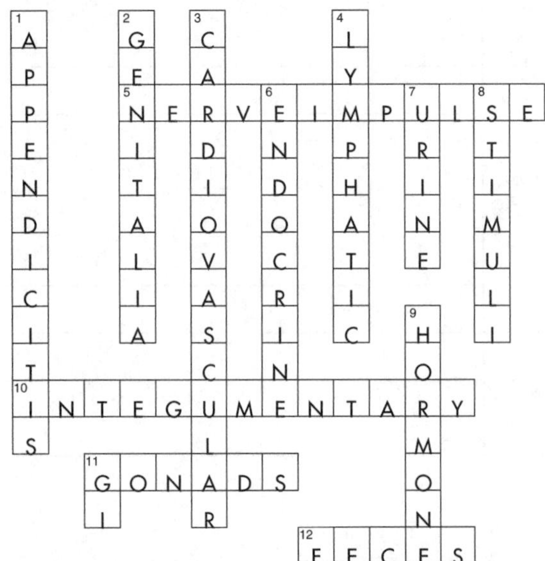

Check your knowledge

Multiple choice

1. D, p. 76
2. C, p. 77
3. C, p. 81
4. B, p. 71
5. D, p. 72
6. A, p. 72
7. B, p. 78
8. A, p. 75
9. A, p. 76
10. C, p. 71

Matching

11. C, p. 72
12. D, p. 76
13. H, p. 76
14. G, p. 81
15. B, p. 78
16. F, p. 78
17. I, p. 82
18. E, p. 77
19. J, p. 74
20. A, p. 76

CHAPTER 5
THE INTEGUMENTARY SYSTEM AND BODY MEMBRANES

Select the best answer

1. B, p. 90
2. D, p. 91
3. C, p. 91
4. A, p. 90
5. B, p. 90
6. D, p. 91
7. C, p. 91
8. C, p. 91

Matching

Group A

9. D, p. 92
10. A, p. 92
11. B, p. 93
12. C, p. 93
13. E, p. 92

Group B

14. A, p. 93
15. D, p. 93
16. E, p. 93
17. C, p. 94
18. B, p. 94

Select the correct term

19. A, p. 93
20. B, p. 94
21. B, p. 94
22. A, p. 93
23. A, p. 93
24. B, p. 94
25. B, p. 94
26. B, p. 94
27. B, p. 94
28. A, p. 93 (Fig. 5-3)

Fill in the blanks

29. Protection, temperature regulation, and sense organ activity, p. 99
30. Melanin, p. 93
31. Lanugo, p. 95
32. Hair papillae, p. 95
33. Lunula, p. 96
34. Arrector pili, p. 95
35. Light touch, p. 96
36. Eccrine, p. 97
37. Apocrine, p. 97
38. Sebum, p. 97

Circle the correct answer

39. Will not, p. 101
40. Will, p. 101
41. Will not, p. 101
42. 11, p. 100
43. Third, p. 101

Unscramble the words

44. Epidermis
45. Keratin
46. Hair
47. Lanugo
48. Dehydration
49. Third degree

Applying what you know

50. 46
51. Pleurisy
52. Fingerprints

53. WORD FIND

S	U	D	O	R	I	F	E	R	O	U	S	V	K	R
E	J	U	Q	U	E	S	T	E	C	N	O	H	Y	U
I	S	J	L	M	E	L	A	N	O	C	Y	T	E	H
R	I	M	U	E	N	O	T	I	R	E	P	H	S	B
O	M	K	N	V	A	S	T	R	L	A	N	U	G	O
T	R	G	U	F	G	A	U	C	E	G	O	V	W	D
A	E	A	L	P	R	D	I	O	N	T	F	D	R	N
L	D	V	A	D	M	L	C	P	D	H	S	L	Z	F
I	I	N	Y	N	L	R	L	A	M	E	N	I	R	E
P	P	H	Q	O	N	E	U	X	R	R	F	E	L	G
E	E	Z	F	J	U	M	Y	O	U	U	O	C	C	B
D	Z	P	E	R	J	Y	U	V	F	C	I	I	E	O
G	J	S	I	W	J	S	K	C	D	T	N	O	Z	C
C	O	S	M	Z	M	F	I	B	U	G	U	X	O	J
X	Y	P	M	E	I	W	E	C	V	S	U	G	B	I

Crossword

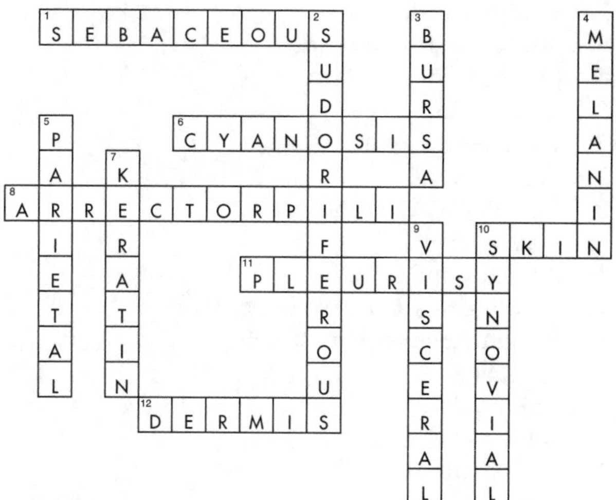

Check your knowledge

Multiple choice

1. A, p. 91
2. B, p. 93
3. A, p. 94
4. D, p. 93
5. B, p. 94
6. D, p. 95
7. B, p. 96
8. B, p. 96
9. C, p. 97
10. B, p. 97

Matching

11. C, p. 92
12. D, p. 90
13. B, p. 91
14. G, p. 91

15. I, p. 91
16. H, p. 93
17. J, p. 95
18. E, p. 95
19. A, p. 96
20. F, p. 97

Completion

21. A, p. 99
22. H, p. 99
23. B, p. 91
24. F, p. 91
25. I, p. 101
26. E, p. 101
27. G, p. 101
28. D, p. 101
29. J, p. 97
30. C, p. 97

Longitudinal section of the skin

1. Dermal papilla
2. Stratum corneum
3. Stratum germinativum
4. Openings of sweat ducts
5. Sweat gland
6. Cutaneous nerve
7. Papilla of hair
8. Lamillar (Pacini) corpuscle
9. Hair follicle
10. Arrector muscle
11. Tactile (Meissner) corpuscle
12. Subcutaneous tissue
13. Dermis
14. Epidermis
15. Sebaceous (oil) gland
16. Hair shaft

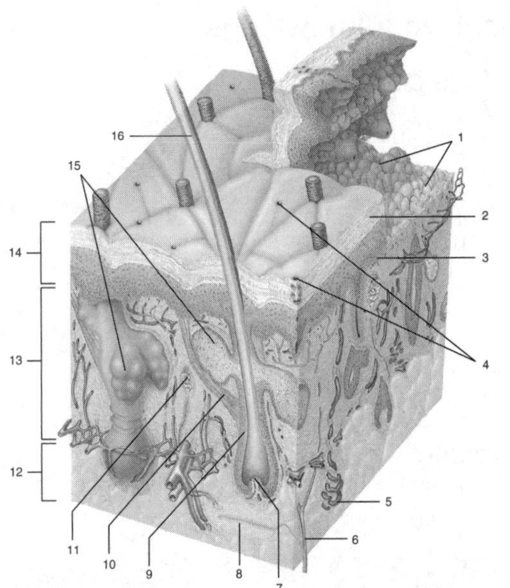

"Rule of Nines" for estimating skin surface burned

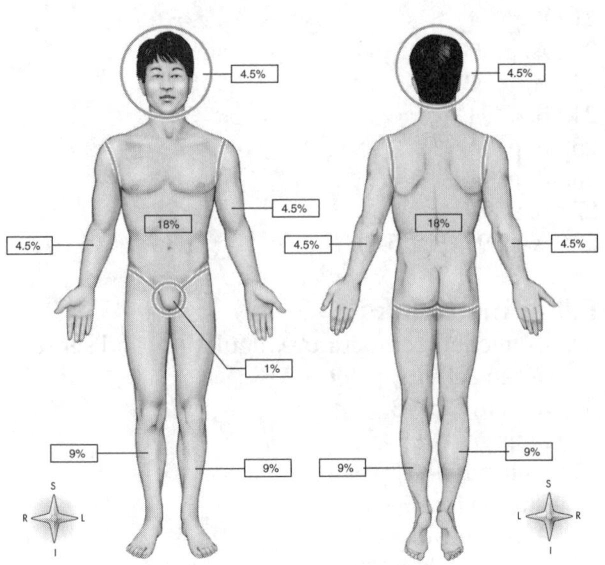

CHAPTER 6 THE SKELETAL SYSTEM

Fill in the blanks

1. 4, p. 110
2. Medullary cavity, p. 110
3. Articular cartilage p. 110
4. Endosteum, p. 111
5. Hemopoiesis, p. 110
6. Red bone marrow, p. 110
7. Periosteum, p. 110
8. Elderly white females, p. 115
9. Calcium, p. 110
10. Move, p. 110

Matching

Group A

11. D, p. 111
12. B, p. 111
13. E, p. 111
14. A, p. 112
15. C, p. 112

Group B

16. D, p. 112
17. A, p. 112
18. E, p. 111
19. B, p. 112
20. C, p. 111

True or false
21. T
22. Epiphyses, not diaphyses, p. 115
23. Osteoblasts, not osteoclasts, p. 113
24. T
25. Increase, not decrease, p. 114
26. Juvenile, not adult, p. 115
27. Diaphysis, not articulation, p. 115
28. T
29. Ceases, not begins, p. 115
30. T

Multiple choice
31. A, p. 123
32. D, p. 117
33. A, p. 121
34. D, p. 121
35. C, p. 123
36. C, p. 126
37. D, p. 124
38. D, p. 126
39. A, p. 126
40. B, p. 117
41. A, p. 121
42. B, p. 124
43. B, p. 122
44. B, p. 124
45. C, p. 124
46. A, p. 126
47. D, p. 117
48. C, p. 121
49. C, p. 117

Circle the one that does not belong
50. Coxal bone (all others refer to the spine)
51. Axial (all others refer to the appendicular skeleton)
52. Maxilla (all others refer to the cranial bones)
53. Ribs (all others refer to the shoulder girdle)
54. Vomer (all others refer to the bones of the middle ear)
55. Ulna (all others refer to the coxal bone)
56. Ethmoid (all others refer to the hand and wrist)
57. Nasal (all others refer to cranial bones)
58. Anvil (all others refer to the cervical vertebra)

Choose the correct term
59. A, p. 127
60. B, p. 127
61. B, p. 127
62. A, p. 127
63. B, p. 127

Matching
64. C, p. 117
65. G, p. 122
66. J, L, M, and K, p. 126
67. N, p. 126
68. I, p. 124
69. A, p. 117
70. P, p. 126
71. D, B, p. 117
72. F, p. 117
73. H, Q, p. 124
74. O, T, p. 126
75. R, p. 117
76. S, E, p. 117

Circle the correct answer
77. Diarthroses, p. 128
78. Synarthrotic, p. 128
79. Diarthrotic, p. 129
80. Ligaments, p. 129
81. Articular cartilage, p. 129
82. Least movable, p. 133
83. Largest, p. 135
84. 2, p. 130
85. Mobility, p. 132
86. Pivot, p. 130

Unscramble the words
87. Vertebrae
88. Pubis
89. Scapula
90. Mandible
91. Phalanges
92. Pelvic girdle

Applying what you know
93. The bones are responsible for the majority of our blood cell formation. The disease condition of the bones might be inhibiting the production of blood cells for Mrs. Perine.
94. Epiphyseal cartilage is present only while a child is still growing. It becomes bone in adulthood. It is particularly vulnerable to fractures in childhood and preadolescence.
95. Osteoporosis

96. WORD FIND

A R T I C U L A T I O N N U T
M M L T N I N G U I H J N C G
P R P E R I O S T E U M A N B
H V P G U A T B M E O P R F G
I N V R N O B O F S M H X E R
A G J O A J P E T O E O H T Q
R U R B X O E E C A S G I S B
T S S Y I M O Q N U O O L X Q
H J I E A B P U N Q L E Q K S
R I S I L U C I L A N A C X R
O I N A M A S Q M A Q K E C T
S T S A L C O E T S O U I D G
E T S Y F W L N M P U F N U F
S B H Q H L O U S A R X I T V
R P M P A F M G X K D S L G A

Crossword

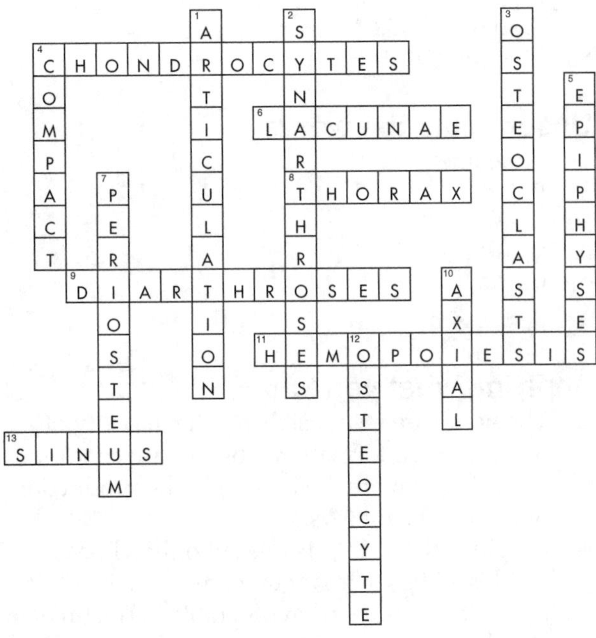

Check your knowledge

Multiple choice

1. A, p. 110
2. C, p. 110
3. A, p. 110
4. C, p. 116
5. C, pp. 124 and 126
6. D, p. 112
7. C, p. 119
8. C, p. 122
9. D, p. 124 and Table 6-5
10. A, p. 128

Matching

11. G, p. 128
12. B, p. 110
13. I, p. 111
14. J, p. 117
15. E, p. 122
16. H, p. 117
17. A, p. 124
18. C, p. 128
19. F, p. 130
20. D, p. 132

Longitudinal section of long bone

1. Articular cartilage
2. Cancellous (spongy) bone
3. Epiphyseal line
4. Red marrow cavities
5. Compact bone
6. Medullary cavity
7. Endosteum
8. Yellow marrow
9. Periosteum
10. Diaphysis
11. Epiphysis

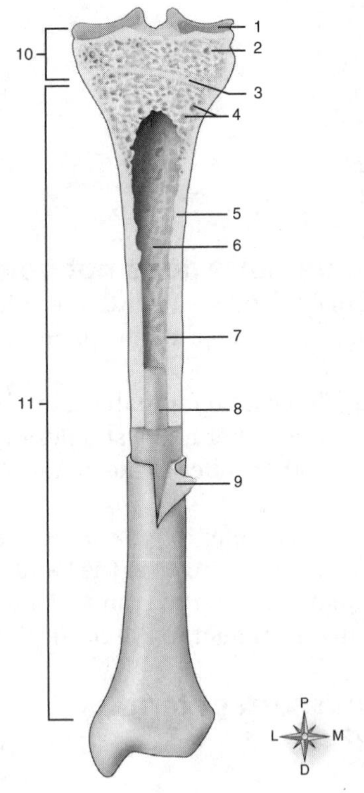

Anterior view of skeleton

1. Frontal bone
2. Nasal bone
3. Zygomatic bone
4. Sternum
5. Ribs
6. Vertebrae
7. Ilium
8. Pubis
9. Ischium
10. Greater trochanter
11. Phalanges
12. Metatarsals
13. Tarsals
14. Fibula
15. Tibia
16. Patella
17. Femur
18. Phalanges
19. Metacarpals
20. Carpals
21. Ulna
22. Radius
23. Humerus
24. Xiphoid process
25. Costal cartilage
26. Scapula
27. Manubrium
28. Clavicle
29. Mandible
30. Maxilla

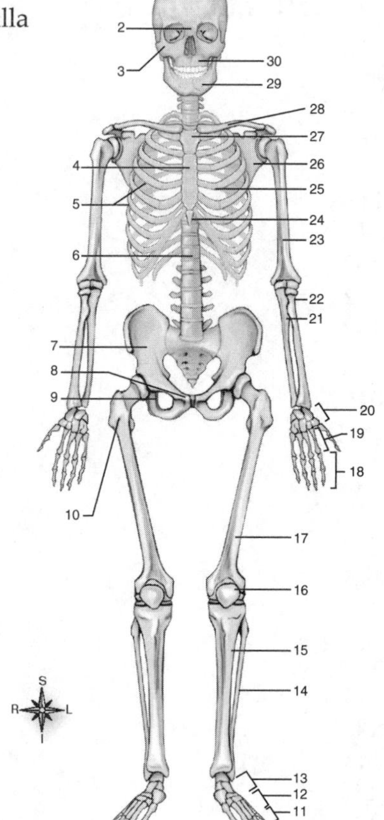

Posterior view of skeleton

1. Clavicle
2. Acromion process
3. Scapula
4. Ribs
5. Humerus
6. Ulna
7. Radius
8. Carpals
9. Metacarpals
10. Phalanges
11. Ilium
12. Ischium
13. Pubis
14. Coxal (hip) bone
15. Calcaneus (a tarsal bone)
16. Metatarsal bones
17. Phalanges
18. Tarsals
19. Fibula
20. Tibia
21. Femur
22. Sacrum
23. Lumbar vertebrae
24. Thoracic vertebrae
25. Cervical vertebrae
26. Occipital bone
27. Parietal bone

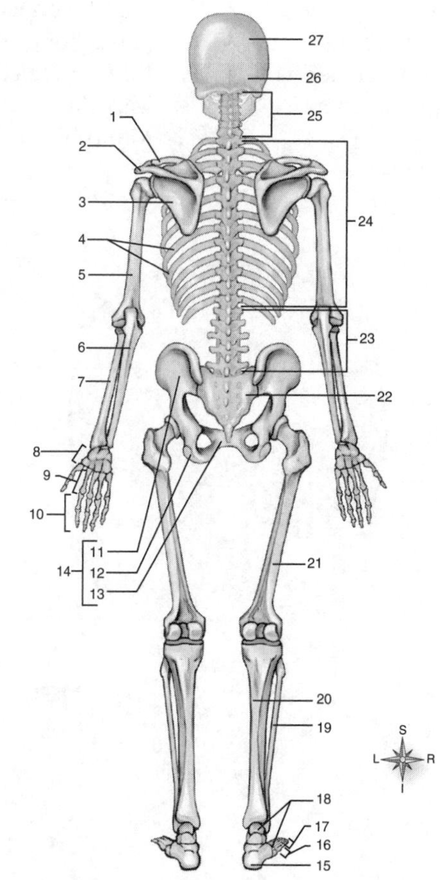

Skull viewed from the right side

1. Parietal bone
2. Squamous suture
3. Occipital bone
4. Lambdoidal suture
5. Temporal bone
6. External auditory canal
7. Mastoid process
8. Coronal suture
9. Frontal bone
10. Sphenoid bone
11. Ethmoid bone
12. Nasal bone
13. Zygomatic bone
14. Maxilla
15. Mandible

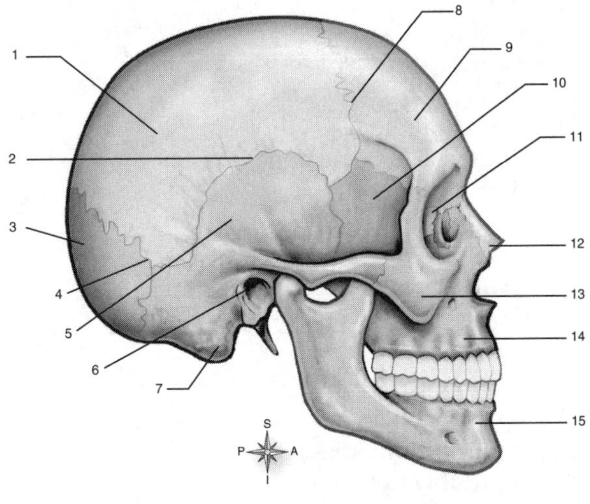

Skull viewed from the front

1. Sphenoid bone
2. Ethmoid bone
3. Lacrimal bone
4. Zygomatic bone
5. Vomer
6. Frontal bone
7. Parietal bone
8. Nasal bone
9. Inferior concha
10. Maxilla
11. Mandible

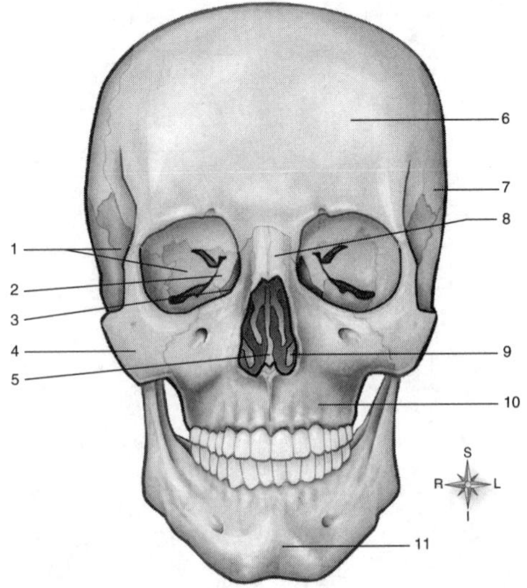

Structure of a diarthrotic joint

1. Bone
2. Periosteum
3. Blood vessel
4. Nerve
5. Articular cartilage
6. Joint cavity
7. Joint capsule
8. Articular cartilage
9. Synovial membrane

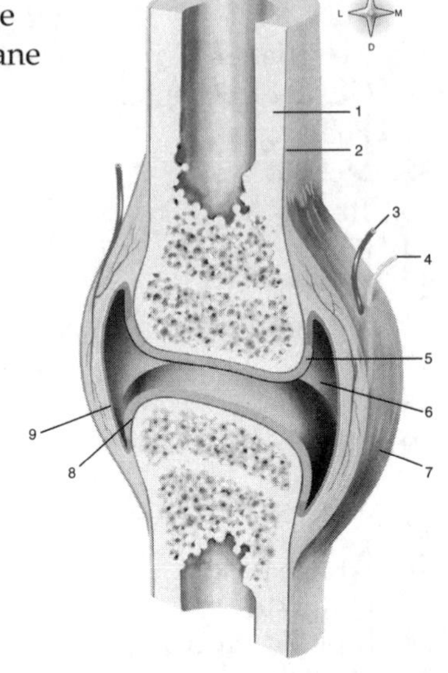

CHAPTER 7
THE MUSCULAR SYSTEM

Select the correct term

1. A and B, p. 142
2. B, p. 142
3. C, p. 142
4. C, p. 142
5. A, p. 142
6. B, p. 142
7. C and B, p. 142
8. A, p. 142
9. C, p. 142
10. C, p. 142

Matching

Group A

11. D, p. 143
12. B, p. 143
13. A, p. 143
14. E, p. 143
15. C, p. 143

Group B

16. E, p. 143
17. C, p. 143
18. B, p. 143
19. A, p. 143
20. D, p. 143

Fill in the blanks

21. Pulling, p. 145
22. Insertion, p. 145
23. Insertion, origin, p. 145
24. Prime mover, p. 146
25. Antagonists, p. 146
26. Synergist, p. 146
27. Tonic contraction, p. 146
28. Muscle tone, p. 146
29. Hypothermia, p. 147
30. ATP, p. 147

True or false

31. Neuromuscular junction, p. 148
32. T
33. T
34. Oxygen debt, p. 147
35. "All or none," p. 149
36. Lactic acid, p. 147
37. T
38. T
39. Skeletal muscle, p. 148
40. T

Circle the correct answer

41. A, p. 149
42. B, p. 149
43. B, p. 150
44. C, p. 150
45. D, p. 150
46. A, p. 149
47. B, p. 149
48. C, p. 149
49. B, p. 150
50. D, p. 150

Circle the correct answer

51. A, p. 151
52. D, p. 152
53. C, p. 152
54. A, p. 152
55. D, p. 152
56. C, p. 152

Select the best choice or choices

57. C, p. 154
58. F, A, and D, pp. 154 and 156
59. F and B, pp. 154 and 156
60. A, p. 154
61. C, p. 154
62. B and F, pp. 154 and 156
63. A, p. 154
64. A and D, pp. 154 and 156
65. B, p. 154
66. B, p. 154
67. A and E, p. 156
68. B, p. 156
69. D, p. 156

Unscramble the words

70. Flexion
71. Actin
72. Eversion
73. Origin
74. Sarcomere
75. Extension

Applying what you know

76. Bursitis
77. Deltoid area
78. Tendon

79. WORD FIND

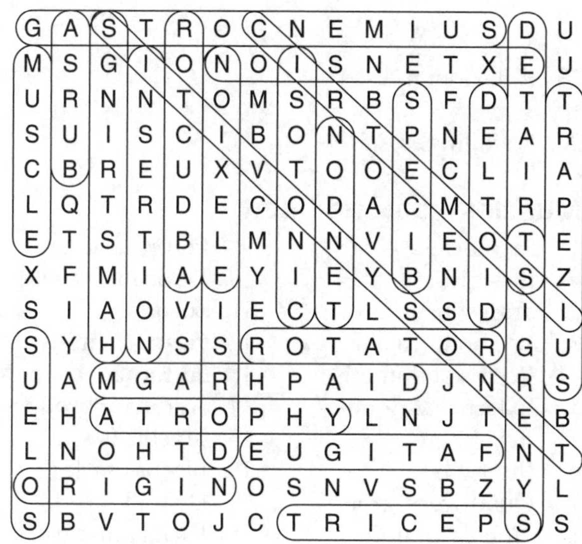

Crossword

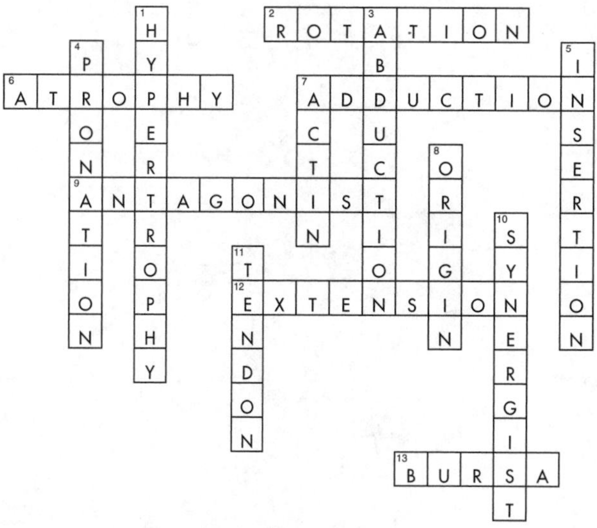

Check your knowledge

Multiple choice

1. D, p. 150
2. A, p. 150
3. C, p. 149
4. B, p. 148
5. A, p. 146
6. B, p. 144
7. D, p. 147
8. A, p. 143
9. A, p. 142
10. C, p. 158

True or false

11. T
12. T
13. F, myosin, p. 143
14. F, posterior, p. 155
15. T
16. T
17. T
18. F, flexion, p. 151
19. T
20. F, smiling, p. 154

Muscles—anterior view

1. Sternocleido-mastoid
2. Trapezius
3. Pectoralis major
4. Rectus abdominis
5. External abdominal oblique
6. Iliopsoas
7. Quadriceps group
8. Tibialis anterior
9. Peroneus longus
10. Peroneus brevis
11. Soleus
12. Gastrocnemius
13. Sartorius
14. Adductor group
15. Brachialis
16. Biceps brachii
17. Deltoid
18. Facial muscles

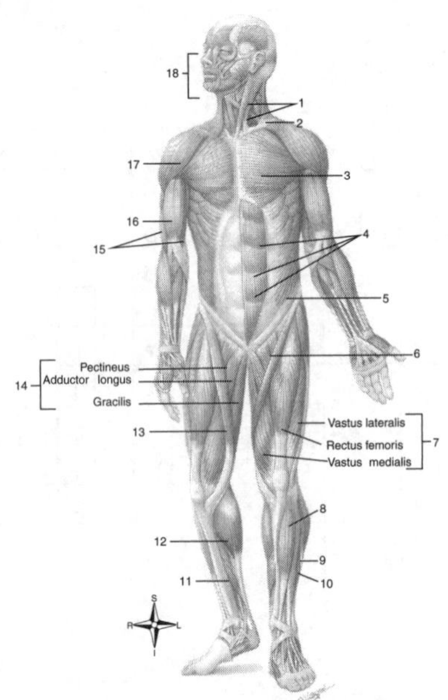

Muscles—posterior view

1. Trapezius
2. External abdominal oblique
3. Gluteus maximus
4. Adductor magnus
5. Soleus
6. Peroneus brevis
7. Peroneus longus
8. Gastrocnemius
9. Hamstring group
10. Latissimus dorsi
11. Triceps brachii
12. Deltoid
13. Sternocleido-mastoid

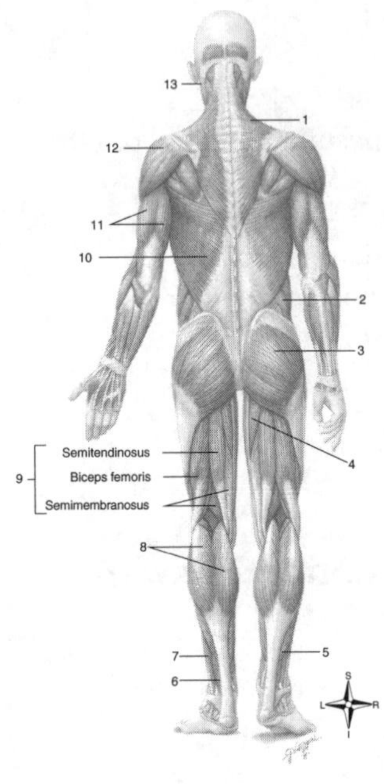

CHAPTER 8 THE NERVOUS SYSTEM

Matching

Group A

1. B, p. 168
2. C, p. 168
3. D, p. 168
4. A, p. 168

Group B

5. B, p. 168
6. D, p. 168
7. C, p. 168
8. A, p. 169
9. F, p. 171
10. E, p. 171

Select the correct term

11. A, p. 168
12. B, p. 169
13. B, p. 170
14. A, p. 168
15. A, p. 168

16. B, p. 170
17. B, p. 170
18. A, p. 168
19. B, p. 173
20. A, p. 169

Fill in the blanks

21. Two-neuron arc, p. 171
22. Sensory, interneurons, and motor neurons, p. 171
23. Receptors, p. 172
24. Synapse, p. 172
25. Reflex, p. 173
26. Withdrawal reflex, p. 173
27. Ganglion, p. 172
28. Interneurons, p. 173
29. "Knee jerk," p. 172
30. Gray matter, p. 173

Circle the correct answer

31. Do not, p. 174
32. Increases, p. 174
33. Excess, p. 174
34. Postsynaptic, p. 174
35. Presynaptic, p. 174
36. Neurotransmitter, p. 176
37. Communicate, p. 174
38. Specifically, p. 176
39. Sleep, p. 176
40. Pain, p. 176

Circle the correct answer

41. E, p. 176
42. D, p. 177
43. A, p. 177
44. E, p. 179
45. E, p. 179
46. D, p. 179
47. B, p. 180
48. E, p. 182
49. B, p. 181
50. D, p. 181
51. D, p. 179
52. B, p. 180
53. A, p. 182
54. D, p. 180
55. C, p. 180

True or false

56. 17 to 18 inches, p. 183
57. Bottom of the first lumbar vertebra, p. 183
58. Lumbar punctures, p. 187
59. Spinal tracts, p. 184
60. T
61. One general function, p. 184
62. Anesthesia, p. 185

Circle the one that does not belong

63. Ventricles (all others refer to meninges)
64. CSF (all others refer to the arachnoid)
65. Pia mater (all others refer to the cerebrospinal fluid)
66. Choroid plexus (all others refer to the dura mater)
67. Brain tumor (all others refer to a lumbar puncture)

68. Fill in the missing areas on the chart below.

NERVE		CONDUCT IMPULSES	FUNCTION
I	Olfactory		
II			Vision
III		From brain to eye muscles	
IV	Trochlear		
V			Sensations of face, scalp, and teeth, chewing movements
VI		From brain to external eye muscles	
VII		Sense of taste; contractions of muscles of facial expression	
VIII	Vestibulocochlear		
IX		From throat and taste buds of tongue to brain; also from brain to throat muscles and salivary glands	
X	Vagus		
XI			Shoulder movements; turning movements of head
XII	Hypoglossal		

Select the correct term
69. A, p. 187
70. B, p. 189
71. A, p. 187
72. B, p. 195
73. B, p. 188
74. A, p. 187
75. B, p. 188
76. B, p. 189

Matching
77. D, p. 189
78. E, p. 190
79. F, p. 190
80. B, p. 191
81. A, p. 190
82. C, p. 190

Circle the correct answer
83. C, p. 192
84. B, p. 192
85. B, p. 193
86. D, p. 193
87. A, p. 193
88. A, p. 194

Select the correct term
89. B, p. 193
90. A, p. 193
91. A, p. 193
92. B, p. 193
93. A, p. 193
94. B, p. 193
95. A, p. 193
96. A, p. 193
97. B, p. 193
98. B, p. 193

Fill in the blanks
99. Acetylcholine, p. 194
100. Adrenergic fibers, p. 194
101. Cholinergic fibers, p. 194
102. Homeostasis, p. 194
103. Heart rate, p. 195
104. Decreased, p. 195

Unscramble the words
105. Neurons
106. Synapse
107. Autonomic
108. Smooth muscle
109. Sympathetic

Applying what you know

110. Right
111. Hydrocephalus
112. Sympathetic
113. Parasympathetic
114. Sympathetic; No, the digestive process is not active during sympathetic control. Bill may experience nausea, vomiting, or discomfort because of this factor. See p. 193

115. WORD FIND

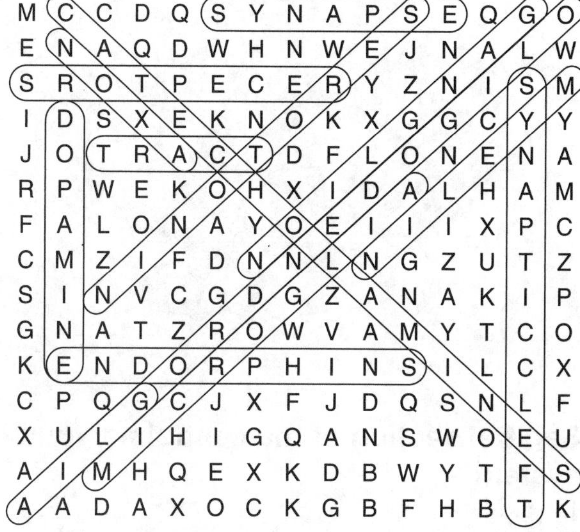

Crossword

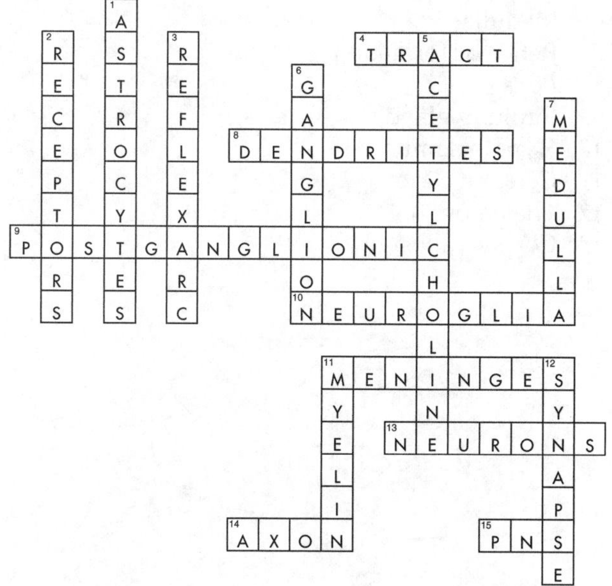

Check your knowledge

Multiple choice

1. D, p. 168
2. B, p. 169
3. A, p. 170
4. B, p. 171
5. A, p. 172
6. D, p. 174
7. D, p. 176
8. C, p. 169
9. C, p. 185
10. D, p. 189

Matching

11. C, p. 173
12. A, p. 180
13. J, p. 182
14. H, p. 185
15. B, p. 189
16. I, p. 188
17. F, p. 191
18. E, p. 193
19. D, p. 194
20. G, p. 180

Neuron

1. Dendrites
2. Cell body
3. Mitochondrion
4. Nucleus
5. Axon
6. Schwann cell
7. Node of Ranvier
8. Nucleus of Schwann cell
9. Myelin sheath
10. Axon
11. Cell membrane of axon
12. Neurilemma (sheath of Schwann cell)

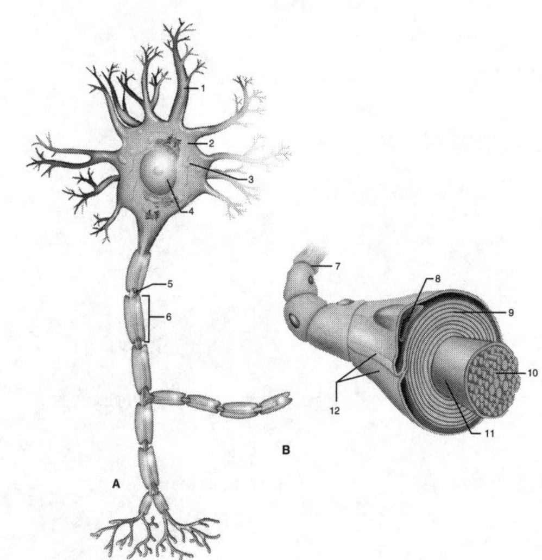

Cranial nerves
1. Olfactory nerve
2. Trigeminal nerve
3. Glossopharyngeal nerve
4. Hypoglossal nerve
5. Accessory nerve
6. Vagus nerve
7. Vestibulocochlear nerve
8. Facial nerve
9. Abducens nerve
10. Oculomotor nerve
11. Optic nerve
12. Trochlear nerve

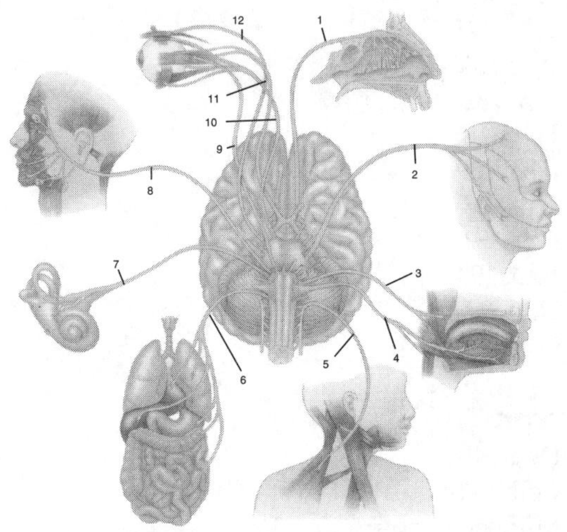

Neural pathway involved in the patellar reflex
1. Dorsal root ganglion
2. Sensory neuron
3. Stretch receptor
4. Patella
5. Patellar tendon
6. Quadriceps muscle
7. Motor neuron
8. Monosynaptic synapse
9. Gray matter
10. Interneuron

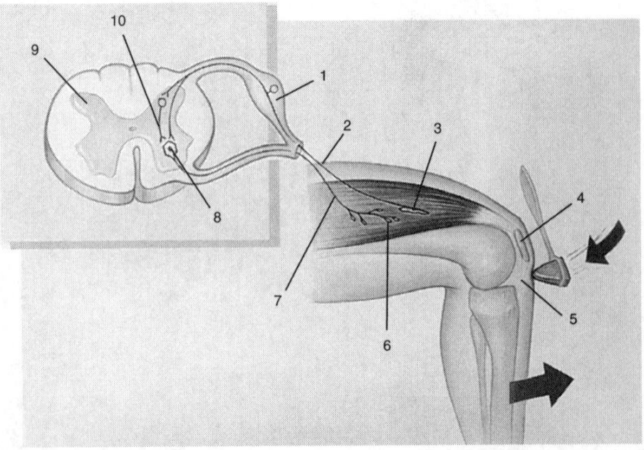

The cerebrum
1. Occipital lobe
2. Temporal lobe
3. Lateral fissure
4. Frontal lobe
5. Central sulcus
6. Parietal lobe

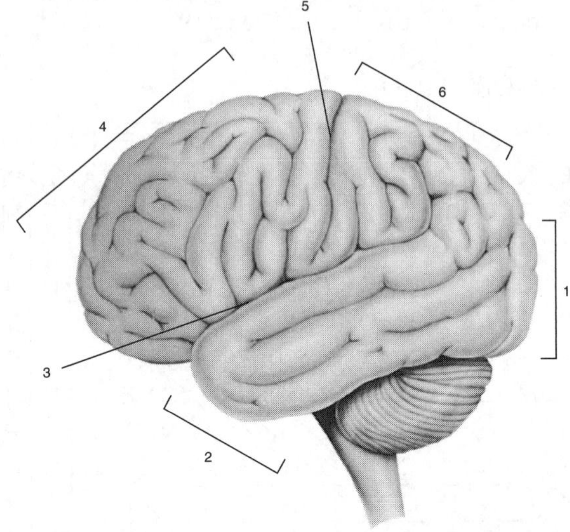

Sagittal section of the central nervous system
1. Skull
2. Pineal gland
3. Cerebellum
4. Midbrain
5. Spinal cord
6. Medulla
7. Reticular formation
8. Pons
9. Pituitary gland
10. Hypothalamus
11. Cerebral cortex
12. Thalamus
13. Corpus callosum

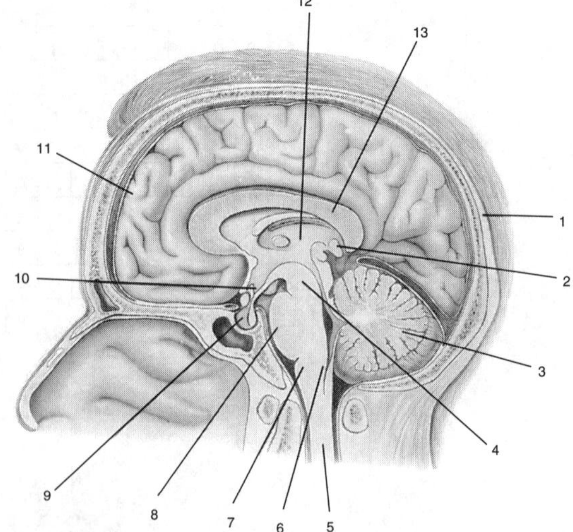

Autonomic conduction paths

1. Axon of somatic motor neuron
2. Cell body of somatic motor neuron
3. White matter
4. Spinal cord
5. Gray matter
6. Cell body of preganglionic neuron
7. Dorsal root
8. Ventral root
9. Axon of preganglionic sympathetic neuron
10. Axon of postganglionic neuron
11. Sympathetic ganglion
12. Collateral ganglion
13. Axon of postganglionic sympathetic neuron

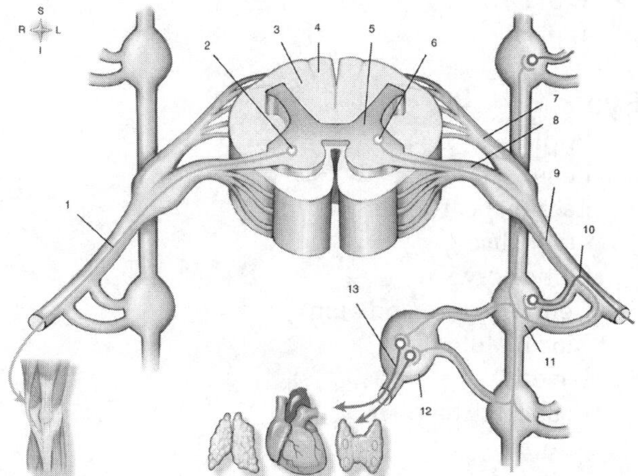

CHAPTER 9 SENSE ORGANS

Matching

1. D, p. 206
2. B, p. 206
3. A, p. 206
4. E, p. 206
5. C, p. 206

Circle the correct answer

6. C, p. 208
7. E, p. 209
8. B, p. 208
9. C, p. 209
10. E, p. 209
11. D, p. 210
12. A, p. 210
13. B, p. 210
14. C, p. 210
15. B, p. 211
16. D, p. 210
17. A, p. 210
18. D, p. 212

Select the correct term

19. B, p. 214
20. C, p. 215
21. B, p. 214
22. A, p. 214
23. C, p. 215
24. A, p. 214
25. C, p. 215
26. B, p. 214
27. B, p. 214
28. C, p. 215

Fill in the blanks

29. Auricle; external auditory canal, p. 214
30. Eardrum, p. 214
31. Ossicles, p. 214
32. Oval window, p. 214
33. Otitis media, p. 214
34. Vestibule, p. 215
35. Mechanoreceptors, p. 215
36. Crista ampullaris, p. 215

Circle the correct answer

37. Papillae, p. 216
38. Cranial, p. 218
39. Mucus, p. 218
40. Memory, p. 218
41. Chemoreceptors, p. 216

Unscramble the words

42. Auricle
43. Sclera
44. Papilla
45. Conjunctiva
46. Pupils

Applying what you know

47. External otitis
48. Cataracts
49. The eustachian tube connects the throat to the middle ear and provides a perfect pathway for the spread of infection.
50. Olfactory

51. WORD FIND

M	E	C	H	A	N	O	R	E	C	E	P	T	O	R
H	R	A	T	B	Q	I	R	T	B	N	H	M	A	E
P	F	T	Y	R	O	T	C	A	F	L	O	X	R	C
G	U	A	Y	I	N	A	I	H	C	A	T	S	U	E
G	P	R	A	C	E	R	U	M	E	N	O	P	X	P
I	E	A	I	P	O	Y	B	S	E	R	P	K	D	T
W	L	C	P	L	Y	N	E	Y	K	E	I	T	O	O
C	Q	T	O	I	B	R	J	B	S	F	G	L	M	R
Z	U	S	R	C	L	E	O	U	J	R	M	N	N	S
F	D	M	E	O	H	L	Q	T	N	A	E	Y	I	S
H	I	D	P	N	D	L	A	M	A	C	N	X	S	Z
A	M	L	Y	E	S	S	E	E	D	T	T	M	Z	H
D	D	M	H	S	F	E	X	A	Y	I	S	I	I	A
J	C	G	N	J	T	I	S	L	P	O	G	U	V	J
P	H	G	Y	A	K	H	S	U	C	N	I	S	G	A

Crossword

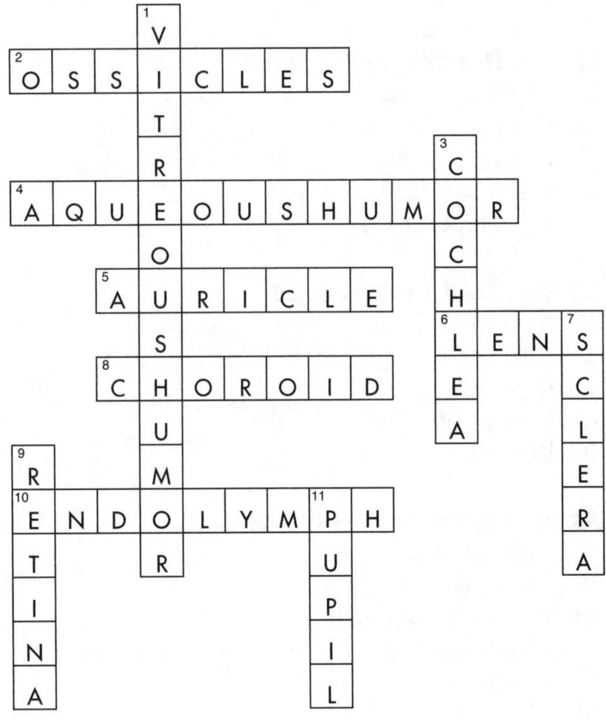

Check your knowledge

Multiple choice

1. A, p. 206
2. B, p. 212
3. A, p. 215
4. C, p. 212
5. B, p. 214
6. B, p. 215
7. D, p. 208
8. B, p. 210
9. D, p. 214
10. A, p. 210

True or false

11. T, p. 205
12. F, Window of the eye, p. 208
13. T, p. 209
14. F, Cataract, p. 210
15. T, p. 209
16. T, p. 212
17. T, p. 214
18. T, p. 214
19. T, p. 216
20. T, p. 209

Eye

1. Pupil
2. Lens
3. Lacrimal caruncle
4. Optic disc
5. Optic nerve
6. Central artery and vein
7. Macula lutea
8. Fovea
9. Posterior chamber
10. Sclera
11. Choroid
12. Retina
13. Ciliary body
14. Lower lid
15. Iris
16. Anterior chamber
17. Cornea

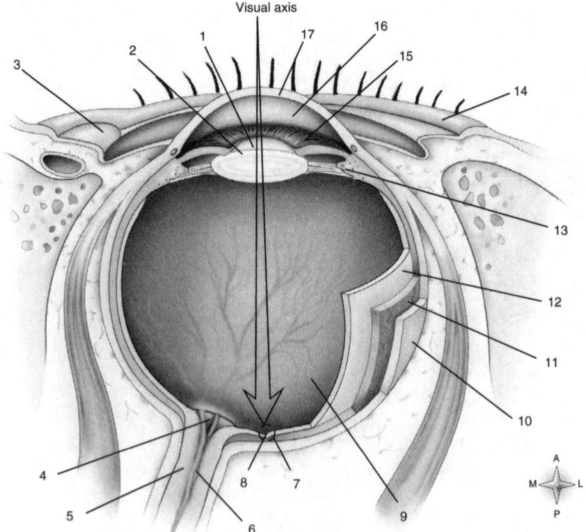

Ear

1. Auricle
2. Temporal bone
3. External auditory meatus
4. Tympanic membrane
5. Semicircular canals
6. Oval window
7. Facial nerve
8. Vestibular nerve
9. Cochlear nerve
10. Cochlea
11. Vestibule
12.. Auditory tube
13. Stapes
14. Incus
15. Malleus

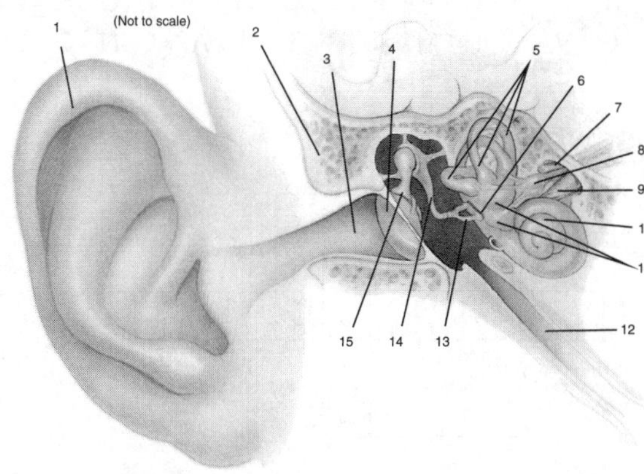

CHAPTER 10 ENDOCRINE SYSTEM

Matching

Group A

1. D, p. 226
2. C, p. 226
3. E, p. 226
4. A, p. 226
5. B, p. 226

Group B

6. E, p. 229
7. C, p. 230
8. A, p. 226
9. D, p. 225
10. B, p. 225

Fill in the blanks

11. First messengers, p. 226
12. Endocrine glands, p. 226
13. Target organs, p. 226
14. Cyclic AMP, p. 226
15. Second messenger, p. 226
16. Communication, p. 226
17. Target cells, p. 226

Circle the correct answer

18. B, p. 231
19. E, p. 231
20. D, p. 231
21. D, p. 231
22. A, p. 232
23. C, p. 232
24. C, p. 232
25. B, p. 231
26. A, p. 231
27. A, p. 231
28. D, p. 232
29. B, p. 232
30. A, p. 233
31. C, p. 233
32. C, p. 233

Select the correct term

33. A, p. 231
34. B, p. 231
35. B, p. 233
36. C, p. 234
37. A, p. 233
38. C, p. 234
39. A, p. 231
40. A, p. 231
41. A, p. 233
42. C, p. 233

Circle the correct answer

43. Below, p. 234
44. Calcitonin, p. 234
45. Iodine, p. 234
46. Do not, p. 234
47. Thyroid, p. 234
48. Decrease, p. 235
49. Hypothyroidism, p. 235
50. Cretinism, p. 235
51. PTH, p. 236
52. Increase, p. 236

Fill in the blanks

53. Adrenal cortex; adrenal medulla, p. 236
54. Corticoids, p. 236
55. Mineralocorticoids, p. 236
56. Glucocorticoids, p. 237
57. Sex hormones, p. 237
58. Gluconeogenesis, p. 237
59. Blood pressure, p. 237
60. Epinephrine; norepinephrine, p. 238
61. Stress, p. 238
62. Addison disease, p. 239

Select the correct term

63. A, p. 236
64. A, p. 237
65. B, p. 239
66. A, p. 239
67. B, p. 238
68. A, p. 237
69. A, p. 238

Circle the term that does not belong

70. Beta cells (all others refer to glucagon)
71. Glucagon (all others refer to insulin)
72. Thymosin (all others refer to female sex glands)
73. Chorion (all other refer to male sex glands)
74. Aldosterone (all others refer to the thymus)
75. ACTH (all others refer to the placenta)
76. Semen (all others refer to the pineal gland)

Matching

Group A

77. E, p. 240
78. C, p. 240
79. B, p. 241
80. D, p. 241
81. A, p. 241

Group B

82. E, p. 243
83. A, p. 243
84. B, p. 243
85. C, p. 241
86. D, p. 242

Unscramble the words

87. Corticoids
88. Diuresis
89. Glucocorticoids
90. Steroids
91. Stress

Applying what you know

92. She was pregnant.
93. Adrenal cortex (This source of testosterone may produce secondary male characteristics if unattended to at this young age.)
94. Oxytocin

95. WORD FIND

S	S	I	S	E	R	U	I	D	M	E	S	I	T	W
N	D	N	X	E	B	A	M	E	D	E	X	Y	M	I
I	I	G	O	N	R	S	G	X	T	I	I	Y	V	B
D	O	M	S	I	N	I	T	E	R	C	C	U	Q	D
N	C	X	S	R	T	N	B	O	T	V	M	Y	O	M
A	I	M	E	C	L	A	C	R	E	P	Y	H	I	X
L	T	Y	R	O	I	E	Z	Q	R	T	J	V	K	F
G	R	E	T	D	P	S	N	I	L	D	J	M	X	N
A	O	O	S	N	I	D	K	I	N	K	S	P	P	O
T	C	P	R	E	T	I	O	G	R	I	F	M	X	G
S	L	M	H	Y	P	O	G	L	Y	C	E	M	I	A
O	A	J	L	H	O	R	M	O	N	E	O	T	G	C
R	C	E	L	T	S	E	L	C	N	P	N	X	U	U
P	I	O	S	W	R	T	X	C	G	U	L	O	E	L
G	G	V	Y	H	M	S	H	Y	K	A	K	N	Q	G

Crossword

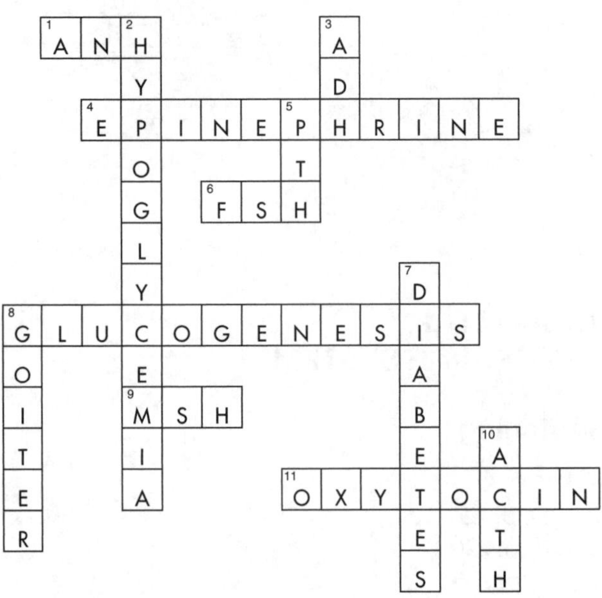

Check your knowledge

Multiple choice

1. A, p. 225
2. C, p. 231
3. D, p. 231
4. C, p. 232
5. D, p. 232
6. D, p. 232
7. B, p. 234
8. D, p. 238
9. D, p. 243
10. B, p. 242

Matching
11. J, p. 228
12. G, p. 230
13. H, p. 231
14. I, p. 235
15. B, p. 234
16. F, p. 234
17. A, p. 240
18. D, p. 241
19. E, p. 243
20. C, p. 231

Endocrine glands
1. Pineal
2. Hypothalamus
3. Pituitary
4. Thyroid
5. Thymus
6. Adrenals
7. Pancreas (islets)
8. Ovaries (female)
9. Testes (male)
10. Parathyroids

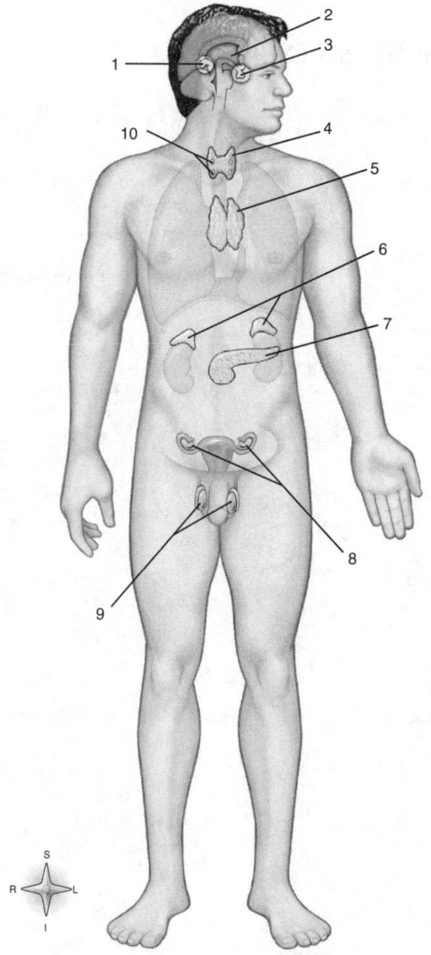

CHAPTER 11 BLOOD

Circle the correct answer
1. E, p. 251
2. D, p. 252
3. D, p. 252
4. B, p. 252
5. C, p. 253
6. A, p. 255
7. B, p. 255
8. D, p. 253
9. C, p. 257
10. D, p. 255
11. A, p. 255
12. B, p. 259
13. B, p. 260
14. B, p. 253
15. E, p. 254
16. B, p. 253
17. C, p. 253
18. D, p. 253
19. D, p. 256
20. D, p. 256
21. B, p. 257
22. D, p. 254
23. B, p. 257
24. C, p. 257
25. B, p. 257
26. A, p. 260
27. E, p. 260

Fill in the missing areas
28.

Blood Type	Antigen	Antibody
A	A	
B		Anti-A
AB	A, B	
O		Anti-A, Anti-B

Fill in the blanks
29. Antigen, p. 260
30. Antibody, p. 260
31. Agglutinate, p. 260
32. Erythroblastosis fetalis, p. 262
33. Rhesus monkey, p. 261
34. RhoGAM, p. 263
35. AB positive, p. 261

Unscramble the words

36. Phagocyte
37. Thrombin
38. Antigen
39. Fibrin
40. Typing

Applying what you know

41. No. If Mrs. Lassiter had a negative Rh factor and her husband had a positive Rh factor, it would set up the strong possibility of erythroblastosis fetalis.
42. Both procedures assist the clotting process.

43. WORD FIND

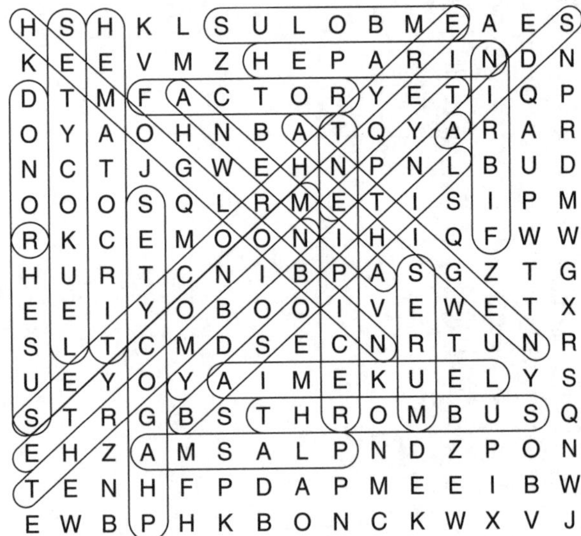

Crossword

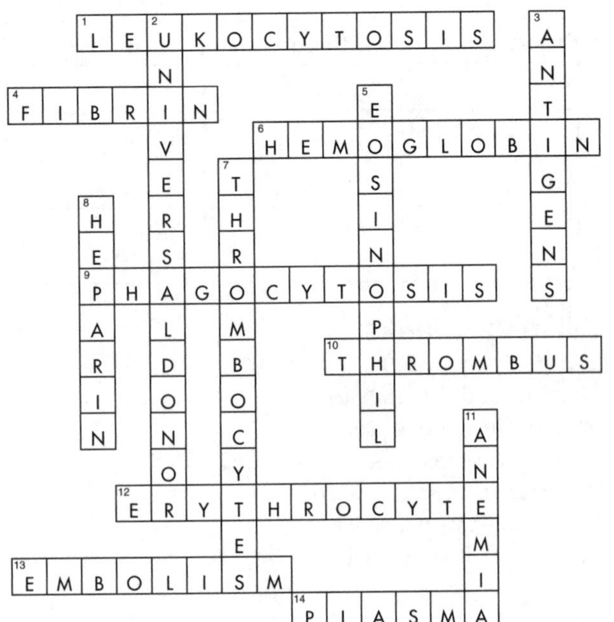

Check your knowledge

Multiple choice

1. B, p. 251
2. B, p. 252
3. A, p. 253
4. A, p. 255
5. D, p. 259
6. A, p. 256
7. A, p. 260
8. D, p. 260
9. C, p. 262
10. B, p. 263

Matching

11. D, p. 251
12. F, p. 254
13. H, p. 253
14. A, p. 255
15. G, p. 256
16. C, p. 257
17. B, p. 257
18. E, p. 255
19. I, p. 257
20. J, p. 260

Human Blood Cells

BODY CELL	FUNCTION
Erythrocyte	Oxygen and carbon dioxide transport
Neutrophil	Immune defense (phagocytosis)
Eosinophil	Defense against parasites
Basophil	Inflammatory response and heparin secretion
B lymphocyte	Antibody production (precursor of plasma cells)
T lymphocyte	Cellular immune response
Monocyte	Immune defenses (phagocytosis)
Thrombocyte	Blood clotting

Blood Typing

Recipient's blood		Reactions with donor's blood			
RBC antigens	Plasma antibodies	Donor type O	Donor type A	Donor type B	Donor type AB
None (Type O)	Anti-A Anti-B				
A (Type A)	Anti-B				
B (Type B)	Anti-A				
AB (Type AB)	(none)				

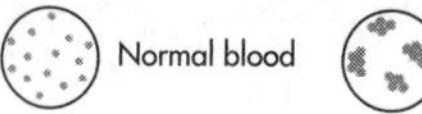

CHAPTER 12
THE CARDIOVASCULAR SYSTEM

Fill in the blanks
1. CPR, p. 270
2. Interatrial septum, p. 270
3. Atria, p. 270
4. Ventricles, p. 270
5. Myocardium, p. 270
6. Endocarditis, p. 270
7. Bicuspid or mitral; tricuspid, p. 274
8. Pulmonary circulation, p. 274
9. Coronary embolism or coronary thrombosis, p. 275
10. Myocardial infarction, p. 275
11. Sinoatrial, p. 277
12. P; QRS complex; T, p. 279
13. Repolarization, p. 279

Choose the correct term
14. A, p. 272
15. K, p. 270
16. G, p. 274
17. C, p. 271
18. D, p. 274
19. F, p. 270
20. H, p. 275
21. B, p. 276
22. E, p. 277
23. I, p. 273
24. J, p. 279
25. L, p. 270
26. M, p. 272

Matching
27. D, p. 280
28. B, p. 280
29. C, p. 279
30. G, p. 280
31. A, p. 281
32. E, p. 280
33. F, p. 279

Multiple choice
34. D, p. 280
35. C, p. 280
36. B, p. 281
37. A, p. 280
38. B, p. 279
39. B, p. 285
40. D, p. 286
41. B, p. 287
42. B, p. 288
43. A, p. 288
44. D, p. 280
45. A, p. 281

True or false
46. Highest in arteries, lowest in veins, p. 289
47. Blood pressure gradient, p. 289
48. Stop, p. 290
49. High, p. 290
50. Decreases, p. 290
51. T
52. T
53. T
54. Stronger will increase, weaker will decrease, p. 291
55. Contract, p. 292
56. Relax, p. 292
57. Artery, p. 293
58. T
59. T
60. Brachial, p. 293

Unscramble the words
61. Systemic
62. Venule
63. Artery
64. Pulse
65. Vessel

Applying what you know
66. Coronary bypass surgery
67. Artificial pacemaker
68. The endocardial lining can become rough and abrasive to red blood cells passing over its surface. As a result, a fatal blood clot may be formed.
69. Dan may be hemorrhaging. The heart beats faster during hemorrhage in an attempt to compensate for blood loss.

70. WORD FIND

```
Y H Y S I S O B M O R H T A R
L A C I L I B M U O A Y N I Y
E E S Y S T E M I C C G D E U
M V E N U L E D D C I X M D I
E Y M U I R T A R N L E C G Y
N O I T A Z I R A L O P E D N
U D L A T R O P C I T A P E H
S I U K M U E T O E S L U P U
R P N F Y C B E D R A L Z P J
D S A H T I T V N L I I B D W
Q U R O I V A Q E O D A K R K
K C R M P G A I G N D D Z Y J
Y I Y R I N E A F Z L Q S P X
S R M I C C Q O A W U N H O K
P T A V H H Z L H I J J X K Z
```

Crossword

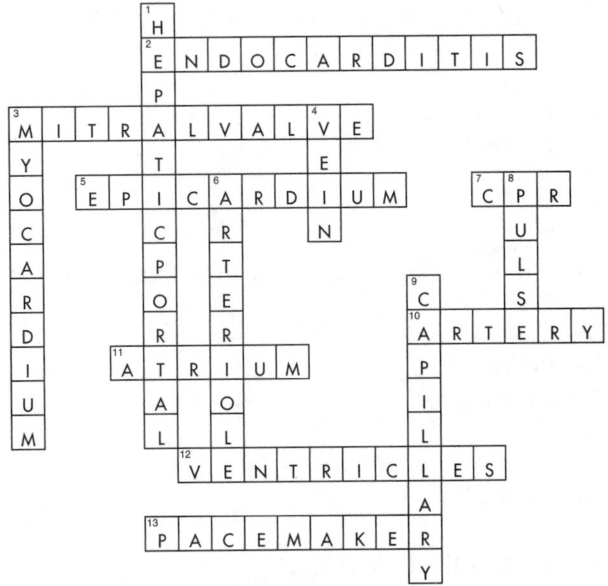

Check your knowledge

Multiple choice

1. A, p. 270
2. C, p. 274
3. B, p. 274
4. A, p. 277
5. A, p. 280
6. D, p. 279
7. C, p. 289
8. D, p. 287
9. C, p. 276
10. C, p. 281

Matching

11. F, p. 270
12. G, p. 270
13. H, p. 272
14. I, p. 274
15. J, p. 280
16. B, p. 277
17. C, p. 270
18. A, p. 292
19. D, p. 293
20. E, p. 273

The heart

1. Left common carotid artery
2. Left subclavian artery
3. Arch of aorta
4. Left pulmonary artery
5. Left atrium
6. Left pulmonary veins
7. Great cardiac vein
8. Branches of left coronary artery and cardiac vein
9. Left ventricle
10. Apex
11. Right ventricle
12. Right atrium
13. Right coronary artery and cardiac vein
14. Right pulmonary veins
15. Ascending aorta
16. Right pulmonary artery
17. Superior vena cava
18. Brachiocephalic trunk

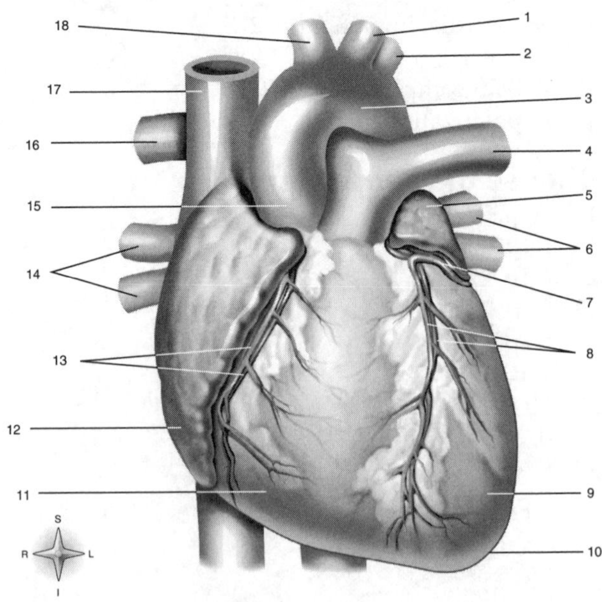

Conduction system of the heart

1. Aorta
2. Pulmonary artery
3. Pulmonary veins
4. Mitral (bicuspid) valve
5. Purkinje fibers
6. Right and left branches of AV bundle (bundle of His)
7. Left ventricle
8. Inferior vena cava
9. Right ventricle
10. Tricuspid valve
11. Atrioventricular (AV) node
12. Sinoatrial (SA) node or pacemaker
13. Superior vena cava

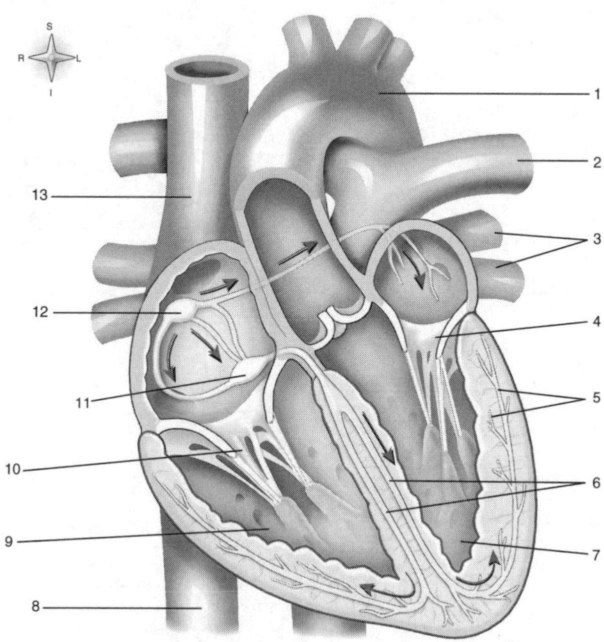

Fetal circulation

1. Aortic arch
2. Abdominal aorta
3. Common iliac artery
4. Internal iliac arteries
5. Umbilical arteries
6. Fetal umbilicus
7. Umbilical cord
8. Fetal side of placenta
9. Maternal side of placenta
10. Umbilical vein
11. Hepatic portal vein
12. Ductus venosus
13. Inferior vena cava
14. Foramen ovale
15. Superior vena cava
16. Ascending aorta
17. Pulmonary trunk
18. Ductus arteriosus

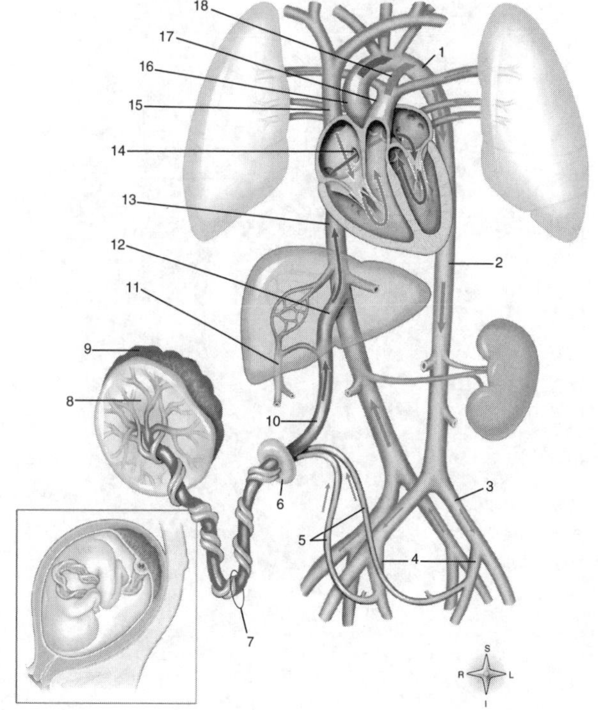

Hepatic portal circulation

1. Inferior vena cava
2. Stomach
3. Gastric vein
4. Spleen
5. Pancreatic vein
6. Splenic vein
7. Gastroepiploic vein
8. Descending colon
9. Inferior mesenteric vein
10. Small intestine
11. Appendix
12. Ascending colon
13. Superior mesenteric vein
14. Pancreas
15. Duodenum
16. Hepatic portal vein
17. Liver
18. Hepatic veins

Principal arteries of the body

1. Right common carotid
2. Brachiocephalic
3. Right coronary
4. Axillary
5. Brachial
6. Superior mesenteric
7. Abdominal aorta
8. Common iliac
9. Internal iliac
10. External iliac
11. Deep femoral
12. Femoral
13. Popliteal
14. Anterior tibial
15. Occipital
16. Facial
17. Internal carotid
18. External carotid
19. Left common carotid
20. Left subclavian
21. Arch of aorta
22. Pulmonary
23. Left coronary
24. Aorta
25. Splenic
26. Renal
27. Celiac
28. Inferior mesenteric
29. Radial
30. Ulnar

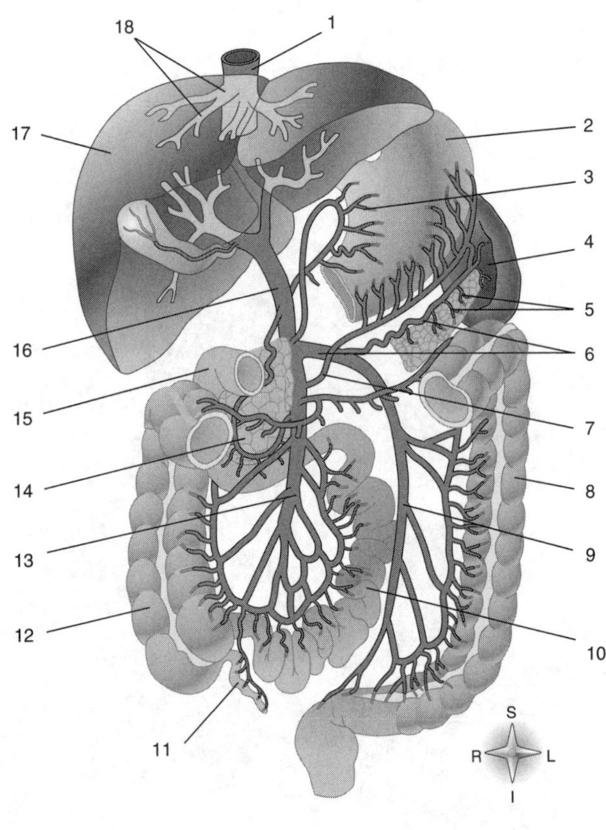

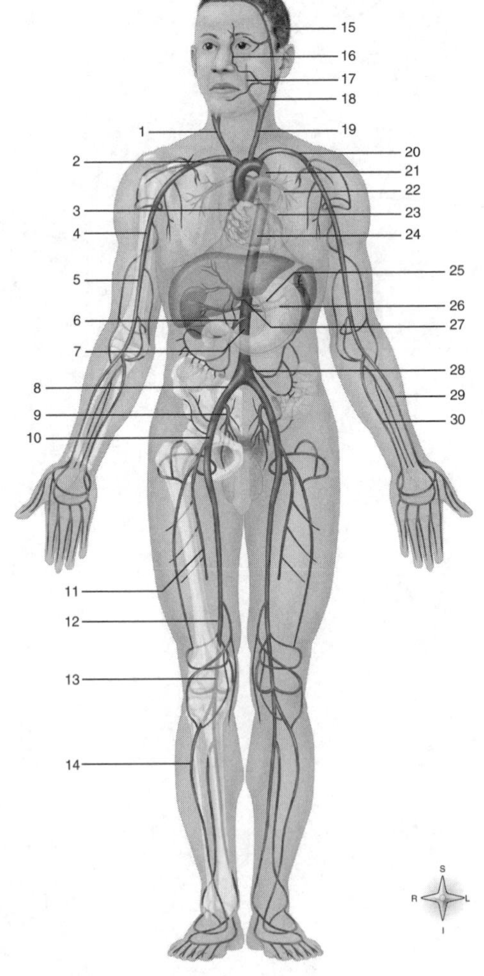

Principal veins of the body

1. Right brachiocephalic
2. Right subclavian
3. Superior vena cava
4. Right pulmonary
5. Small cardiac
6. Inferior vena cava
7. Hepatic
8. Hepatic portal
9. Superior mesenteric
10. Median cubital
11. Common iliac
12. External iliac
13. Femoral
14. Great saphenous
15. Fibular (peroneal)
16. Anterior tibial
17. Posterior tibial
18. Occipital
19. Facial
20. External jugular
21. Internal jugular
22. Left brachiocephalic
23. Left subclavian
24. Axillary
25. Cephalic
26. Great cardiac
27. Basilic
28. Brachial veins
29. Long thoracic
30. Splenic
31. Inferior mesenteric
32. Ulnar vein
33. Radial vein
34. Common iliac
35. Internal iliac
36. Digital veins
37. Femoral
38. Popliteal

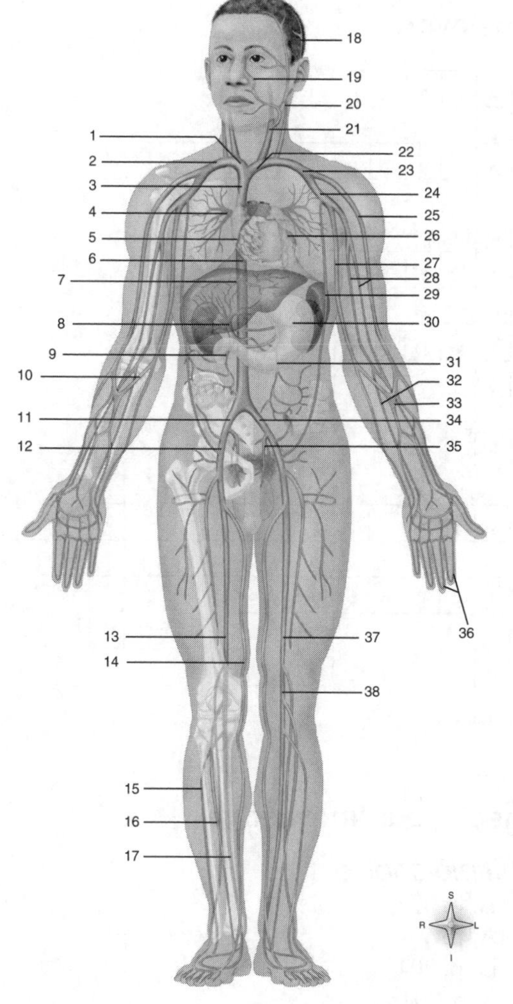

Normal ECG deflections

1. Atrial depolarization
2. Ventricular depolarization
3. Ventricular repolarization

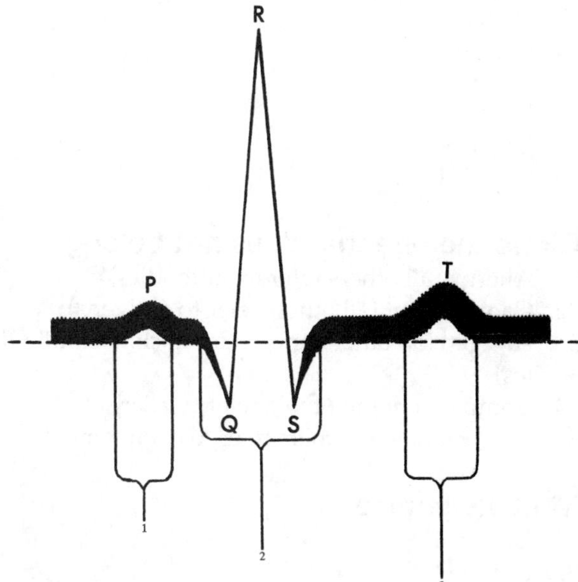

CHAPTER 13
THE LYMPHATIC SYSTEM AND IMMUNITY

Fill in the blanks

1. Lymph, p. 302
2. Interstitial fluid, p. 302
3. Lymphatic capillaries, p. 302
4. Right lymphatic duct; thoracic duct, p. 302
5. Cisterna chyli, p. 302
6. Lymph nodes, p. 304
7. Afferent, p. 304
8. Efferent, p. 305

Select the correct term

9. B, p. 307
10. C, p. 307
11. C, p. 307
12. A, p. 306
13. C, p. 307
14. A, p. 307
15. A, p. 306

Matching

16. C, p. 308
17. A, p. 310
18. E, p. 309
19. B, p. 310
20. D, p. 310

Choose the correct term

21. C, p. 307
22. D, p. 307
23. E, p. 313
24. A, p. 310
25. H, p. 310
26. B, p. 310
27. I, p. 310
28. F, p. 311
29. J, p. 313
30. G, p. 311

Circle the one that does not belong

31. Allergy (all others refer to antibodies)
32. Complement (all others refer to antigens)
33. Antigen (all others refer to monoclonal antibodies)
34. Complement (all others refer to allergy)
35. Monoclonal (all others refer to complement)

Multiple choice

36. D, p. 314
37. D, p. 314
38. C, p. 314
39. B, p. 306
40. C, p. 314
41. C, p. 314
42. E, p. 314
43. E, p. 314
44. C, p. 315
45. E, p. 315
46. E, p. 415
47. D, p. 318
48. E, p. 315
49. A, p. 315
50. B, p. 316

Fill in the blanks

51. Stem cell, p. 314
52. Liver and bone marrow; bone marrow, p. 314
53. Plasma cells, p. 315
54. Thymus gland, p. 315
55. Azidothymidine or AZT, p. 318
56. AIDS, p. 318
57. Vaccine, p. 318

Unscramble the words

58. Complement
59. Immunity
60. Clones
61. Interferon
62. Memory cells

Applying what you know

63. Interferon would possibly decrease the severity of the chickenpox virus.
64. AIDS
65. Baby Phelps had no means of producing T cells, thus making him susceptible to several diseases. Isolation was a means of controlling his exposure to these diseases.

66. WORD FIND

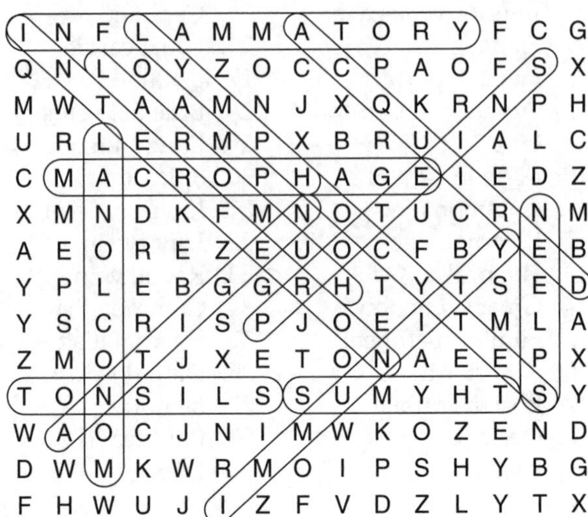

Crossword

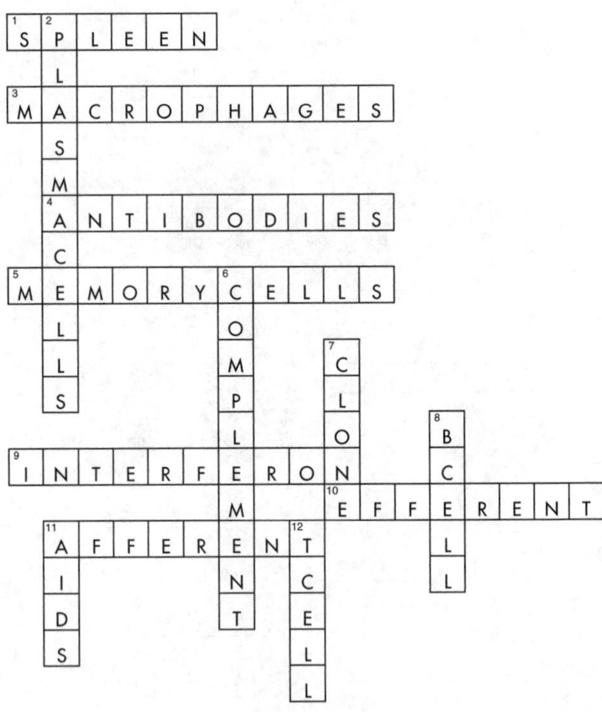

Check your knowledge

Multiple choice

1. A, p. 302
2. A, p. 307
3. D, p. 304
4. B, p. 304

5. D, p. 307
6. B, p. 307
7. D, p. 310
8. D, p. 316
9. D, p. 308
10. C, p. 310

Matching

11. E, p. 305
12. D, p. 307
13. I, p. 308
14. H, p. 309
15. G, p. 310
16. B, p. 307
17. A, p. 310
18. J, p. 313
19. C, p. 315
20. F, p. 314

Principal organs of the lymphatic system

1. Tonsils
2. Submandibular nodes
3. Axillary lymph nodes
4. Thymus
5. Thoracic duct
6. Spleen
7. Cisterna chyli
8. Inguinal lymph nodes
9. Popliteal lymph nodes
10. Lymph vessels
11. Red bone marrow
12. Right lymphatic duct
13. Cervical lymph nodes

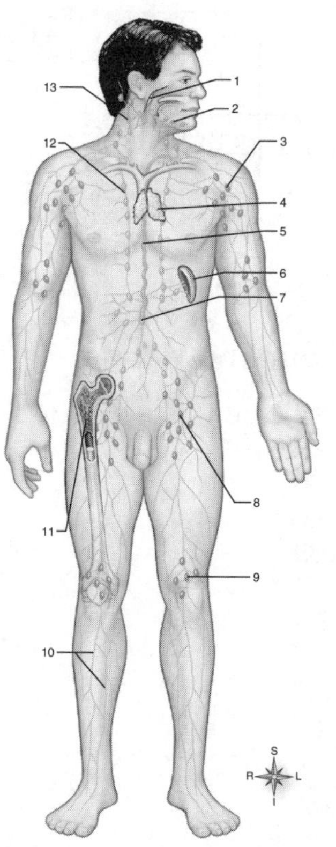

CHAPTER 14 THE RESPIRATORY SYSTEM

Matching

1. J, p. 325
2. G, p. 327
3. A, p. 326
4. I, p. 331
5. B, p. 325
6. F, p. 328
7. C, p. 328
8. H, p. 327
9. D, p. 327
10. E, p. 325

Fill in the blanks

11. Air distributor, p. 325
12. Gas exchanger, p. 325
13. Filters, p. 325
14. Warms, p. 325
15. Humidifies, p. 325
16. Nose, p. 326
17. Pharynx, p. 326
18. Larynx, p. 326
19. Trachea, p. 326
20. Bronchi, p. 326
21. Lungs, p. 326
22. Alveoli, p. 326
23. Diffusion, p. 326
24. Respiratory mucosa, p. 328
25. Goblet, p. 328

Circle the one that does not belong

26. Oropharynx (the others refer to the nose)
27. Conchae (the others refer to paranasal sinuses)
28. Epiglottis (the others refer to the pharynx)
29. Uvula (the others refer to the adenoids)
30. Larynx (the others refer to the eustachian tubes)
31. Tonsils (the others refer to the larynx)
32. Eustachian tube (the others refer to the tonsils)
33. Pharynx (the others refer to the larynx)

Choose the correct term

34. A, p. 328
35. B, p. 329
36. A, p. 329
37. A, p. 329
38. A, p. 328
39. B, p. 330
40. B, p. 330
41. C, p. 331

Fill in the blanks

42. Trachea, p. 331
43. Cartilage (C-rings), p. 332

44. Suffocation, p. 332
45. Primary bronchi, p. 332
46. Alveolar sacs, p. 333
47. Apex, p. 334
48. Pleura, p. 334
49. Pleurisy, p. 334
50. Pneumothorax, p. 334

True or false

51. Breathing, p. 337
52. Expiration, p. 337
53. Down, p. 338 (review Chapter 3)
54. Internal, p. 338
55. T
56. 1 pint, p. 341
57. T
58. Vital capacity, p. 341
59. T

Circle the correct answer

60. E, p. 336
61. C, p. 340
62. C, p. 340
63. B, p. 337
64. D, p. 342
65. D, p. 342
66. D, p. 342

Matching

67. E, p. 342
68. B, p. 343
69. G, p. 344
70. A, p. 344
71. F, p. 344
72. D, p. 344
73. C, p. 344

Unscramble the words

74. Pleurisy
75. Bronchitis
76. Epistaxis
77. Adenoids
78. Inspiration

Applying what you know

79. During the day Mr. Gorski's cilia are paralyzed because of his heavy smoking. They use the time when Mr. Gorski is asleep to sweep accumulations of mucus and bacteria toward the pharynx. When he awakes, these collections are waiting to be eliminated.
80. Swelling of the tonsils or adenoids caused by infection may make it difficult or impossible for air to travel from the nose into the throat. The individual may be forced to breathe through the mouth.

81. WORD FIND

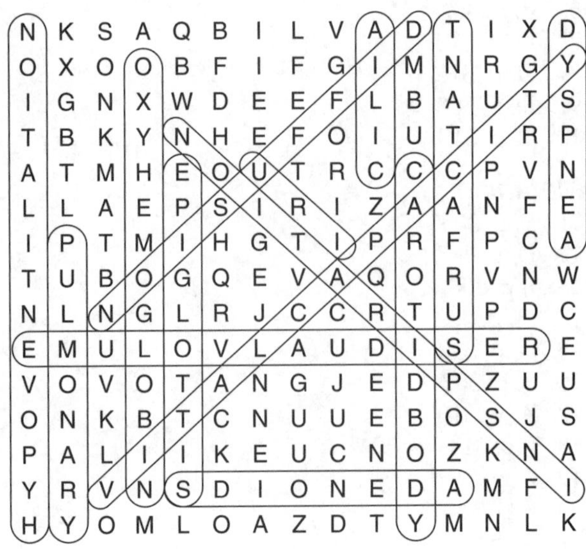

Crossword

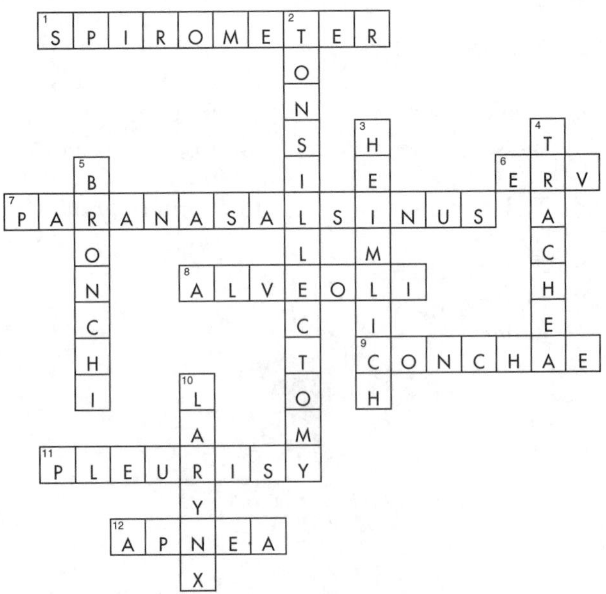

Check your knowledge

Multiple choice

1. A, p. 326
2. B, p. 330
3. D, p. 325
4. B, p. 332
5. A, p. 337
6. D, p. 334
7. A, p. 336
8. C, p. 342
9. D, p. 344
10. B, p. 342

Matching

11. E, p. 327
12. I, p. 327
13. A, p. 328
14. G, p. 331
15. D, p. 332
16. B, p. 341
17. C, p. 343
18. H, p. 344
19. F, p. 344
20. J, p. 334

Sagittal view of head and neck

1. Sphenoidal air sinus
2. Pharyngeal tonsil (adenoids)
3. Opening of auditory (eustachian) tube
4. Nasopharynx
5. Soft palate
6. Uvula
7. Palatine tonsil
8. Oropharynx
9. Epiglottis (part of larynx)
10. Laryngopharynx
11. Esophagus
12. Trachea
13. Vocal cords (part of larynx)
14. Thyroid cartilage (part of larynx)
15. Hyoid bone
16. Lingual tonsil
17. Hard palate
18. Inferior concha
19. Middle nasal concha of ethmoid
20. Superior nasal concha of ethmoid
21. Nasal bone
22. Frontal sinus

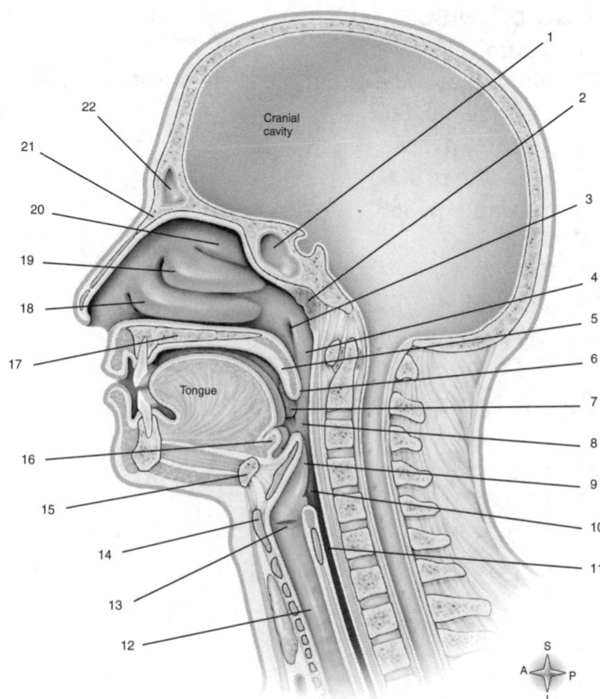

Respiratory organs

1. Nasal cavity
2. Nasopharynx
3. Oropharynx
4. Laryngopharynx
5. Pharynx
6. Larynx
7. Trachea
8. Bronchioles
9. Left and right primary bronchi
10. Alveolar duct
11. Alveolar sac
12. Capillary
13. Alveoli

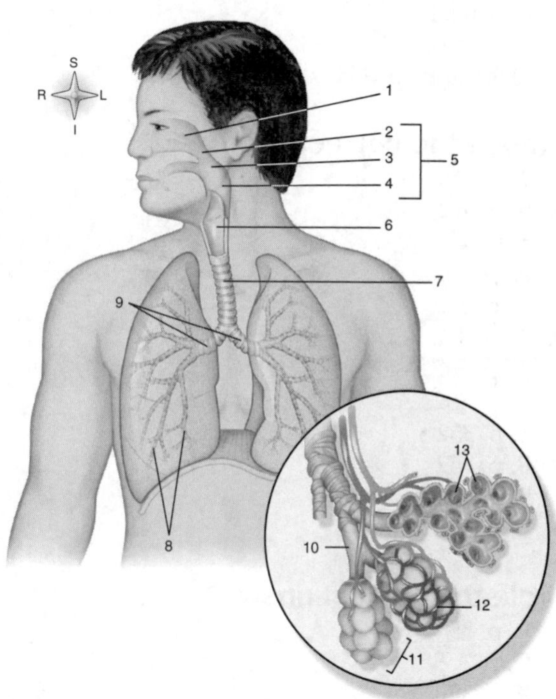

Pulmonary ventilation volumes

1. Total lung capacity
2. Inspiratory reserve volume
3. Tidal volume
4. Expiratory reserve volume
5. Residual volume
6. Vital capacity

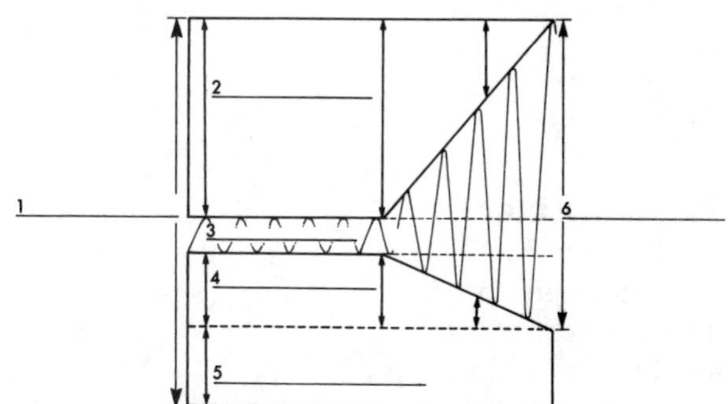

CHAPTER 15
THE DIGESTIVE SYSTEM

Fill in the blanks

1. Gastrointestinal tract or GI tract, p. 351
2. Mechanical, p. 352
3. Chemical, p. 352
4. Feces, p. 353
5. Digestion, p. 352
6. Absorption, p. 352
7. Mouth; anus, p. 353
8. Lumen, p. 353
9. Mucosa, p. 353
10. Submucosa, p. 353
11. Peristalsis, p. 353
12. Serosa, p. 353
13. Mesentery, p. 355

Choose the correct term

14. A, p. 352
15. B, p. 352
16. B, p. 352
17. A, p. 352
18. A, p. 352
19. A, p. 352
20. A, p. 352
21. A, p. 352
22. B, p. 352
23. B, p. 352
24. B, p. 352
25. B, p. 352

Circle the correct answer

26. E, p. 355
27. C, p. 355
28. E, p. 356
29. D, p. 355
30. B, p. 355
31. C, p. 355
32. D, p. 355
33. D, p. 356
34. D, p. 355
35. A, p. 358
36. C, p. 357
37. A, p. 358
38. A, p. 356
39. B, p. 356
40. C, p. 358

Fill in the blanks

41. Pharynx, p. 358
42. Esophagus, p. 352
43. Stomach, p. 359
44. Cardiac sphincter, p. 359
45. Chyme, p. 359
46. Fundus, p. 360
47. Body, p. 360
48. Pylorus, p. 360
49. Pyloric sphincter, p. 360
50. Small intestine, p. 360

Matching

51. D, p. 360
52. J, p. 359
53. G, p. 359
54. A, p. 359
55. H, p. 359
56. B, p. 359
57. C, p. 360
58. E, p. 362
59. I, p. 359
60. F, p. 360

Circle the correct answer

61. C, p. 360
62. B, p. 360 and pp. 361 and 362
63. A, p. 363
64. A, p. 364
65. B, p. 362
66. E, p. 363
67. D, p. 362
68. D, p. 363 ; review Chapter 10 (hormones circulate in blood)
69. B, p. 364
70. C, p. 363

True or false

71. Vitamin K, p. 365
72. No villi are present in the large intestine, p. 365
73. Diarrhea, p. 365
74. Cecum, p. 366
75. Hepatic, p. 366
76. Sigmoid, p. 366
77. T
78. T
79. Parietal, p. 367
80. Mesentery, p. 368

Circle the correct answer

81. B, p. 353
82. D, p. 353
83. C, p. 353
84. C, p. 369
85. C, p. 370

86. Fill in the blank areas on the chart below.

DIGESTIVE JUICES AND ENZYMES	SUBSTANCE DIGESTED (OR HYDROLYZED)	RESULTING PRODUCT
Saliva		
	1. Starch (polysaccharide)	
Gastric juice		
		2. Partially digested proteins
Pancreatic juice		
		3. Peptides and amino acids
	4. Fats emulsified by bile	
	5. Starch	
Intestinal enzymes		
	6. Peptides	
7. Sucrase		
	8. Lactose (milk sugar)	
		9. Glucose

Unscramble the words

87. Bolus
88. Chyme
89. Papilla
90. Peritoneum
91. Lace apron

Applying what you know

92. Ulcer
93. Pylorospasm
94. Basal metabolic rate or protein-bound iodine to determine thyroid function

95. WORD FIND

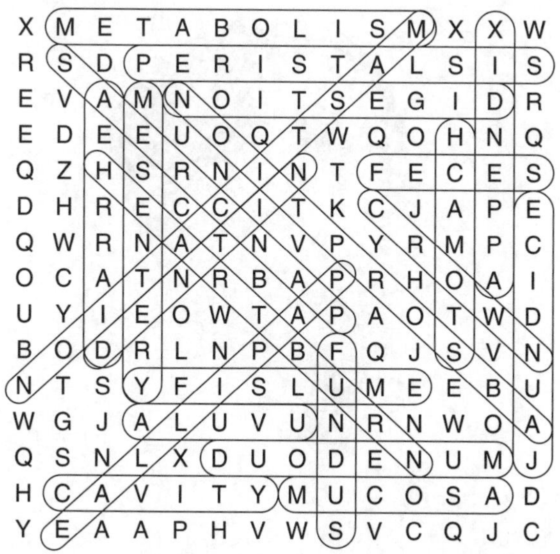

Crossword

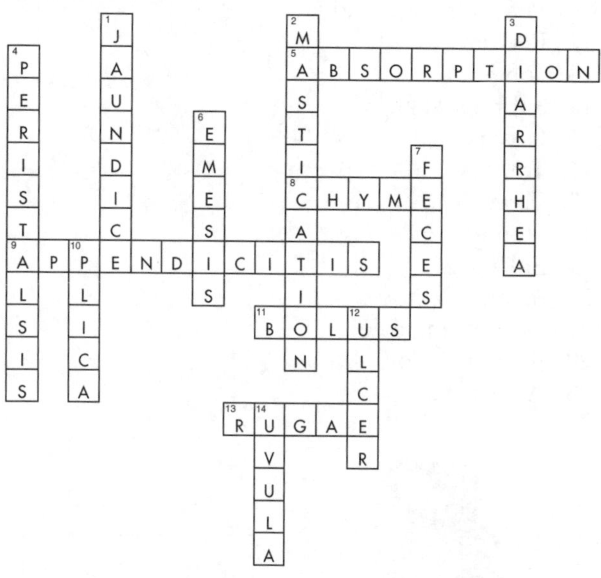

Check your knowledge

Multiple choice

1. A, p. 351
2. C, p. 353
3. A, p. 352
4. B, p. 356
5. B, p. 357
6. B, p. 358
7. B, p. 360
8. C, p. 359

9. C, p. 362
10. A, p. 364

Completion

11. Ileocecal valve, p. 365
12. Sigmoid colon, p. 365
13. Cecum, p. 367
14. Mesentery, p. 368
15. Mechanical digestion, p. 368
16. Monosaccharides, p. 369
17. Amino acids, p. 370
18. Fatty acids, glycerol, p. 370
19. Absorption, p. 371
20. Maltase, sucrase, lactase, p. 369

Digestive organs

1. Parotid gland
2. Submandibular gland
3. Pharynx
4. Esophagus
5. Diaphragm
6. Transverse colon
7. Hepatic flexure
8. Ascending colon
9. Ilium
10. Cecum
11. Vermiform appendix
12. Rectum
13. Tongue
14. Sublingual gland
15. Larynx
16. Trachea
17. Liver
18. Stomach
19. Spleen
20. Splenic flexure
21. Descending colon
22. Sigmoid colon
23. Anal canal

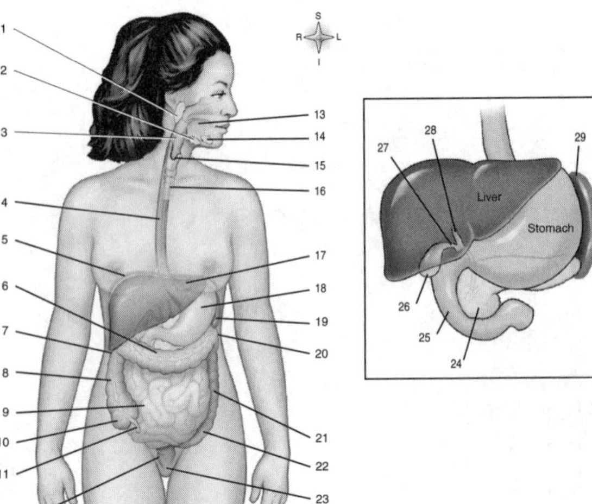

Tooth

1. Cusp
2. Enamel
3. Dentin
4. Pulp cavity with nerves and vessels
5. Gingiva
6. Root canal
7. Peridontal membrane
8. Cementum
9. Bone
10. Root
11. Neck
12. Crown

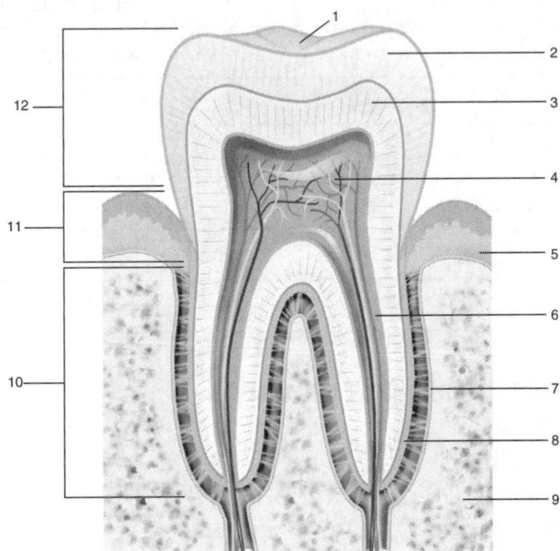

The salivary glands

1. Parotid gland
2. Parotid duct
3. Submandibular gland
4. Submandibular duct
5. Sublingual gland

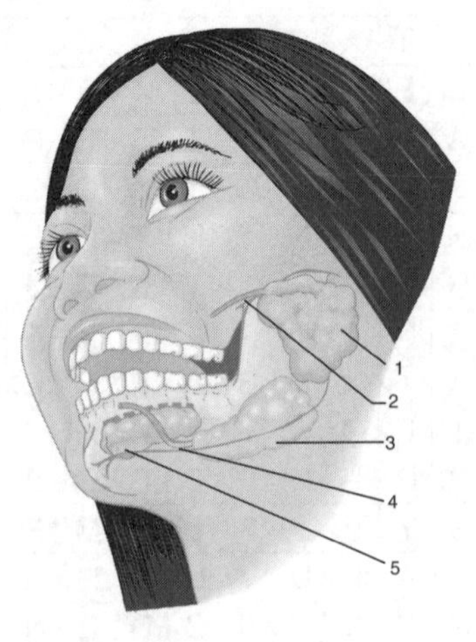

Stomach

1. Gastroesophageal sphincter
2. Esophagus
3. Gastroesophageal opening
4. Lesser curvature
5. Pylorus
6. Pyloric sphincter
7. Duodenum
8. Rugae
9. Greater curvature
10. Submucosa
11. Mucosa
12. Oblique muscle layer
13. Circular muscle layer
14. Longitudinal muscle layer
15. Serosa
16. Body
17. Fundus

Gallbladder and bile ducts

1. Corpus (body) of gallbladder
2. Neck of gallbladder
3. Cystic duct
4. Liver
5. Minor duodenal papilla
6. Major duodenal papilla
7. Duodenum
8. Sphincter muscles
9. Superior mesenteric artery and vein
10. Pancreatic duct
11. Pancreas
12. Common bile duct
13. Common hepatic duct
14. Right and left hepatic ducts

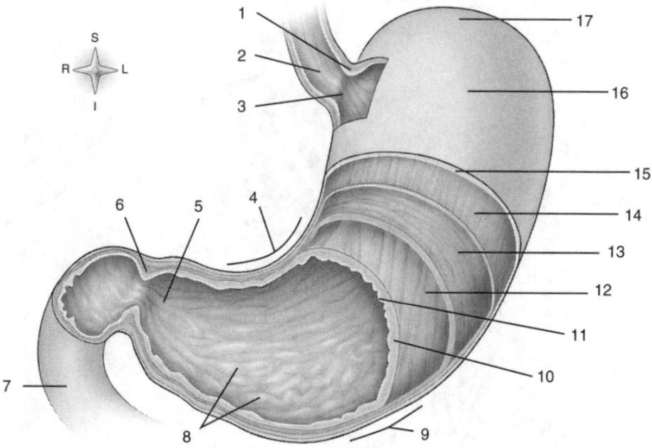

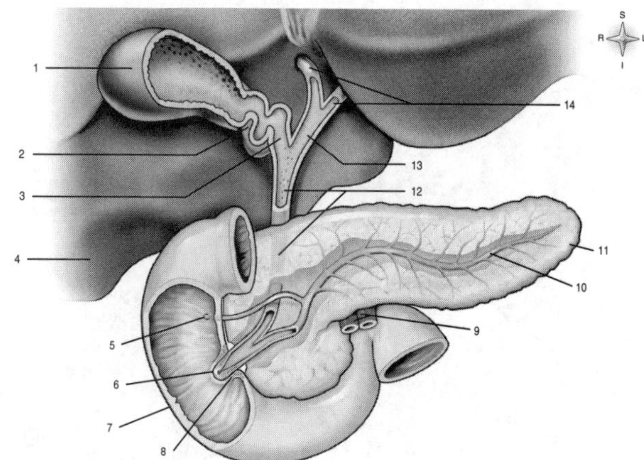

The small intestine

1. Mesentery
2. Serosa
3. Longitudinal muscle
4. Circular muscle
5. Muscularis
6. Submucosa
7. Plica (fold)
8. Lymph nodule
9. Mucosa
10. Segment of jejunum
11. Microvilli
12. Epithelial cell
13. Single villus
14. Mucosa
15. Microvilli
16. Submucosa
17. Lacteal (lymph capillary)
18. Artery and vein

Large intestine

1. Aorta
2. Splenic vein
3. Superior mesenteric artery
4. Splenic (left colic) flexure
5. Inferior mesenteric artery and vein
6. Descending colon
7. Sigmoid colon
8. Rectum
9. Mesentery
10. Ileum
11. Vermiform appendix
12. Cecum
13. Ileocecal valve
14. Ascending colon
15. Hepatic (right colic) flexure
16. Transverse colon
17. Inferior vena cava
18. Portal vein

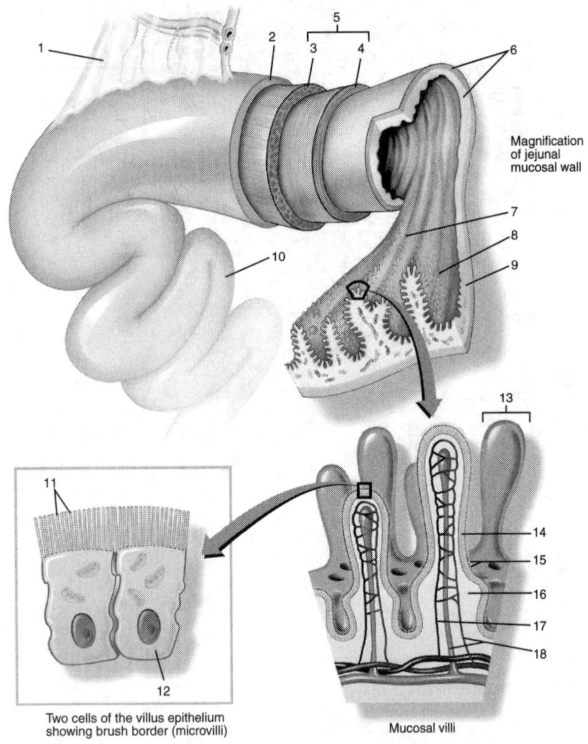

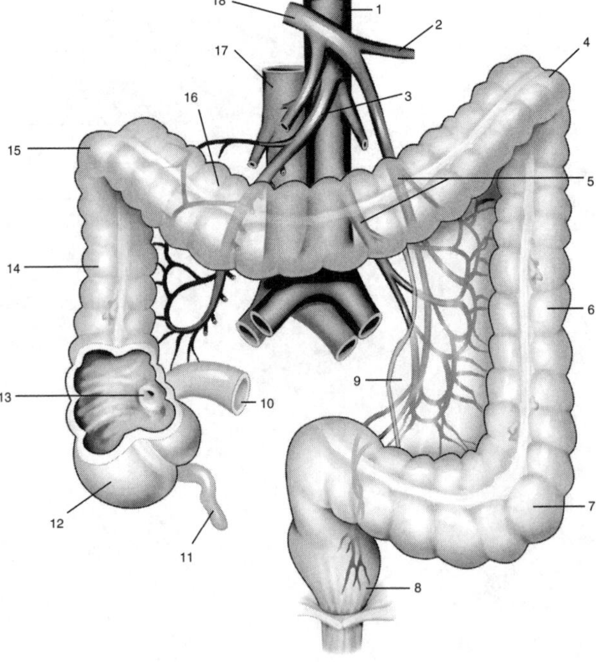

CHAPTER 16
NUTRITION AND METABOLISM

Fill in the blanks
1. Bile, p. 380
2. Prothrombin, p. 380
3. Fibrinogen, p. 380
4. Iron, p. 380
5. Hepatic portal vein, p. 380

Matching
6. B, p. 382
7. A, p. 380
8. C, p. 382
9. D, p. 384
10. E, p. 384
11. A, p. 380
12. E, p. 384
13. A, p. 381

Circle the one that does not belong
14. Bile (all others refer to carbohydrate metabolism)
15. Amino acids (all others refer to fat metabolism)
16. M (all other refer to vitamins)
17. Iron (all others refer to protein metabolism)
18. Insulin (all others tend to increase blood glucose)
19. Folic acid (all others are minerals)
20. Ascorbic acid (all others refer to the B-complex vitamins)

Circle the correct answer
21. C, p. 384
22. A, p. 384
23. C, p. 386
24. B, p. 387
25. B, p. 387
26. A, p. 387
27. C, p. 387
28. D, p. 387
29. A, p. 387

Unscramble the words
30. Liver
31. Catabolism
32. Amino
33. Pyruvic
34. Evaporation

Applying what you know
35. Weight loss; anorexia nervosa
36. Iron; meat, eggs, vegetables, and legumes
37. She was carbohydrate loading or glycogen loading which allows the muscles to sustain aerobic exercise for up to 50% longer than usual.

38. WORD FIND

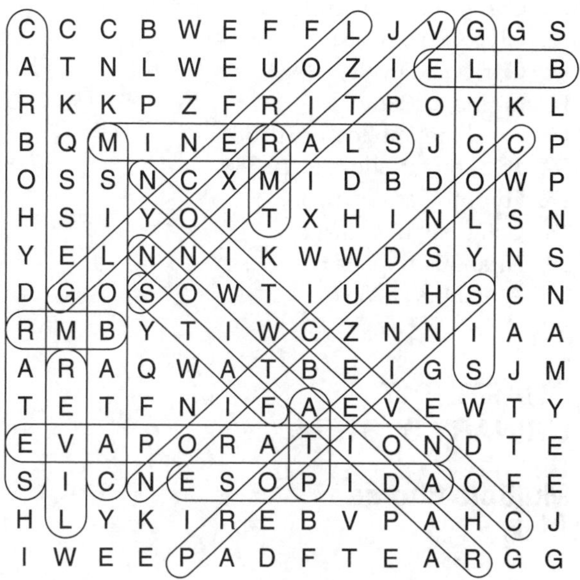

Crossword

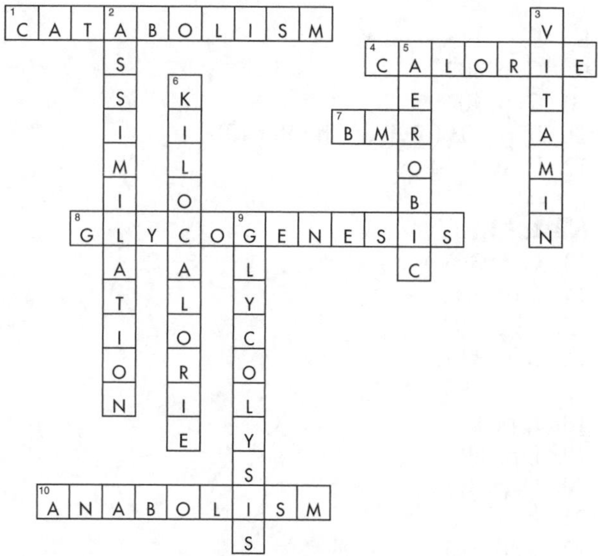

Check your knowledge

Multiple choice
1. B, p. 379
2. A, p. 381
3. C, p. 381
4. C, p. 382
5. B, p. 382

6. B, p. 382
7. A, p. 384
8. A, p. 386
9. B, p. 387
10. D, p. 380

Completion

11. Carbohydrates, p. 380
12. Glycolysis, p. 381
13. Citric acid cycle, p. 381
14. Iodine, p. 386
15. Basal metabolic rate, p. 384
16. Total metabolic rate, p. 384
17. Hypothalamus, p. 387
18. Catabolism, p. 379
19. Anabolism, p. 379
20. A, E, D, K, p. 384

CHAPTER 17
URINARY SYSTEM

Multiple choice

1. E, p. 395
2. C, p. 396
3. E, p. 396
4. C, p. 396
5. E, p. 403
6. C, p. 401
7. B, p. 401
8. E, p. 396
9. C, p. 402
10. C, p. 402
11. B, p. 403 (review Chapter 10)
12. D, p. 403

Matching

13. G, p. 396
14. I, p. 399
15. H, p. 394
16. B, p. 395
17. K, p. 396
18. F, p. 396
19. J, p. 396
20. D, p. 395
21. L, p. 396
22. C, p. 395
23. M, p. 400
24. A, p. 395

Indicate which organ is identified

25. B, p. 404
26. C, p. 405
27. A, p. 404
28. B, p. 404
29. C, p. 405
30. C, p. 405
31. A, p. 403
32. C, p. 404
33. B, p. 404
34. A, p. 404
35. B, p. 404

Fill in the blanks

36. Renal colic, p. 404
37. Mucous membrane, p. 404
38. Renal calculi, p. 406
39. Ultrasound, p. 406
40. Reduced, p. 405
41. Renal pelvis, p. 396
42. Semen, p. 405
43. Urinary meatus, p. 405

Fill in the blanks

44. Micturition, p. 405
45. Urination, p. 405
46. Voiding, p. 405
47. Internal urethral, p. 405
48. Exit, p. 405
49. Striated, p. 405
50. Voluntary, p. 405
51. Emptying reflex, p. 405
52. Urethra, p. 405
53. Retention, p. 405
54. Suppression, p. 405
55. Overactive bladder, p. 406

Unscramble the words

56. Calyx
57. Voiding
58. Papilla
59. Glomerulus
60. Pyramids

Applying what you know

61. Polyuria
62. Residual urine is often the cause of repeated cystitis.
63. A high percentage of catheterized patients develop cystitis, often due to poor aseptic technique when inserting the catheter.

64. WORD FIND

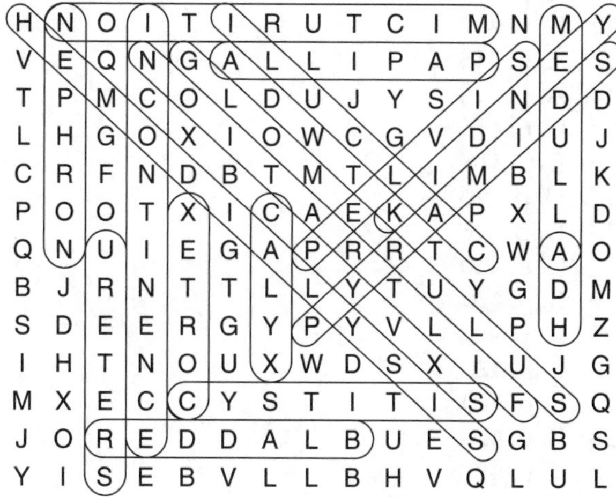

Crossword

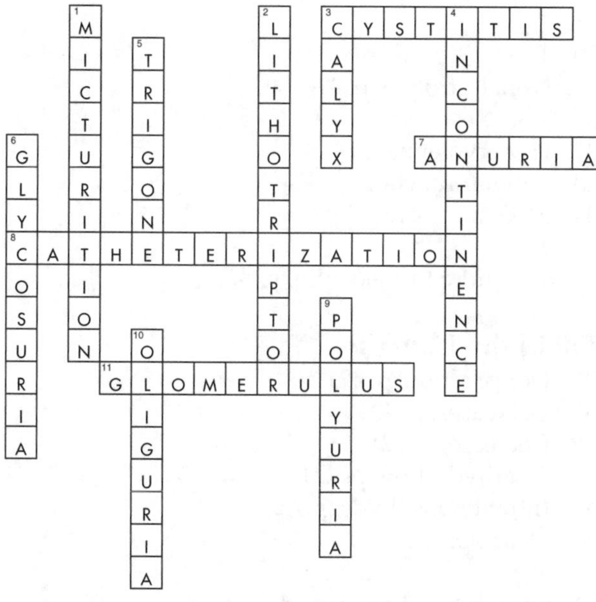

Check your knowledge

Multiple choice

1. D, p. 395
2. B, p. 396
3. D, p. 396
4. A, p. 400
5. C, p. 402
6. C, p. 406
7. B, p. 403
8. C, p. 403
9. B, p. 404
10. A, p. 400

Matching

11. E, p. 394
12. C, p. 396
13. F, p. 396
14. D, p. 398
15. J, p. 402
16. H, p. 400
17. A, p. 405
18. G, p. 405
19. I, p. 396
20. B, p. 395

Urinary system

1. Urinary bladder
2. Ureter
3. Right kidney
4. Twelfth rib
5. Liver
6. Adrenal gland
7. Spleen
8. Renal artery
9. Renal vein
10. Left kidney
11. Abdominal aorta
12. Inferior vena cava
13. Common iliac artery and vein
14. Urethra

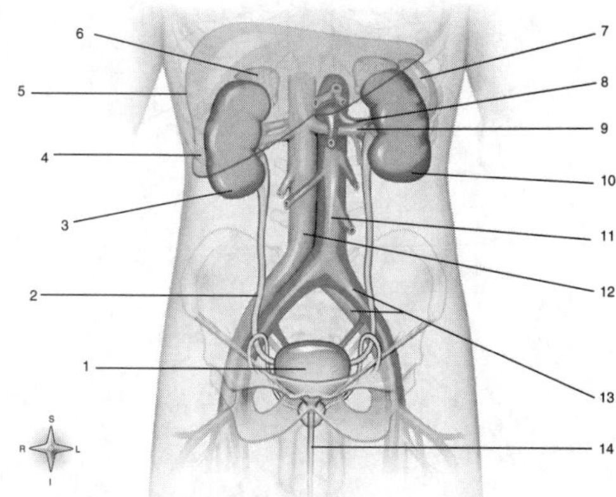

Kidney

1. Interlobular arteries
2. Renal column
3. Renal sinus
4. Hilum
5. Renal pelvis
6. Renal papilla of pyramid
7. Ureter
8. Medulla
9. Medullary pyramid
10. Major calyces
11. Minor calyces
12. Cortex
13. Capsule (fibrous)

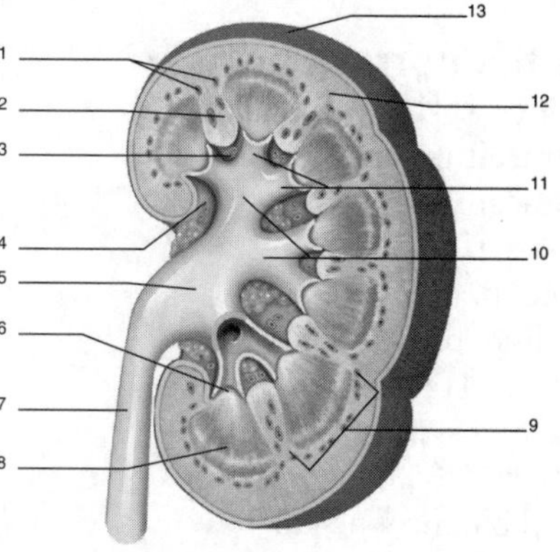

Nephron

1. Proximal convoluted tubule
2. Collecting duct
3. Descending limb of Henle's loop
4. Ascending limb of Henle's loop
5. Descending limb of Henle's loop
6. Artery and vein
7. Distal convoluted tubule
8. Peritubular capillaries
9. Afferent arteriole
10. Juxtaglomerular (JG) apparatus
11. Efferent arteriole
12. Glomerulus
13. Bowman capsule
14. Renal corpuscle

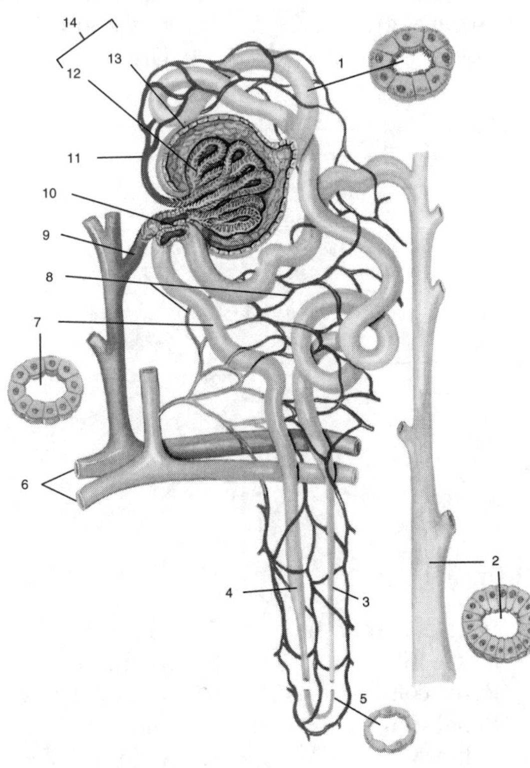

Multiple choice

11. A, p. 417
12. D, p. 417
13. A, p. 418
14. A, p. 418
15. C, p. 416
16. E, p. 416
17. D, p. 416
18. D, p. 418
19. C, p. 420
20. B, p. 420
21. D, p. 421
22. E, p. 420
23. B, p. 420
24. B, p. 420
25. B, p. 421
26. E, p. 419

True or false

27. Catabolism, p. 416
28. T
29. T
30. Nonelectrolyte, p. 417
31. T
32. Hypervolemia, p. 419
33. Tubular function, p. 421
34. 2400 ml, p. 416
35. T
36. 1000 mEq to 1300 mEq, p. 420

Fill in the blanks

37. Dehydration, p. 421
38. Decreases, p. 421
39. Decrease, p. 421
40. Overhydration, p. 421
41. Intravenous fluids, p. 421
42. Heart, p. 421

Unscramble the words

43. Edema
44. Fluid
45. Ion
46. Intravenous
47. Volume

Applying what you know

48. Ms. Titus could not accurately measure water intake created by foods or catabolism, nor could she measure output created by lungs, skin, or the intestines.
49. A careful record of fluid intake and output should be maintained and the patient should be monitored for signs and symptoms of electrolyte and water imbalance.

CHAPTER 18
FLUID AND ELECTROLYTE BALANCE

Circle the correct answer

1. Inside, p. 415
2. Extracellular, p. 415
3. Extracellular, p. 415
4. Lower, p. 413
5. More, p. 414
6. Decline, p. 414
7. Less, p. 414
8. Decreases, p. 414
9. 55%, p. 413
10. Fluid balance, p. 413

50. WORD FIND

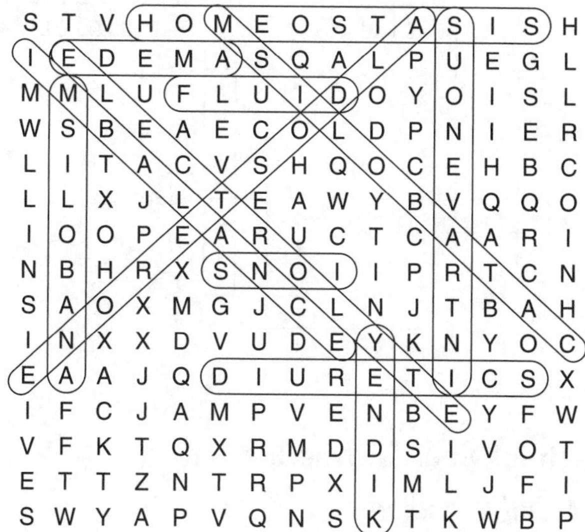

Crossword

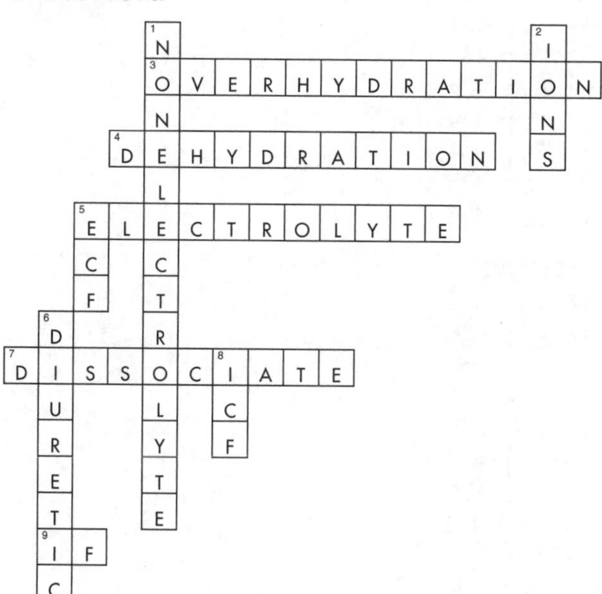

Check your knowledge

Multiple choice

1. A, p. 414
2. D, p. 416
3. D, p. 415
4. C, p. 416
5. A, p. 421
6. B, p. 419
7. D, p. 420
8. A, p. 419
9. A, p. 415
10. D, p. 416

Completion

11. E, p. 415
12. B, p. 415
13. A, p. 417
14. J, p. 413
15. D, p. 421
16. C, p. 413
17. F, p. 419
18. G, p. 421
19. H, p. 421
20. I, p. 420
21. O, p. 419
22. L, p. 415
23. M, p. 417
24. N, p. 418
25. K, p. 417

CHAPTER 19
ACID-BASE BALANCE

Choose the correct term

1. B, p. 428
2. A, p. 428
3. A, p. 428
4. B, p. 428
5. B, p. 428
6. B, p. 428
7. B, p. 428
8. A, p. 428
9. B, p. 428
10. B, p. 428

Multiple Choice

11. E, p. 429
12. E, p. 429
13. A, p. 429
14. E, p. 431
15. C, p. 431
16. D, p. 431
17. C, p. 432
18. B, p. 432
19. D, p. 432
20. E, p. 434
21. E, p. 434

True or false

22. Buffer (instead of heart), p. 429
23. Buffer pairs, p. 429
24. T
25. T
26. Alkalosis, p. 432
27. Kidneys, p. 432
28. T
29. Kidneys, p. 434
30. Lungs, p. 434

Matching

31. E, p. 435
32. G, p. 432
33. F, p. 435
34. A, p. 434
35. I, p. 435
36. B, p. 434
37. H, p. 434
38. C, p. 434
39. D, p. 434
40. J, p. 434

Unscramble the words

41. Fluids
42. Bicarbonate
43. Base
44. Fixed
45. Hydrogen
46. Buffer

Applying what you know

47. Normal saline contains chloride ions, which replace bicarbonate ions and thus relieve the bicarbonate excess which occurs during severe vomiting.
48. Most citrus fruits, although acid-tasting, are fully oxidized during metabolism and have little effect on acid-base balance. Cranberry juice is one of the few exceptions.
49. Milk of magnesia. It is a base. Milk is slightly acidic (see chart, p. 428).

50. WORD FIND

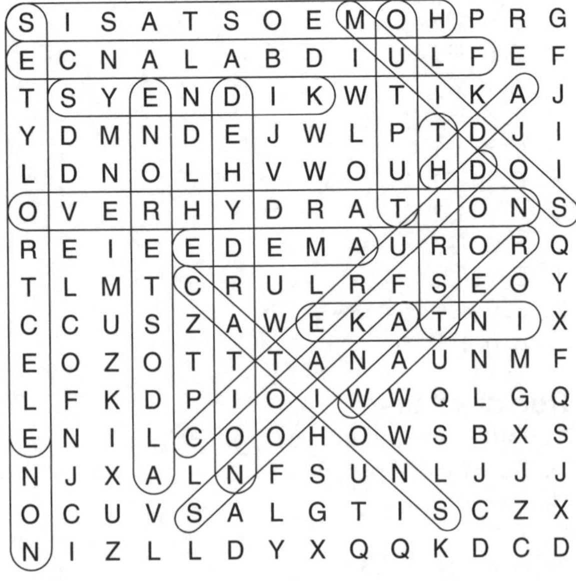

Crossword

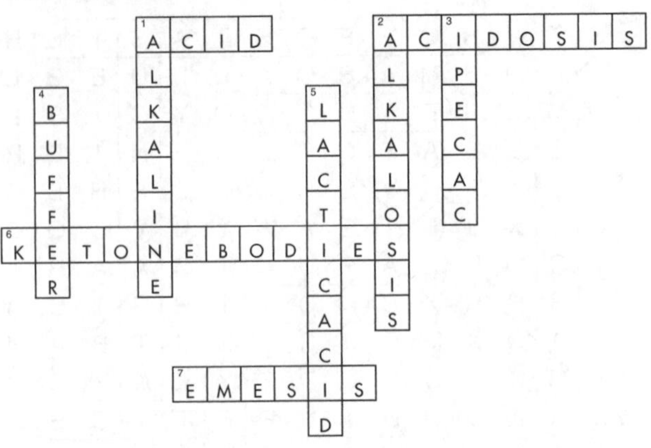

Check your knowledge

Multiple choice

1. A, p. 434
2. C, p. 428
3. A, p. 429
4. D, p. 431
5. A, p. 435
6. D, p. 429
7. D, p. 434
8. D, p. 434
9. D, p. 435
10. A, p. 436

Matching

11. G, p. 428
12. C, p. 428
13. I, p. 429
14. E, p. 431
15. F, p. 429
16. A, p. 432
17. B, p. 429
18. D, p. 432
19. J, p. 434
20. H, p. 434

CHAPTER 20
THE REPRODUCTIVE SYSTEMS

Matching

Group A

1. D, p. 442
2. C, p. 442
3. E, p. 441
4. B, p. 442
5. A, p. 441

Group B

6. C, p. 442
7. A, p. 442

8. D, p. 441
9. B, p. 442
10. E, p. 442

Multiple choice

11. B, p. 443
12. C, p. 443
13. A, p. 443
14. D, p. 447
15. E, p. 443
16. D, p. 446
17. C, p. 446
18. C, p. 443
19. A, p. 446
20. B, p. 447

Fill in the blanks

21. Testes, p. 442
22. Spermatozoa or sperm, p. 443
23. Ovum, p. 441
24. Testosterone, p. 443
25. Interstitial cells, p. 443
26. Masculinizing, p. 446
27. Anabolic, p. 446

Choose the correct term

28. B, p. 447
29. H, p. 448
30. G, p. 448
31. A, p. 447
32. F, p. 448
33. C, p. 447
34. I, p. 447
35. E, p. 448
36. D, p. 448
37. J, p. 449

Matching

38. D, p. 450
39. C, p. 450
40. B, p. 450
41. A, p. 450
42. E, p. 450

Select the correct term

43. A, p. 455
44. B, p. 450
45. A, p. 455
46. B, p. 450
47. A, p. 455
48. A, p. 455
49. A, p. 455
50. B, p. 450

Fill in the blanks

51. Gonads, p. 451
52. Oogenesis, p. 451
53. Meiosis, p. 451
54. One-half or 23, p. 452
55. Fertilization, p. 452
56. 46, p. 452
57. Estrogen, p. 452
58. Progesterone, p. 452
59. Secondary sexual characteristics, p. 452
60. Menstrual cycle, p. 452
61. Puberty, p. 452

Select the correct term

62. A, p. 453
63. B, p. 453
64. C, p. 454
65. B, p. 453
66. A, p. 452; C, p. 454
67. B, p. 452
68. A, p. 452
69. A, p. 452
70. C, p. 454
71. B, p. 458

Matching

Group A

72. D, p. 454
73. E, p. 454
74. B, p. 454
75. C, p. 454
76. A, p. 454

Group B

77. E, p. 455
78. A, p. 455
79. D, p. 455
80. B, p. 455
81. C, p. 455

True or false

82. Menarche, p. 455
83. One, p. 456
84. 14, p. 456
85. Menstrual period, p. 456
86. T, p. 456
87. Anterior, p. 456

Matching

88. B, p. 458
89. A, p. 456
90. B, p. 456
91. B, p. 456
92. A, p. 458

Unscramble the words

93. Vulva
94. Testes
95. Menses
96. Fimbriae
97. Prepuce
98. Vestibule

Applying what you know

99. Yes. The testes are not only essential organs of reproduction, but are also responsible for the "masculinizing" hormone. Without this hormone, Mr. Belinki will have no desire to reproduce.
100. Sterile—The sperm count may be too low to reproduce but the remaining testicle will produce enough masculinizing hormone to prevent impotency.
101. The uterine tubes are not attached to the ovaries and infections can exit at this area and enter the abdominal cavity.
102. Yes. Yes. Without the hormones from the ovaries to initiate the menstrual cycle, Mrs. Harlan will no longer have a menstrual cycle and can be considered to be in menopause (cessation of menstrual cycle).
103. No. Delceta still will have her ovaries which are the source of her hormones, she will not experience menopause due to this procedure.

104. WORD FIND

```
M K O V I D U C T S E D H G
S E I R A V O I F U T G L L
I N H Z H M P M K O H I C W
D D V A S D E F E R E N S H
I O A C C I P J V E H Y D S
H M G R R B M N X F G Y I O
C E I O O E Z Y T I C S T E
R T N S T P S D D N O V A D
O R A O U W E B A I J S M Z
T I C M M E Y N E M D L R V
P U A E U D G M I E H I E H
Y M O T C E T A T S O R P B
R P E E R M N E G O R T S E
C O W P E R S I N X K E A P
```

Crossword

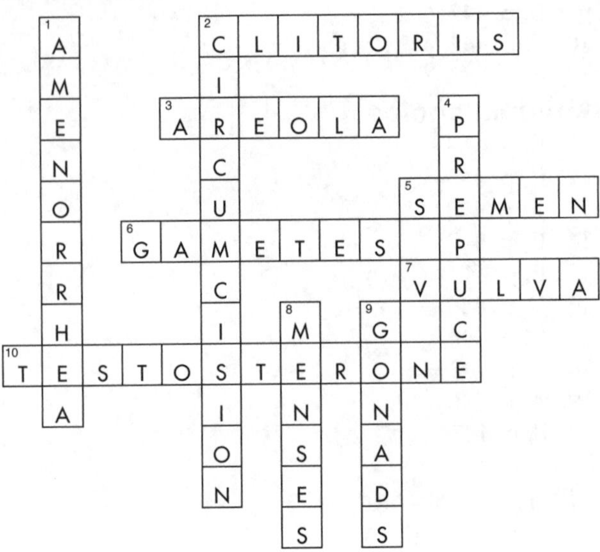

Check your knowledge

Multiple choice

1. A, p. 442
2. D, p. 446
3. D, p. 448
4. C, p. 447
5. C, p. 448
6. A, p. 451
7. B, p. 452
8. C, p. 455
9. A, p. 443
10. D, p. 459

Matching

11. C, p. 441
12. A, p. 443
13. H, p. 446
14. G, p. 448
15. F, p. 442
16. E, p. 458
17. B, p. 444
18. D, p. 455
19. J, p. 454
20. I, p. 455

Male reproductive organs

1. Seminal vesicle
2. Ejaculatory duct
3. Prostate gland
4. Rectum
5. Bulbourethral (Cowper's gland)
6. Anus
7. Scrotum
8. Testis
9. Epididymis
10. Foreskin
11. Penis
12. Urethra
13. Ductus deferens
14. Urinary bladder
15. Ureter

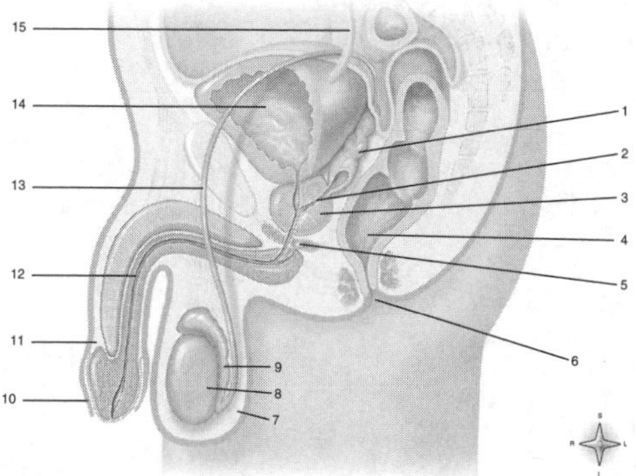

Tubules of testis and epididymis

1. Ductus (vas) deferens
2. Nerves and blood vessels in the spermatic cord
3. Epididymis
4. Seminiferous tubules
5. Testis
6. Tunica albuginea
7. Lobule
8. Septum

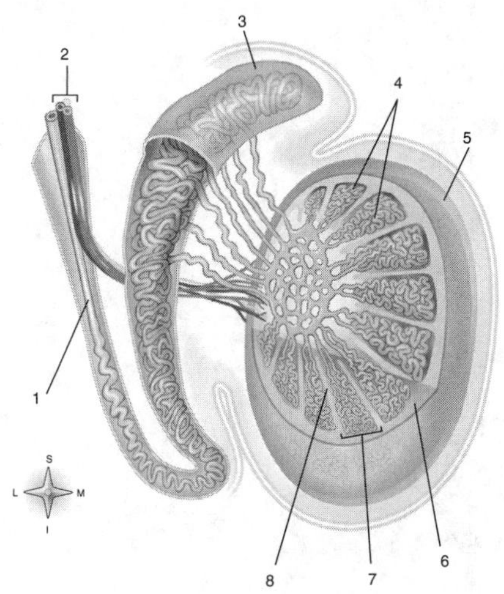

Vulva

1. Mons pubis
2. Pudendal fissure
3. Labium majus
4. Frenulum (of clitoris)
5. Opening of lesser vestibular (Skene) gland
6. Orifice of vagina
7. Hymen
8. Frenulum (of labia)
9. Posterior commissure (of labia)
10. Anus
11. Perineum
12. Greater vestibular (Bartholin) gland
13. Vestibule (clitoral bulb)
14. Vestibule
15. External urinary meatus
16. Labium minus
17. Clitoris (glans)
18. Foreskin (prepuce)

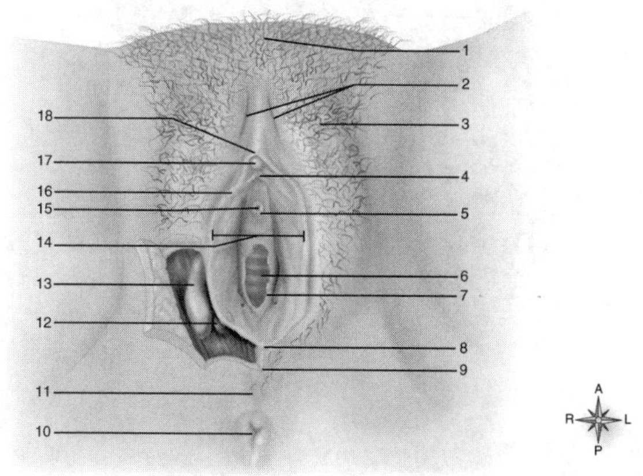

Breast

1. Clavicle
2. Pectoralis major muscle
3. Intercostal muscles
4. Nipple pores
5. Lactiferous duct
6. Alveoli
7. Suspensory ligaments of Cooper

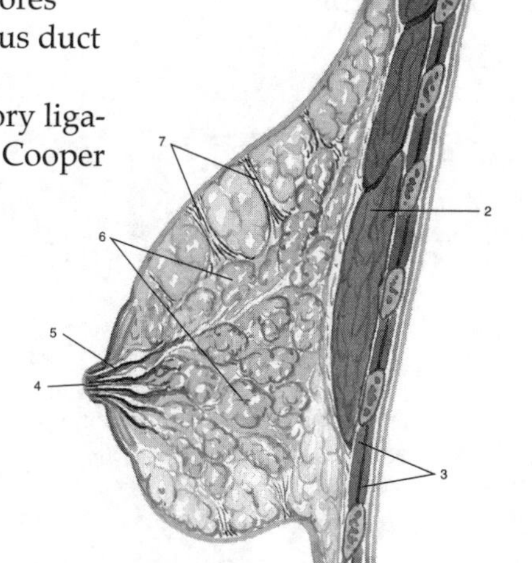

Female pelvis
1. Uterine tube (fallopian tube)
2. Ovary
3. Body of uterus
4. Fundus of uterus
5. Urinary bladder
6. Symphysis pubis
7. Urethra
8. Clitoris
9. Vagina
10. Labium minus
11. Labium majus
12. Rectum
13. Cervix
14. Ureter

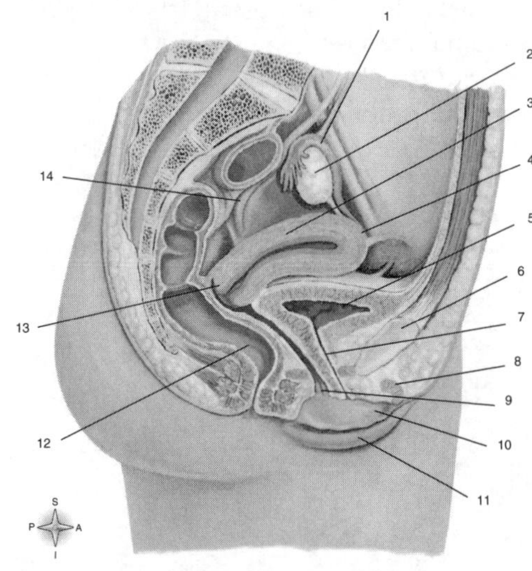

Uterus and adjacent structures
1. Fundus
2. Body of uterus
3. Cervix
4. Vagina
5. Cervical canal
6. Perimetrium
7. Myometrium
8. Endometrium

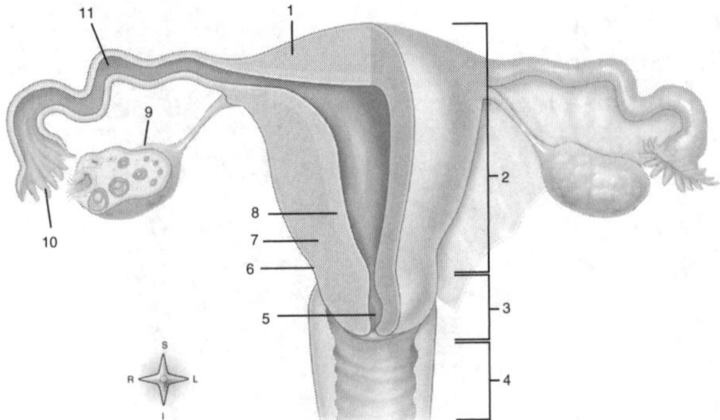

9. Ovary
10. Fimbriae
11. Uterine (fallopian) tube

CHAPTER 21
GROWTH AND DEVELOPMENT

Fill in the blanks
1. Conception, p. 467
2. Birth, p. 467
3. Embryology, p. 468
4. Oviduct, fallopian tube, or uterine tube, p. 468
5. Zygote, p. 468
6. Morula, p. 468
7. Blastocyst, p. 468
8.. Amniotic cavity, p. 468
9. Chorion, p. 468
10. Placenta, p. 468

Matching
11. G, p. 471
12. F, p. 472
13. C, p. 478
14. B, p. 472
15. A, p. 471
16. H, p. 474
17. E, p. 477
18. D, p. 473
19. I, p. 471
20. J, p. 478

Multiple choice
21. E, p. 476
22. E, p. 477
23. E, p. 478
24. A, p. 478
25. B, p. 478
26. C, p. 478
27. B, p. 478
28. D, p. 478
29. E, p. 478
30. D, p. 479
31. C, p. 478
32. C, p. 479
33. C, p. 479
34. C, p. 479
35. E, p. 479

Matching
36. F, p. 476
37. A, p. 478
38. C, p. 479
39. H, p. 478
40. D, p. 479

41. B, p. 477
42. E, p. 479
43. G, p. 477
44. I, p. 480

Fill in the blanks

45. Lipping, p. 481
46. Osteoarthritis, p. 481
47. Nephron, p. 482
48. Barrel chest, p. 482
49. Atherosclerosis, p. 482
50. Arteriosclerosis, p. 482
51. Hypertension, p. 482
52. Presbyopia, p. 481
53. Cataract, p. 481
54. Glaucoma, p. 481

Unscramble the words

55. Infancy
56. Postnatal
57. Organogenesis
58. Zygote
59. Childhood
60. Fertilization

Applying what you know

61. Normal
62. Only about 40% of the taste buds present at age 30 remain at age 75.
63. A significant loss of hair cells in the organ of Corti causes a serious decline in ability to hear certain frequencies.
64. WORD FIND

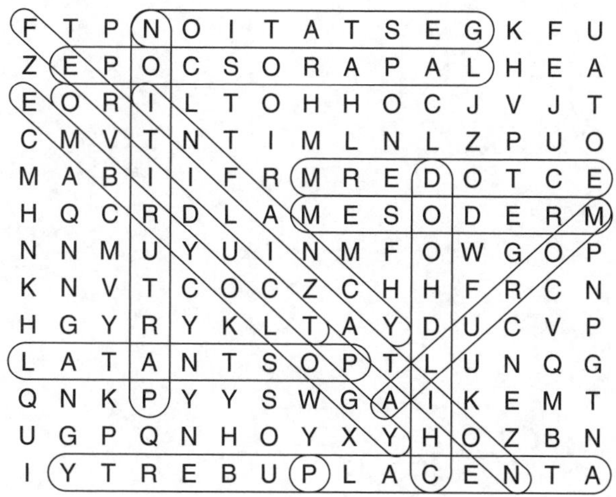

Crossword

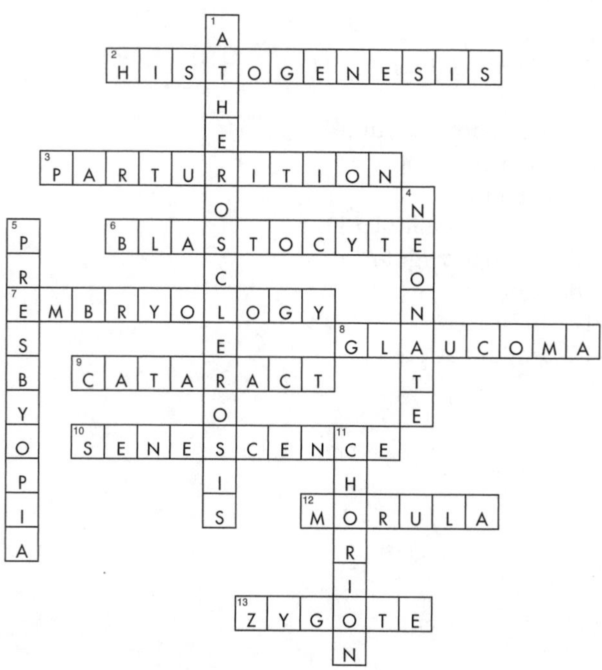

Check your knowledge

Multiple choice

1. C, p. 467
2. D, p. 468
3. D, p. 468
4. A, p. 468
5. D, p. 471
6. D, p. 472
7. C, p. 476
8. A, p. 472
9. C, p. 478
10. B, p. 480

Matching

11. E, p. 468
12. G, p. 468
13. C, p. 470
14. I, p. 480
15. H, p. 474
16. D, p. 477
17. J, p. 481
18. F, p. 481
19. A, p. 480
20. B, p. 477

Fertilization and implantation

1. Ovary
2. Developing follicles
3. Corpus luteum
4. Fimbriae
5. Discharged ovum
6. Spermatozoa
7. First mitosis
8. Uterine (fallopian) tube
9. Divided zygote
10. Morula
11. Blastocyst
12. Implantation

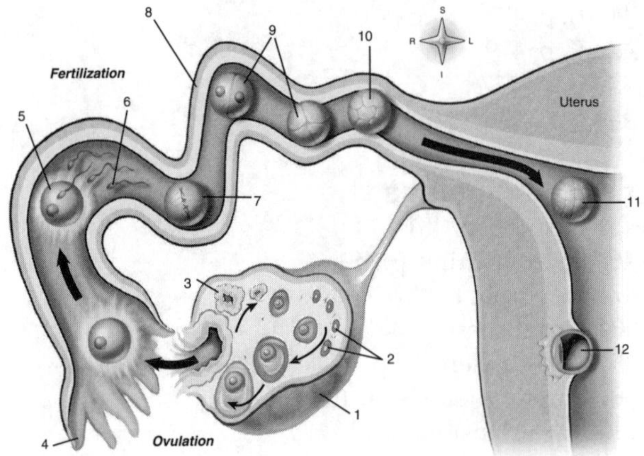

Notes

Notes

Notes

Notes

Notes

Notes

Notes

Notes